Healthcare in Latin America

# HEALTHCARE IN LATIN AMERICA

HISTORY, SOCIETY, CULTURE

· · · · · · · · · · · · · · · · ·

Edited by

**David S. Dalton and
Douglas J. Weatherford**

University of Florida Press
Gainesville

Publication of this work made possible by a Sustaining the Humanities through the American Rescue Plan grant from the National Endowment for the Humanities.

Copyright 2022 by David S. Dalton and Douglas J. Weatherford
All rights reserved
Published in the United States of America.

27  26  25  24  23  22    6  5  4  3  2  1

Library of Congress Cataloging-in-Publication Data
Names: Dalton, David S., editor. | Weatherford, Douglas, editor.
Title: Healthcare in Latin America : history, society, culture / edited by
  David S. Dalton and Douglas J. Weatherford.
Description: 1. | Gainesville : University of Florida Press, 2022. |
  Includes bibliographical references and index. | Summary: "Illustrating
  the diversity of disciplines that intersect within global health
  studies, contributors to this volume explore the development and
  representation of public health in Latin American countries"— Provided
  by publisher.
Identifiers: LCCN 2021055330 (print) | LCCN 2021055331 (ebook) | ISBN
  9781683402619 (hardback) | ISBN 9781683403258 (paperback) | ISBN
  9781683402763 (pdf) | ISBN 9781683403135 (ebook)
Subjects: LCSH: Medical care—Latin America—History. | Medical care—Latin
  America—Social conditions. | Public health—Latin America—History. |
  Public health—Latin America—Social conditions. | Medical policy—Latin
  America. | BISAC: MEDICAL / History | HISTORY / Latin America / General
Classification: LCC RA450.5 .H44 2022  (print) | LCC RA450.5  (ebook) | DDC
  362.1098—dc23/eng/20211122
LC record available at https://lccn.loc.gov/2021055330
LC ebook record available at https://lccn.loc.gov/2021055331

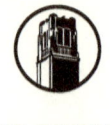

University of Florida Press
2046 NE Waldo Road
Suite 2100
Gainesville, FL 32609
http://upress.ufl.edu

# Contents

List of Figures  vii
List of Tables  ix
Acknowledgments  xi

Introduction: Healthcare in Latin America; History, Society, Culture  1
   *David S. Dalton and Douglas J. Weatherford*

## Part I. Healthcare in Mexico

1. Healers and Doctors: A History of the Healing Occupations in Mexico  19
   *Jethro Hernández Berrones*

2. A Systematic Approach to Health and Development in Mexico over the Last Century  40
   *Katherine E. Bliss*

3. Health after Internal Migration within Mexico: The Role of Age at Migration, Motivations, and Place of Origin and Destination  51
   *Gabriela León-Pérez*

4. Practicing Medicine in Post-Revolution Mexico: The Case of John Steinbeck and Emilio Fernández  69
   *Douglas J. Weatherford*

## Part II. Healthcare in United States Latino/a/x Communities

5. Colonial Care: Medicalizing Latino/a Bodies in the United States, 1894–1970s  91
   *Benny J. Andrés Jr.*

6. Healthcare in the US Latinx Community: Challenges, Disparities, and Opportunities  117
   *Christopher D. Mellinger*

7. Eugenics and Doubly Marginalized Mexican and Chicana Women: Forced Sterilizations in Renee Tajima-Peña's *No más bebés/No More Babies*  130
   *David S. Dalton*

## Part III. Healthcare in Central America and the Caribbean

8. Cuba and the Cuban Healthcare System   143
   *Katherine Hirschfeld*

9. Disaster Preparedness and Management in Cuba: A Health-Based Approach   157
   *Emily J. Kirk*

10. Stories of Giving Birth in Central America: Class, Race, and Politics in Women's Health   169
    *Sophie Esch and Alicia Z. Miklos*

## Part IV. Healthcare in the Andean Region

11. A Revolution in Healthcare? The Politics of Public Health in Postrevolutionary Bolivia   187
    *Nicole L. Pacino*

12. Maternal and Child Health in the Andean Region   202
    *Renata Forste*

13. Transness and Disability in Discourses of Access to Healthcare in the Colombian Press (2000–2019)   218
    *Javier E. García León and David L. García León*

14. Biomedicine and Ancestral Knowledges: *Vengo volviendo* and Healthcare Services in Ecuador   241
    *Manuel F. Medina*

## Part V. Healthcare in the Southern Cone

15. Health Systems in Argentina and Chile: A Comparative History   259
    *Eric D. Carter*

16. Health as a Right in Brazil and Argentina   278
    *Carlos S. Dimas*

17. The Politics and Medical Discourse of Intersexuality in Argentina through Film: Lucía Puenzo's *XXY*   296
    *Javier Barroso*

List of Contributors   309
Index   315

# Figures

4.1. In *The Forgotten Village* a female student looks through a microscope in a school in Mexico City   75

4.2. *The Forgotten Village* overflows with images of learning environments   76

4.3. In *Río Escondido* Rosaura prepares the long line of patients for their inoculation   78

4.4. The doctor's tools of the trade are laid out with almost religious admiration in *Río Escondido*   79

4.5. In *Río Escondido* Rosaura stands at the front of the class in the newly opened school   80

4.6. In *La perla/The Pearl* medical instruments and medical practitioners are used to confuse and deceive rather than instruct   83

14.1. Abuela Mariana mixes medicinal herbs   246

14.2. Ismael and Luz driving to distribute Abuela's product   247

# Tables

3.1. Characteristics of Mexican male and female internal migrants (Mexican Family Life Survey, 2002–2012)  60
3.2. Regression models predicting self-rated health after internal migration by gender (Mexican Family Life Survey, 2002–2012)  61
3.3. Regression models predicting depressive symptoms after internal migration by gender (Mexican Family Life Survey, 2002–2012)  63
12.1. Maternal and child health measures, Andean region (2015–2019)  204
12.2. Fertility and reproductive health measures, Andean region (2015–2018)  208
12.3. Percentage of women married or cohabiting, by age (15 to 29 years), Bolivia (1989–2012)  209
12.4. Educational and economic measures, Andean region  212
15.1. Demographic, economic, and health indicators for Argentina and Chile  270

# Acknowledgments

The editors wish to thank the many friends, colleagues, and contributors who helped advance this project during a global pandemic. Additionally, we thank our respective institutions, the University of North Carolina at Charlotte and Brigham Young University, for generous institutional support. This volume was funded, in part, by a subvention grant from the BYU College of Humanities.

Emily J. Kirk published a similar version of her contribution (chapter 9) as "Disaster Preparedness and Management: What Makes the Cuban Approach Different?" in *Disaster Preparedness and Climate Change in Cuba*, edited by Emily J. Kirk, Isabel Story, and Anna Clayfield (7–20). Lanham, MD: Lexington Books, 2021.

# Introduction

## Healthcare in Latin America

### History, Society, Culture

DAVID S. DALTON AND DOUGLAS J. WEATHERFORD

Public health policies across the world came under increased scrutiny in 2020 with the rapid spread of the SARS-CoV-2 virus which led to the COVID-19 pandemic. The disease's spread—and the resulting policies instituted in each country to confront it—highlighted how differing cultural attitudes and approaches to public health produced distinctive results as diverse institutions engaged the outbreak with varying degrees of success.[1] This was particularly true in the Western Hemisphere where the various nations of the Americas employed at-times contradictory strategies to weather both the physical and economic effects of the disease. Indeed, the pandemic presents a valuable springboard for this current volume because it provides a striking example of how state directives and policies shape public health and set the terms through which individual states can/not engage emergency situations.

In many cases, the pandemic laid bare the shortcomings of the Hemisphere's national healthcare systems. In the United States, for example, Black and Latino/a/x populations faced structural barriers to healthcare access that resulted in disproportionately high instances of hospitalization and death (Gold et al. 2020). In some countries, state, local, and federal leaders used the virus to push political agendas. In the early stages of the pandemic in Brazil, for example, the far-right president Jair Bolsonaro called the virus a "media trick" and a "little flu" (Phillips 2020). He lashed out at state and local leaders in places like Rio de Janeiro and São Paolo for imposing quarantines, claiming they were "tricking" Brazilian citizens (Phillips 2020). Infection and death rates climbed throughout the country. At the time of this writing, Brazil's 580,000 reported COVID-related deaths place the country second worldwide, behind only the United States (Worldometer 2021). In Mexico,[2] Luis Miguel Barbos Huerta, governor of Puebla and a member of president Andrés Manuel López Obrador's leftist Morena Party claimed, "if you are rich you are in danger; if you are poor, no; we, the poor, are . . . immune" ["*si son ricos tienen el riesgo; si son pobres no, los pobres estamos . . . inmunes*"] (*La Razón* 2020). This claim reverberated especially well within the system of left-wing austerity that had characterized the López Obrador administration up to that point (see Hanrahan and Fugellie 2019). On the one hand, it played to populist notions of poor and working-class greatness; on the other, the governor implicitly encouraged Mexicans to work rather than quarantine (see Agren 2020). In Ecuador, Guayaquil became arguably the first Latin American city to be overrun by the pandemic. Hospitals overflowed and local officials scrambled to find burial sites for the dead (Valencia and Gaibor del Pino 2020). The COVID pandemic clearly represented exceptional circumstances the likes of which Latin America had not seen since the 1918 Spanish Flu pandemic. Nevertheless, in confronting the crisis, countries throughout the region depended on a healthcare framework established during the previous decades and centuries (see Few 2020).

*Healthcare in Latin America: History, Society, Culture* may not tell the story of the COVID-19 pandemic, but it does reverberate with it. As national leaders discussed the disease publicly, they provided a window into a decades-long context—based on national values, assumptions, policies, and practices—that undergirds each nation's current approach to healthcare. Viewed in this light, any attempt to understand the ongoing efforts of the diverse nations of Latin America to respond to the pandemic requires some understanding of the role of public health in each nation's history and identity. That said, the scope of this volume goes far beyond any single moment. Healthcare has occupied a key position in Latin American thought since the earliest days of the Conquest, when Indigenous and Iberian ways of knowing first came into contact (see Hernández Berrones's chapter in this volume).[3] Although informed by this earlier historic moment, the studies collected in this anthology focus primarily on Latin America's approach to healthcare from the nineteenth century—following each nation's independence from Spain—to the present, with particular emphasis on the twentieth and twenty-first centuries. Furthermore, each chapter reveals that the various nations that make up Latin America view the ability to provide healthcare as a necessary component of governing.

Establishing a robust healthcare system has been one of the principal goals of most Latin American regimes—be they revolutionary or reactionary—in their quest for national betterment. Most of the historiographical studies included in this volume (see Bliss, Hirschfeld, Pacino, Carter, and Dimas) frame healthcare as a public good that governments from all sides of the political spectrum have embraced in their quest for legitimacy. National leaders and their constituents tend to view the state's ability to preserve life as a biopolitical imperative (see Foucault 1994). As such, ensuring the health of all residents is crucial to any regime's ability to stay in power. In many cases, medical ventures have existed alongside paternalistic projects of modernization meant to assimilate Indigenous citizens into contemporary society (Dalton 2018). Regardless of the motivation, these countries have taken seriously—with varying degrees of success—their responsibility to ensure public health. As economic and political conditions throughout the region have shifted, many voices have begun to question the exact role of government in administering healthcare. By the end of the twentieth century (and into the twenty-first), neoliberal reforms began to call for greater privatization of the medical sector (see Bliss, Carter, and Dimas in this book). That said, such approaches have remained controversial throughout the region. In the end, Latin American governments continue to draw support from the citizenry by proving their ability to meet their particular country's public health needs. Healthcare as a topic is not limited to political and medical discourse, however, and through the years Latin American writers, artists, and filmmakers have engaged health issues with motivations that range from the aesthetic to the activist. In recognition of the prominence of public health in Latin American artistic expressions, this volume includes several chapters that explore the issue in a variety of cinematic endeavors from Mexico and the United States to Ecuador and Argentina.

*Healthcare in Latin America: History, Society, Culture* builds on a range of studies focused on health services in the Americas, including Katherine E. Bliss's (2001) *Compromised Positions: Prostitution, Public Health, and Gender Politics in Revolutionary Mexico City*, Eric D. Carter's (2012) *Enemy in the Blood: Malaria, Environment, and Development in Argentina*, and Nicole Pacino's (2013) doctoral thesis "Prescription for a Nation: Public Health in Post-Revolutionary Bolivia, 1952–1964." Bliss (2001) discusses the intersections of gender, health, and hygiene in postrevolutionary Mexico. In so doing, she identifies the ideological role that public health played in constructing a modern, postrevolutionary order. Pacino (2013) echoes these sentiments in her own work in Bolivia when she argues that "the MNR's [Movimiento Nacional Revolucionario/National Revolutionary Movement] Health Ministry largely focused its efforts on expanding modern medical care to the country to consolidate power and institutionalize ideas about revolutionary change" (36). Carter (2012) identifies a similar modernizing quality to public health in Argentina; he explains, "to hygienists, malaria served to symbolize the danger, backwardness, and decay of northwestern environment and society" (170).

Most of the essays in this volume—particularly those dedicated to historiography and cultural studies—build on the work of the aforementioned authors, and others, by bringing into play the paradigm of modernization and development. Viewed in this light, this volume answers the call of Marcos Cueto and Steven Palmer (2014) to "promote a fluid dialogue among, on the one hand, historians and health researchers, administrators, and activists, and, on the other hand, between historians of medicine and those who focus on Latin American social and political history" (2). In bringing together the work of social scientists, historians, and cultural theorists, *Healthcare in Latin America: History, Society, Culture* facilitates precisely this sort of conversation. In doing so, it also captures the flavor of public health across the diverse countries of the region. The volume is divided into five sections that engage different regions of Latin America: Mexico, the United States (US Latino/a/x), Central America and the Caribbean, the Andean region, and the Southern Cone. Each section of this book includes at least three chapters that examine a particular subregion's healthcare situation from distinct disciplinary angles. In each case, the first chapter is strongly historiographical and generally broad in scope, thus allowing it to function as an overview of the region. That chapter is followed by essays that are more specific in nature, and that offer eclectic perspectives on each region's approach to healthcare through the social sciences and humanistic methods. The eclectic nature of this volume is one of its assets that should appeal to a broad audience. The quality and significance of the research will attract experts in the fields of public health, history, the social sciences, cultural studies, and Latin American studies. Additionally, all chapters have been written with accessibility in mind. Indeed, the focus on innovative, but comprehensible, multidisciplinary chapters makes this volume a valuable resource for instructors tasked with creating and teaching interdisciplinary healthcare courses at both the undergraduate and graduate levels.

The decision to base the book's organization on geography reflects long-standing beliefs within Latin American studies that different regions face distinct realities based on a combination of demographic and environmental factors.[4] Furthermore, this organization allows us to approach healthcare systematically in different parts of Latin America, where local conditions have produced distinctive outcomes. Nonetheless, the anthology offers readings beyond the more obvious geographic one. For example, an instructor using the volume as part of a healthcare-based course could easily assign readings based on a methodological approach, favoring chapters on historiographical, the social sciences, or cultural studies topics. This may prove especially valuable to an audience more interested in a specific disciplinary lens. Additionally, the attentive reader will notice that the eclectic nature of the anthology is challenged by the presence of a variety of consequential themes that reappear throughout various chapters: eugenics, women's health, healthcare and modernization, universal healthcare, health and sexuality, linguistic barriers to healthcare, public health, and national identity, among others. Ultimately, *Healthcare in Latin America: History, Society, Culture* is a valuable resource as it tracks how specific national and regional conditions have contributed to healthcare practices and outcomes throughout Latin America. In the pages that follow, we provide a brief overview of the sections and chapters that comprise this volume.

**Part 1: Healthcare in Mexico**

Mexico is a country where Indigenous and European cultures have both coexisted and competed with each other since the earliest days of the Conquest. This dynamic manifests itself especially clearly in the case of healthcare, where disagreements surrounding "popular medicine" and "professional medicine" have abounded for centuries (Glasco 2010, 62–65). The chapters in this section focus primarily on healthcare from Independence to the present. The republican state took its mandate to provide adequate care to its population seriously; what is more, the Mexican populace demanded that the state fulfill its commitment to public health in order to maintain legitimacy. Many scholars argue that the Revolution of 1910 emerged in part due to socioeconomic frustrations among Indigenous citizens that included grievances about access to healthcare (Knight 1990, 76). The postrevolutionary regime aimed to quell class- and race-based tensions by ensuring access to vaccinations, antibiotics, and medical doctors (Kapelusz-Poppi 2001, 261–67).

One facet of national attempts to improve public health was the continued professionalization of the medical vocation. Indeed, Jethro Hernández Berrones's chapter tracks the creation of a professional medical apparatus from the arrival of the first Spanish colonizers to the mid-twentieth century. As he shows, by the end of the nineteenth century, the federal government had taken upon itself the task of licensing medics. Nevertheless, and particularly in rural areas, national healthcare efforts continued to compete with Indigenous healing practices. Given the institutional support for professionalizing the practice of medicine—which the state saw as key to overseeing the modernization of the nation—it is not surprising that the state-sponsored artistic movements—including muralism and filmmaking—that flourished in the decades following the Revolution would present modern medicine in triumphalist, pro-government terms. Douglas J. Weatherford discusses one example of this tendency in a chapter that discusses the representation of medical progress in postrevolutionary Mexico in the works and collaborations of the iconic Mexican director Emilio Fernández and North American Nobel laureate John Steinbeck. Similar to Diego Rivera, who revered healthcare advances through murals on the nation's walls, Fernández and Steinbeck used cinema to convey a nationalist discourse that didactically invited viewers, along with on-screen protagonists, to participate in the advances of medical modernity.

The priorities and aims of the Mexican state evolved in the decades following the Revolution. Katherine E. Bliss tracks the shifting goals of the national healthcare apparatus in her chapter. As she shows, during the first half of the twentieth century, the state viewed healthcare primarily as a means to promote economic development and to secure political support. By the 1940s, the country began to institute programs aimed at uplifting the urban poor, and, by 2012, it achieved universal coverage. Despite these gains, healthcare inequality persists in Mexico, a disparity that is especially pronounced within the country's Indigenous populations that often live far from major urban centers with their higher concentration of hospitals and doctors (Barber, Stefano, and Gertler 2007; Smith-Oka 2015). This relative lack of access to healthcare underscores the difficult socioeconomic conditions that have led many Indigenous Mexican peoples to consider migrating to urban centers where they have greater opportunities and better access to services like healthcare. Gabriela León-Pérez engages directly with this reality as she tracks the health of internal migrants after leaving their homes and moving to other parts of the country. She shows that health is an important indicator to consider as we discuss issues like internal mobility in the country.

## Part 2: Healthcare in US Latino/a/x Communities

This section stretches traditional understandings of what constitutes Latin American healthcare by including the experiences of Latin American diasporic communities in the United States. The decision to include these groups is not unprecedented, of course, as scholarship on Latin America over the last several decades has been more likely to include the United States due to its expansive Latino/a/x populations (see Mignolo 2005,

135–41). The various contributors to this volume use a variety of terms to designate people of Latin American descent who live in the United States: US Latino; US Latino/a; US Latinx; US Latino/a/x. This variation reflects both the key differences of each term and the unsettled nature of current debates surrounding how best to accurately and respectfully refer to this diverse population.[5] Each of these terms has advantages, but each is also problematic. It is not our intention, as editors of this volume, to delve into this debate, and, as such, we chose to allow individual contributors to determine how best to navigate these labels in their respective chapters. The term US Latino/a/x (and its variants) can apply to people with very different ethnic, racial, socioeconomic, and even linguistic identities (United States Census 2020). The majority of Latin American diasporic communities in the United States have historically come from Mexico, Central America, and the Caribbean. The former two demographics have traditionally inhabited the US Southwest (Zuñiga and Hernández-León 2005, xii-xiv), while those from the Caribbean have generally lived along the East Coast, particularly in Miami and New York City (McHugh et al. 1997; Grasmuck and Pessar 1991, 18–50; Rodríguez 1997). That said, there have been many exceptions (see Acosta-Belén and Santiago 2006, 54). Furthermore, as we enter the third decade of the twenty-first century, Latino/a/x populations in the United States have expanded beyond these traditional regions and inhabit states throughout the country (see Zuñiga and Hernández-León 2005). Also worth noting is the fact that an increasing number of immigrants to the United States come from South American countries, particularly Venezuela and Colombia.

Given the broad nature of what it means to be Latino/a/x, it can be difficult to identify a singular healthcare experience for people of Latin American descent in the United States. Nevertheless, there are certain factors that tend to hold true across these populations. For example, many members of the US Latino/a/x community have often been seen as "other" and have existed on the periphery of their country of residence. Benny J. Andrés Jr. examines this marginalization through public health practices in Puerto Rico and along the US-Mexico border—often aggressively eugenicist in nature—that were developed in large measure by colonial physicians returning from service in the island territories of an expanding empire who often viewed Latino/a/x bodies as dysgenic and diseased. Christopher D. Mellinger follows with a chapter that presents an overview of the social science literature specific to healthcare disparities in the US Latino/a/x community, with emphasis placed on the challenges, among others, of health literacy and access to health services. The section concludes with a study by David

S. Dalton that highlights an example of how some medical practitioners in the United States have taken advantage of linguistic barriers to implement eugenicist projects. Dalton analyzes Renee Tajima-Peña's 2015 documentary film *No más bebés/No More Babies*, which discusses the infamous cases of forced sterilization that occurred at the Los Angeles County-USC Medical Center in California during the 1960s and 1970s.

## Part 3: Healthcare in Central America and the Caribbean

The region of Central America and the Caribbean is one of great contrasts. While some countries provide excellent healthcare to their citizens, others do not. Perhaps no Latin American country has touted its gains in public health more visibly than the Revolutionary regime in Cuba. Indeed, since the 1959 Revolution that brought them to power, Fidel Castro and his brother Raúl (followed recently by Miguel Díaz-Canel) have focused on public health as a key site for investment. For example, Cuba has incentivized the study of medicine to deliberately create an oversupply of medical doctors. This practice has allowed the island nation to send thousands of doctors abroad every year—at a price—to help other countries with their own public health emergencies and initiatives (see J. Kirk 2015; J. Kirk and Erisman 2009). These endeavors have received praise from many parts of the international community for providing needed aid to developing nations. At the same time, they have also come under scrutiny due to the minimal compensation that medical practitioners receive for their services (see Hirschfeld's chapter in this book for a discussion). In any case, as Katherine Hirschfeld shows in her informative overview of the history of healthcare in Cuba, a competent public health agenda—at least in appearance—lies at the heart of state projects of national and international legitimacy. By contextualizing Revolutionary gains alongside improvements that were already in place prior to the Revolution, Hirschfeld gauges the veracity of the healthcare claims of the Revolutionary regime. Given the Cuban state's emphasis on healthcare, it should come as no surprise that the government views a wide array of issues through the lens of public health. Along those lines, Emily J. Kirk provides an innovative reading of the Cuban healthcare system by showing how that nation envisions disaster preparedness as a public health matter. When compared to the inadequate handling of natural disasters in Puerto Rico, Haiti, and even mainland United States, Kirk suggests Cuba's investment in disaster preparedness stands out. What is more, she asserts that these successes reflect the fact that state officials recognize public health as a primary goal in the decision-making process.

In Central America, revolutionary leaders like Nicaraguan president Daniel Ortega Saavedra viewed public health as key to their juntas, and, in the 1970s and 1980s before the collapse of the Soviet Union, Ortega was willing to coordinate with Moscow in an attempt to improve national health results (Paszyn 2000, 45). That said, the various nations of Central America have had very different experiences and results regarding healthcare. Costa Rica and Panama have both achieved near-universal healthcare, with Costa Rica boasting one of the most effective healthcare systems in the world (see Unger et al. 2008; Clark 2013). At the same time, countries like Guatemala, Honduras, Nicaragua, El Salvador, and Belize have generally struggled to produce equitable healthcare results due to myriad factors (see George et al. 2009, 106–13; Barillier and Jaegers 2020). In 2015, for example, 43.7 percent of El Salvador residents reported having no health insurance (Pérez-Cuevas et al. 2017, 820). Throughout Central America, a person's access to medical care often reflects a combination of their racial and ethnic identity, and socioeconomic condition. The healthcare disparities among the countries of the region can be seen with particular clarity in the realm of childbirth. Indeed, the final chapter of this section, authored by Sophie Esch and Alicia Z. Miklos, examines literary and print-media depictions of childbirth, maternal care, and women's health in Guatemala, El Salvador, and Nicaragua. The authors demonstrate how racial and patriarchal attitudes continue to define the healthcare options available to expectant mothers throughout the region.

## Part 4: Healthcare in the Andean Region

The Andean region includes the countries of Perú, Ecuador, Bolivia, Colombia, and Venezuela.[6] Despite unique qualities that define each of these countries, shared realities like the geographical (the Andes mountains) and the cultural (including thriving Indigenous cultures) place them in this important Latin American subregion. Andean nations have enjoyed few moments of social and political stability since the arrival of the first Spaniards in the 1530s. The Conquest proved particularly brutal in this northern part of South America, and the poverty, exploitation, and racial divisions that followed continue to plague the area. Substandard health indicators and unequal access to quality healthcare are only two of the many measures that illustrate the struggles that the Andean region continues to face as it looks to improve the lives of its citizens.

When it comes to socioeconomic and public health standards, the landlocked nation of Bolivia traditionally has lagged behind its Andean neighbors and most other countries of the Western Hemisphere. This difficult reality, combined with several attempts—sometimes successful—to improve this situation make Bolivia an intriguing focus of investigation, and two of the four chapters of this section (by Pacino and Forste) focus on this nation with a relatively higher number of Indigenous Peoples. Bolivia is of interest as well since healthcare reforms have developed largely alongside a history of political and social upheaval. That is particularly true over the thirteen-year far-left presidency (2006–2019) of Evo Morales, Bolivia's first Indigenous president and a (not always effective) proponent of increased healthcare access, especially for the nation's poor. His resignation in November 2019 after allegations of voter fraud has left observers wondering about the future of health delivery in that nation. Morales and his Movement for Socialism party [Movimiento al Socialismo] were not the first political coalition to promise improved healthcare only to be removed from office (see Pacino's article in this volume for a review of Bolivia's 1952 Revolution). To be sure, political instability and corruption throughout the Andean region—from Hugo Chávez and Nicolás Maduro in Venezuela to the long list of former presidents like Alberto Fujimori incarcerated in Peru in recent years—have all made sustained improvements to healthcare difficult.

There are bright spots in the Andean region, of course. Colombia emerged recently from a decades-long civil war between a conservative state and the leftist Revolutionary Armed Forces of Colombia [Fuerzas Armadas Revolucionarias de Colombia]. As a result, many health statistics have improved both in that country and throughout the region. In her chapter Renata Forste highlights some of the advances in maternal and child health in the Andean region, while also pointing out the continued need for improvements to support women and children. Alongside these advances, scholars and activists are highlighting emerging challenges. In this volume, for example, Javier E. García León and David L. García León examine access to healthcare for trans and disabled individuals as represented in recent Colombian media. Such forward-looking trends are tempered by a mounting desire to look back. The Andean region has seen numerous movements—whether political, cultural, or artistic—intent on elevating the area's Indigenous heritage (see, among others, the efforts of José Carlos Mariátegui in Peru). In this volume, for example, Manuel F. Medina explores the desire to retain and celebrate ancestral knowledges, including in the realm of healthcare, as seen in a recent Ecuadorian film. Ultimately, the studies included in this section draw attention to the struggles of the healthcare industry in the Andean region, while celebrating a collection of nations that continues a fight for improved living standards and opportunities.

## Part 5: Healthcare in the Southern Cone

As its name implies, the Southern Cone is composed of those nations located geographically in the cone-shaped tip of South America: Brazil, Paraguay, Uruguay, Argentina, and Chile. Despite their proximity, these countries boast diverse identities, be they linguistic (Portuguese, Spanish, and Guaraní, among other languages) or geographic (from the high Andes and the low flat Pampas to the arid Sertão and the verdant Amazonia). In a recent listing of the wealthiest nations of South America (Gross Domestic Product or GDP per capita), the top spot was taken by the Southern Cone country of Uruguay, followed immediately by Chile, Argentina, and Brazil (Nag 2019; see also Oelsner 2005, 5–6). These four countries rank well on the Human Development Report 2019 distributed by the United Nations Development Programme, and they boast strong life expectancy rates and high standards of living. Paraguay, a country with few major cities and a history of isolation and war is by far the poorest country in the region and faces problems distinct from its neighbors. Just the Paraguayan War [Guerra contra la Triple Alianza], for example, that occurred in the nineteenth century is said to have cost the nation over 50 percent of its population. Despite the relative wealth of much of the Southern Cone, all five nations suffered violent military dictatorships during the second half of the twentieth century. During the 1980s and 1990s, top generals negotiated transitions to democracy in each of these countries that secured their own self-preservation on the one hand, while ensuring civilian leadership on the other. These democracies have faced serious issues, but the various nations of the Southern Cone have managed to transition peacefully between right- and left-leaning governments for several decades.

These transitions, as might be expected, have been accompanied by impassioned debate about the role of the state in healthcare delivery and by attempts by politicians, medical professionals, and academic investigators to survey the successes and failures of national health initiatives. Two of the three researchers featured in this section are part of that endeavor. They base their research on comparative studies of the healthcare models established by neighboring states from the early twentieth century to the beginning of the twenty-first century. Eric D. Carter compares the development of national health systems in Chile and Argentina, for example, while Carlos S. Dimas weighs Argentina's efforts to provide universal healthcare against that of Brazil. In a concluding chapter, Javier Barroso offers a humanistic approach to the healthcare debate in the Southern Cone through an analysis of intersexuality in Lucía Puenzo's 2007 film *XXY*.

Ultimately, *Healthcare in Latin America: History, Society, Culture* provides a rich overview of healthcare as it plays out across the multiple countries that comprise Latin America. The volume boasts a wealth of interdisciplinary studies—from history and film studies to the social sciences—to provide both experts and students with diverse avenues to explore the important topic of healthcare in this region of the world. As well, the chapters of this anthology reveal that the chronicle of healthcare in Latin America is deeply enmeshed in the region's diverse political, historical, and cultural identities. As such, *Healthcare in Latin America: History, Society, Culture*'s deeper interrogation of the various national approaches to public health reveals lessons about the region that go well beyond healthcare and get at many of the quintessential questions of Latin American studies more generally.

### Notes

1. For a country-by-country comparison of the response to SARS-CoV-2 throughout the world, see Worldometer (2020).

2. Mexico is another country in the Western Hemisphere that dealt with an especially crippling onslaught of COVID-19. At the time of this writing, it ranks fourth worldwide with 250,000 deaths attributed to the virus (Worldometer 2021).

3. Scholars interested in healthcare prior to Independence should consult Martha Few's (2015) book *For All of Humanity: Mesoamerican and Colonial Medicine in Enlightenment Guatemala* and Christina Ramos's (2022) book *Belam in the New World: A Mexican Madhouse in the Age of Enlightenment* (see also Ramos 2020; 2021).

4. For a discussion of the value—and problems—associated with identifying different "subregions" of Latin America, see Gerald C. Berg (2011).

5. The meanings of terms like Latino, Latina, Latinx (and derivates like Chicano, Chicana, Chicanx) have evolved over time. During the 1960s and 1970s, Latino was generally viewed both as a masculine and gender-neutral term. In the 1980s, women began to call for the spellings Latino/a, Latina/o, Chicano/a, and Chicana/o. These variations would highlight the fact that these communities and movements benefited from work of both men and women. In the early twenty-first century, many groups of Latin American descent in the United States have called for terms like Latinx and Chicanx. They prefer these terms because they are nonbinary and thus include men, women, and nonbinary people (Scharrón-del Río and Aja 2020, 8–10). At the same time, many native speakers of Spanish have pushed back against the "x," viewing it as an imperialistic imposition from English onto Spanish (Guerra and Gilbert Orbea 2015). Still others call for the term Latino/a/x as a compromise that both accounts for the need to move beyond a male/female binary and also respects the linguistic tradition of Spanish speakers (Trujillo-Pagán 2018).

6. Venezuela is not always included in this grouping; meanwhile, Chile and Argentina sometimes are.

## References

Acosta-Belén, Edna, and Carlos E. Santiago. 2006. *Puerto Ricans in the United States: A Contemporary Portrait*. Boulder, CO: Lynne Rienner Publishers.

Agren, David. 2020, 25 Mar. "Coronavirus Advice from Mexico's President: 'Live Life as Usual.'" *The Guardian*.

Barber, Sarah L., Stefano M. Bertozzi, and Paul J. Gertler. 2007. "Variations in Prenatal Care Quality for the Rural Poor in Mexico." *Health Affairs* 26 (2): w310–23.

Barillier, Krya, and Lisa Jaegers. 2020. "Identifying Gaps in OT Services in a Developing Country: Healthcare-Clinic Needs-Assessment in Rural Belize." *American Journal of Occupational Therapy* 74 (4_Supplement_1). https://doi.org/10.5014/ajot.2020.74S1-PO8401

Berg, Gerald C. 2011. "Does Latin America Comprise Transnational 'Subregions'?" *The World Economy* 34 (2): 298–312.

Bliss, Katherine E. 2001. *Compromised Positions: Prostitution, Public Health, and Gender Politics in Revolutionary Mexico City*. University Park: The Pennsylvania State University Press.

Carter, Eric D. 2012. *Enemy in the Blood: Malaria, Environment, and Development in Argentina*. Tuscaloosa: University of Alabama Press.

Clark, Mary A. 2013. "The Final Frontiers of Healthcare Universalisation in Costa Rica and Panama." *Bulletin of Latin American Research* 33 (2): 125–39.

Cueto, Marcos, and Steven Palmer. 2014. *Medicine and Public Health in Latin America*. Cambridge: Cambridge University Press.

Dalton, David S. 2018. *Mestizo Modernity: Race, Technology, and the Body in Postrevolutionary Mexico*. Gainesville: University of Florida Press.

Few, Martha. 2015. *For All of Humanity: Mesoamerican and Colonial Medicine in Enlightenment Guatemala*. Tucson, AZ: University of Arizona Press.

———. 2020. "Epidemics, Indigenous Communities, and Public Health in the COVID-19 Era: Views from Smallpox Innoculation Campaigns in Colonial Guatemala." *Journal of Global History* 15 (3): 380–93.

Foucault, Michel. 1994. "The Birth of Biopolitics." In *The Essential Foucault*, edited by Paul Rabinow and Nikolas Rose, 202–07. New York: The New Press.

George, Asha, Elaine P. Menotti, Dixmer Rivera, Irma Montés, Carmen María Reyes, and David R. Marsh. 2009. "Community Case Management of Childhood Illness in Nicaragua: Transforming Health Systems in Underserved Rural Areas." *Journal of Health Care for the Poor and Underserved* 20 (4): 99–115.

Guerra, Gilbert, and Gilbert Orbea. 2015. "The Argument against the Use of the Term 'Latinx.'" *The Phoenix*, November 19, 2015.

Glasco, Sharon Bailey. 2010. *Constructing Mexico City: Colonial Conflicts over Culture, Space, and Authority*. New York: Palgrave MacMillan.

Gold, Jeremy A.W., Lauren M. Rossen, Farida B. Ahmad, Paul Sutton, Zeyu Li, Phillip P. Salvatore, Jayme P. Coyle, Jennifer DeCuir, Brittney N. Baack, Tonji M. Durant, Kenneth L. Dominguez, S. Jane Henley, Francis B. Annor, Jennifer Fuld, Deborah L. Dee, Achuyt Bhattarai, and Brendan R. Jackson. 2020. "Race, Ethnicity, and Age Trends in

Persons Who Died from COVID-19—United States, May–August 2020." *Morbidity and Mortality Weekly Report* 69 (42): 1517–21.

Grasmuck, Sherri, and Patricia R. Pessar. 1991. *Between Two Islands: Dominican International Migration*. Berkeley: University of California Press.

Hanrahan, Brían, and Paulina Aroch Fugellie. 2019. "Reflections on the Transformation in Mexico." *Journal of Latin American Cultural Studies* 28 (1): 113–37.

Kapelusz-Poppi, Ana María. 2001. "Physician Activists and Development of Rural Health in Post-Revolutionary Mexico." *Radical History Review* 2001 (80): 35–50.

Kirk, John M. 2015. *Healthcare without Borders: Understanding Cuban Medical Internationalism*. Gainesville: University Press of Florida.

Kirk, John M., and Michael H. Erisman. 2009. *Cuban Medical Internationalism: Origins, Evolution and Goals*. New York: Palgrave MacMillan.

Knight, Alan. 1990. "Racism, Revolution, and *Indigenismo*: Mexico, 1910–1940." In *The Idea of Race in Latin America*, edited by Richard Graham, 71–113. Austin: University of Texas Press.

La Razón 2020. "'El riesgo de coronavirus solo es para los ricos. Los pobres somos inmunes': Las polémicas declaraciones del gobernador del Estado mexicano de Puebla sobre el COVID-19 han tenido como efecto que la prensa local investigue su patrimonio." *La Razón*, March 27, 2020. https://www.larazon.es/internacional/20200327/lu44xqevwjekvme6sio4qhrooi.html

McHugh, Kevin, Inés M. Miyares, and Emily H. Skop. 1997. "The Magnetism of Miami: Segmented Paths in Cuban Migration." *The Geographical Review* 87 (4): 504–19.

Mignolo, Walter. 2005. *The Idea of Latin America*. Malden, MA: Blackwell Publishing.

Nag, Oishimaya Sen. 2019. "The Richest Countries in South America." *WorldAtlas*, October 23, 2019. https://www.worldatlas.com/articles/the-richest-countries-in-south-america.html.

Oelsner, Andrea. 2005. *International Relations in Latin America: Peace and Security in the Southern Cone*. New York: Routledge.

Pacino, Nicole. 2013. "Prescription for a Nation: Public Health in Post-Revolutionary Bolivia, 1952–1964." PhD Diss., University of California, Santa Barbara.

Paszyn, Danuta. 2000. *The Soviet Attitude to Political and Social Change in Central America, 1979–90*. New York: Palgrave MacMillan.

Pérez-Cuevas, Ricardo. Federico C. Guanais, Svetlana V. Doubova, Leonardo Pinzón, Luis Tejerina, Diana Pinto Masis, Marcia Rocha, Donna O. Harris, and James Macinko. 2017. "Understanding Public Perception of the Need for Major Change in Latin American Healthcare Systems." *Health Policy and Planning* 32 (6): 816–24.

Phillips, Tom. 2020. "Brazil's Jair Bolsonaro says Coronavirus Crisis is a Media Trick." *The Guardian*, March 23, 2020. https://www.theguardian.com/world/2020/mar/23/brazils-jair-bolsonaro-says-coronavirus-crisis-is-a-media-trick.

Ramos, Christina. 2020. "Caring for *pobres dementes*: Madness, Colonization, and the Hospital de San Hipólito in Mexico City, 1567–1700." *The Americas* 77 (4): 539–71.

———. 2021. "Beyond the Columbian Exchange: Medicine and Public Health in Colonial Latin America." *History Compass* 19 (8): e12682.

———. 2022. *Belam in the New World: A Mexican Madhouse in the Age of Enlightenment*. Chapel Hill: University of North Carolina Press.

Rodríguez, Clara E. 1997. "A Summary of Puerto Rican Migration to the United States." In *Challenging Fronteras: Structuring Latina and Latino Lives in the U.S.*, edited by Mary Romero, Pierrette Honagneu-Sotelo, and Vilma Ortiz, 101–13. New York: Routledge.

Scharrón-del Río, María, and Alan A. Aja. 2020. "*Latinx*: Inclusive Language as Liberation Praxis." *Journal of Latinx Psychology* 8 (1): 7–20.

Smith-Oka, Vania. 2015. "Microaggressions and the Reproduction of Social Inequalities in Medical Encounters in Mexico." *Social Science and Medicine* 143: 9–16.

Trujillo-Pagán, Nicole. 2018. "Crossed out by LatinX: Gender Neutrality and Genderblind Sexism." *Latino Studies* 16 (4): 396–406.

Unger, Jean-Pierre, Pierre de Paepe, René Bultrón, and Werner Soors. 2008. "Costa Rica: Achievements of a Heterodox Health Policy." *American Journal of Public Health* 98 (4): 636–45.

United Nations Development Programme. 2019. *Human Development Report 2019: Beyond Income, Beyond Averages, Beyond Today: Inequalities in Human Development in the 21st Century*. New York. http://hdr.undp.org/sites/default/files/hdr2019.pdf.

United States Census 2020. 2020. Question Asked: Hispanic Origin. https://2020census.gov/en/about-questions/hispanic-origin.html.

Valencia, Alexandria, and Vicente Gaibor del Pino. 2020. "Ecuador Builds Emergency Cemeteries Due to Coronavirus Outbreak." *Reuters*, April 7, 2020. https://www.reuters.com/article/us-health-coronavirus-ecuador/ecuador-builds-emergency-cemeteries-due-to-coronavirus-outbreak-idUSKBN21Q018.

Worldometer. 2020. COVID-19 Coronavirus Pandemic. https://www.worldometers.info/coronavirus/.

Worldometer. 2021. Coronavirus Cases. https://www.worldometers.info/coronavirus/ .

Zuñiga, Víctor, and Rubén Hernández-León. 2005. *New Destinations: Mexican Immigration in the United States*. New York: Russell Sage Foundation.

# PART I

## Healthcare in Mexico

# 1

## Healers and Doctors

### A History of the Healing Occupations in Mexico

JETHRO HERNÁNDEZ BERRONES

The goal of this chapter is twofold. First, it offers an overview of how societies in the territories that we currently call Mexico have organized the transmission of medical knowledge and granted healing authority to those who have this knowledge. In the nineteenth century, medicine began to play a substantial role in the organization of societies of emerging nation-states around the world. By the twentieth century, sociologists interested in understanding this phenomenon identified a new form of social organization that changed the way doctors produced medical knowledge and delivered medical services (Freidson 1970; Hafferty and McKinlay 1993). They referred to it as the medical profession. Using doctors from the United States and the healthcare system they created as a model, Paul Starr (1982) defined the medical profession as a self-conscious, autonomous, and self-regulating group with a set of cohesive values and specialized knowledge that allowed them to dominate the provision of health, expanding and monopolizing its services. If this notion first appealed to professional historians of medicine in the second half of the twentieth century, they soon found its limitations when applied to societies in the past (Burnham 1998; Fee and Brown 2004). The model did not resemble the structure and functioning of medical communities and institutions in the second half of the twentieth century or before the nineteenth century, when physicians did not dominate healthcare. Yet, the very elements of the concept of "profession"—groups of practitioners with shared specialized knowledge—and the provision of health services helped to describe healthcare in these societies. I use the concept of profession and its components as a point of reference to examine the organization of healing occupations in Mexico since precolonial times to the late twentieth century.

The second goal of this paper is to examine healing occupations from the perspective of medical pluralism. Historians of medicine in Latin America have emphasized the peculiar development of the medical profession in this region (Cueto and Palmer 2015). The multiethnic nature of its inhabitants, the region's shared colonial past, the local processes of nation building, and Latin American nations' constant negotiation with outside forces framed the pluralistic nature of health delivery systems and the continuous presence of a mixed group of healers in them. The composition, organization, and history of these pluralist health systems make Latin American countries unique. Consequently, historians Diego Armus (2003) and Marcos Cueto and Steven Palmer (2015) abandoned the term "profession" as an analytical category and focused on healing practices to describe the healing occupations of the region.

In line with this approach, Mexican historians and sociologists have depicted the organization of professional medicine in less triumphalist terms than their counterparts in the United States (Arce Gurza et al. 1982; Castañeda López and Rodríguez de Romo 2007; Cleaves 1985; Martínez Barbosa 2011), in part because medical doctors in Mexico have organized around state institutions since the colonial period. This doctors–state relationship linked doctors' values, training and licensing institutions, and medical labor to state needs, which in turn limited the profession's autonomy, self-regulatory capacities, and control over a market of services. This relationship, however, only applies to a small fraction of healers—usually academically trained ones. Most of the population up to the mid-twentieth century sought healthcare beyond institutions regulated by the state and through healing systems that preserved—to varying degrees—Amerindian or imported African medical traditions. These communities sometimes combined their medical traditions with academic or emerging forms of popular medicine, generating a mosaic of mixed healing traditions and healers. Some contemporary communities still preserve these practices as the first line of care. The history of medical occupations in Mexico is, therefore, a history of medical *mestizaje* [mixtures], where academic and non-academic healing traditions inhabited specific geographic and institutional spaces where they coexisted to provide healthcare through official and unofficial ways. Historically, multiple actors with varying interests defined medical values, training, practice, groups, and services.

This overview emphasizes, then, the pluralist nature of healing occupations in Mexico. Given this scope of seven hundred years, any overview will necessarily be schematic. Nevertheless, my approach offers a framework for understanding individuals and groups that provided healing to Mexicans as well as the changing institutions that regulated these healers' training and practice. The bibliography should help readers identify essential scholarly works that have contributed to the history of healing occupations in Mexico.

## Precolonial Healers

Multiple nomadic groups had established semi-sedentary and sedentary communities throughout Mesoamerica between 2000 and 250 BCE. These communities developed large city-states through 900 CE. The Nahua-speaking people who self-identified as Mexica were one of the last northern groups to migrate to Mexico's central valley. They founded the city of Tenochtitlan in 1325 CE and, over the next two centuries, they grew an empire that exerted military and economic control over the diverse array of ethnic groups inhabiting Mesoamerica and Central America. When Spanish conquistadors arrived on Mesoamerican shores in the early sixteenth century, they documented the cultures of these Mesoamerican societies.

Our understanding of health and healthcare in pre-Columbian societies comes from the analysis of these documentary sources and archaeological excavations. Physical anthropologists have used osteological and demographic information to reconstruct the biological nature of individual and epidemic diseases (Alchon 2003; Márquez Morfín and Hernández Espinosa 2006). Documentary sources offer scholars a window into these societies' ways of explaining, diagnosing, and treating diseases.[1] The study of these sources should be done with caution since they were produced in colonial settings where colonizers' mentalities framed native beliefs and practices as heterodox if not heretical, and native informants may have accommodated their healing systems to European standards. Most scholars agree on the similarities among the different healing cultures of Mesoamerica, though they recognize the variations among different ethnic groups.

Aztecs believed the body was immersed in a cosmos of influences from the natural and supernatural worlds (López Austin 1988, Viesca Treviño 1990). The body was composed by two substances: one dense, material, visual, and subject to accidents of time; and another light, subtle, undetectable, and subject to divisions and reunifications (López Austin, 2017). The realm of subtle substance may penetrate and influence the realm of dense substance, but not the other way around. The body had subtle elements, or souls. Some of them were constitutional and other ones contingent to it, invading it, and altering constitutional souls and dense elements. The *teyolía*, the center of the subtle substance, resided in the heart and remained with the individual from birth to death. The *teyolía* was composed of multiple subdivisions of the same god. These subdivisions gave the individual its essential anthropomorphic characteristics such as ethnicity, town, *callpulli* group or larger familial group, language, customs, and economic specialization. The *tonalli* was a subtle substance imposed at birth by ritual upon the individual. The specific *tonalli* corresponded to a deity governing the Aztec calendar and it concentrated in the head. The *ihíyotl* was the constitutive soul located in the liver that produced desires and appetites. Secondary souls could live in or possess a human body giving them particular attributes. In the body, these interactions expressed as the balance between two antagonistic principles identified with hot and cold. The balance between them defined the state of health. The hot–cold framework guided physicians in the description of disease, the diagnosis, and the selection of therapies in order to restore the balance.

Given the holistic nature of the Aztec healing system, European terms such as medicine and physician provide a limited view of the scope of health and healing in the Aztec world. *Ticiyotl,* roughly translated as medicine, has recently been defined as "a system of extensive networks of actors, materials, and performances that came together to make the restoration and preservation of health possible" (Polanco 2019, 3). Similarly, *Titicih* (plural: *tícitl*), usually translated as sorcerer, healer, or fortuneteller, has been referred to as a ritual specialist that operated within the Aztec cosmos described in the previous paragraph. The distinction avoids anachronistic interpretations of Aztec healing practices in line with the colonizer's religious and naturalistic views of the world.

The *tícitl* acquired knowledge of *ticiyotl* through formal, natural, and supernatural channels. Formal channels included the family and artisan schools called *calmecac* (Andalón González 2016). Natural ways included the consumption of entheogenic substances or near-death experiences (Polanco 2019). Deceased ancestors and deities visited individuals in their dreams or during near-death experiences and granted them the "gift of curing" along with the tools they needed. The *tícitl* engaged in five activities related to healing. They performed rituals to satisfy supernatural forces that they deemed helpful when restoring health. They investigated the causes of disease through *tlapohualiztli*, a term that refers to counting, information, sharing knowledge by a student, uncovering, and also sortilege. It seems that *tícitl* did not interpret texts to diagnose illnesses; rather, they observed patients, consumed entheogens, and/or used objects they created or saw. The list of plants, minerals, animal parts, and rocks that the *tícitl* used for therapeutic purposes is extensive (De Vos 2021; Gimmel 2008). *Tícitl* collected them, prepared concoctions with them, and used them on sick people in a ritualistic manner. Generally, healing occurred domestically. The Nahua described different types of *tícitl* classified based on the type of disease they treated, though strict specialization did not exist. Each class of practitioner had its place and function in the lives of individuals. Specialization as well as social status indicated hierarchies among healers, though a rigid rank system did not exist. Among the large number of *tícitl*, we can find the *tetonalmacani, tetonaltiqui, tetonallaliqui*—the one who restores *tonalli*; the *teapahtiani*—the one who breaks a spell or provides an antidote for a poison; the *tetlacuicuiliqui*—the one who removes a physical representation of the disease from the body; the *techichinami*—the one who sucks the disease out of the body; the *tepoztecpahtiani*—the one who heals what is broken; the one who heals by *teiczaliztli*—a procedure of massaging with the feet; the one who heals by *pacholiztli*—a procedure of massaging children in the chest; the *tepillaliliqui*—the one who helps women conceive; the *tetlaxiliqui*—the one who helps women with abortion; the *texoxotla tícitl*—the one who makes incisions in the body; the *texpatiania*—the one who treats the eyes; the *tenacazpatiani*—the one who treats the ears; and the *tlancopinaliztli*—the one who treats the teeth (Andalón González 2016; López Austin 1967). Pregnancy, childbirth, and the care of newborns belonged exclusively to female midwives.

Indigenous and mestizo communities who survived the acculturation process during the colonial period and after independence (1821) preserved elements of their native healing traditions by word of mouth and in a few codices. To this day, "traditional" healers continue offering this medical knowledge to treat patients in communities situated far from academic and state medical institutions, and sometimes within them (Huber and Sanstrom 2010; Lozoya L. 1986, 1994).

## The Healing Occupations of New Spain

The Spanish Crown ruled in the Americas from the fall of Tenochtitlan in 1521 until the triumph of the revolutions of independence in 1821, in a territory they labeled New Spain. Spaniards viewed the body in humoral terms and the world through the Catholic faith, a holistic view that resembled the one held by the Amerindians. According to Hippocrates (1950), the body had four humors—blood, phlegm, yellow bile, and black bile—that were aligned with four environmental conditions—heat, cold, wetness, and dryness. When in balance, the four humors made the body healthy, but when off balance, the body fell ill. Inherited predispositions, environmental conditions, and personal character contributed to this interplay of forces. The body was also a space of supernatural intervention. Health and disease were usually attributed to grace or sin, divine or demonic intervention, personal grit or weakness, or bodily purification or punishment, all dichotomies delineated by Catholic theology. The similarities between European and Amerindian medicine allowed exchanges and tensions (Foster 1987). Transfers of knowledge were selective and depended on geographic and disciplinary context.

Spanish settlers in New Spain adopted the institutions aimed at regulating medical training that the crown implemented in Spain (Lanning and TePaske 1985). During the early decades, the crown appointed an academically trained physician or surgeon as *protomédico*, an individual who certified medical knowledge, regulated the provision of medicine by physicians, and prosecuted practitioners without the certification. As the colonies matured, new institutions emerged. In 1551, the Crown founded the Royal University in New Spain, which offered the first lecture on medicine in 1578. The Crown created the Tribunal of the Protomedicato in 1646 and linked its functions to the Royal University, unifying the regulation of academic medical instruction and practice. The university granted three degrees in medicine: bachelors, *licenciado* (masters), and doctorate (Hernández Sáenz 1997). Candidates attended lectures in medicine, wrote and defended dissertations, taught medicine, and were examined before obtaining the corresponding degree. Instruction as well as medical books were in Latin and Greek. In the late eighteenth century, candidates were required to attend lectures on clinical medicine. The university offered lectures on medicine and surgery for surgeons and pharmacists, though there were no specific degrees for these occupations. In the late colonial period, the Crown created the Royal College of Surgery and the Royal Botanical Gardens at the demand of surgeons and pharmacists.

Colonial institutions regulating medical practices established very specific requirements for degrees and licenses for the healing occupations. Candidates had to be examined and disclose their academic degree, Catholic baptismal certificate, clean record with the Inquisition, and proof of legitimate ancestry and blood purity (without Jewish, Muslim, or African ancestry) to the Protomedicato in order to obtain a license for practicing (Lanning 1967).[2] In the early nineteenth century, requirements also included two years of clinical internship and a course on medical botany. Pursuing a licensed healing occupation required time as well as social networks and economic resources. For instance, physicians, surgeons, and pharmacists generally inherited their libraries and left their social capital, including patients, to their descendants. However, the actual demography of physicians may have been less socially and racially exclusive than legislation suggests. An important number of mixed-race physicians figure in the archival record, though mixed-race practitioners were usually found practicing phlebotomy, midwifery, and dentistry, the lower ranks of the healing occupations. These practitioners usually learned through apprenticeship and, while these professionals needed a license to practice legally, the Protomedicato neglected to enforce regulations, in part because of the elite's contempt toward practitioners in the lower levels of the colonial healing occupational hierarchy. Criticism and legal oversight, however, allowed these practitioners to fulfill the medical needs of the largest portion of the urban population (Hernández Sáenz 1997). The last category of colonial healers included those who practiced illegally. Medical elites perceived them as competitors and a threat to the social order. They were physicians, surgeons, and pharmacists with partial or complete training, but without a license; phlebotomist, midwives, and dentists who were in regulatory limbo; clergymen who learned from academic and domestic medical manuals and delivered healthcare in their communities; and *curanderos* [healers] with Amerindian or African medical knowledge (Aguirre Beltrán 1963; Quesada 1989).

Colonial demographic landscapes had a socioeconomic and racial gradient reflected in the practice of healing. Academic medicine was elitist and metropolitan. Richer *criollos* [Spaniards born in the Americas] served more as physicians than as phlebotomists or midwives in cities, where the Protomedicato had strong control over medical practice and where Iberians and *criollos* sought medical advice. Below the rank of physician, the Protomedicato was more lenient toward the requirement of purity of blood to grant licenses and the requirement for a license to practice, perhaps because the numbers of Iberians and *criollos* decreased as the Indigenous population and those with African ancestry increased. In towns and villages, the health of most inhabitants of New Spain depended on the skills of low ranked or even unlicensed practitioners. Through their elitism, their incapacity to regulate healers, and their leniency toward popular medicine, colonial institutions created what Gonzalo Aguirre Beltrán (1963) calls "zones of refuge" where many different forms of medical knowledge and practice survived and persisted, adapting, resisting, and challenging academic medicine.

## Healers and Doctors of the Mexican Nation

In the 1810s, inhabitants of the colonies of New Spain, led by *criollos*, rebelled against the Spanish Crown. The independent countries that emerged in the 1820s and 1830s began a long process of political and social reorganization.

Mexico obtained its independence in 1821, but internal political conflicts between royalists and liberals, as well as the struggles against the expansionism of the United States, delayed the establishment of lasting medical institutions for almost half a century, until the heavy-handed stability of the Porfiriato (1876–1910). Medicine changed dramatically in the nineteenth century.

Merging symptomatic descriptions of disease at the bedside with clinical observation of patients and autopsies of corpses at hospitals, physicians made the body—its organs, its tissues, and its cells—the territory of disease. In the morgue, the hospital, the university classroom, and the lab, surgeons and doctors came up with new understandings of the human body that limited the space for metaphysical or religious explanations of life, disease, and death. Advances in chemistry allowed the analysis of medicinal plants and the extraction of chemical compounds with therapeutic properties. Anesthesia opened the doors to surgical procedures without pain. In Europe, Luis Pasteur and Robert Koch proposed the germ theory of disease and Claude Bernard advanced a new experimental method to inquire on the functions of the living body. Yet, besides prophylactic approaches such as smallpox vaccines and hygiene, new therapeutic approaches remained experimental, and therapy consisted mainly of surgery and keeping balance of the six Hippocratic non-naturals: environment, exercise, sleep, diet, excretion of waste, and emotions. As in Europe, the adoption and dissemination of medical knowledge in Mexico was a state-supported process that faced resistance from both physicians and the public. However, by the end of the nineteenth century, Mexico had state-run medical schools, research institutions, and hospitals that adopted the new approaches to medicine in order to treat the diseases of—mostly elite—Mexicans living in cities.

The process of independence just reframed the power disputes between the state and the healing occupations that occurred in the colonial period (Hernández Sáenz 2018). The health of citizens emerged as a field of government's concern and intervention during the century. The increasing authority of municipal health boards and its medical staff undermined the authority of the colonial Protomedicato. New approaches demanded the unification of medicine and surgery, challenging colonial hierarchies in medical education and certification, and creating new ones. Government endorsement of public health and the rise of physician-surgeons as specialists in treating diseases established a new relationship between postcolonial governments and the healing occupations. With the triumph of liberalism in the second half of the nineteenth century, physician-surgeons gained control over the curriculum at medical schools, but they depended on government support for establishing state-of-the-art medical schools, research institutions, and hospitals. Similarly, governments depended on doctors to staff the growing number of medical and sanitary institutions. Therefore, both governments and doctors collaborated in the training, licensing, and employing of health practitioners.

The National School of Medicine [Escuela Nacional de Medicina], located in Mexico City, led medical education in the country in the late nineteenth century (Carrillo and Saldaña 2005; Hernández Sáenz 2018). Other schools in the provinces aspired to recreate the state-of-the-art facilities, academic qualifications of faculty, and, in general, the material resources of the school in the capital. The network of hospitals, medical societies, and research centers in Mexico City contributed to the prestige of physicians from the capital. The secularization of hospitals opened spaces for the anatomical and clinical training that modern medicine demanded. Research institutions kept faculty and students up to date with innovations. This, in turn, promoted curricular renovation and the formation of specialists. In response to the growth and increasing relevance of medicine and the sciences in the life of Mexicans, Gabino Barreda, physician, and the Ministry of Education, introduced Positivism in a newly created National Preparatory School that students attended before enrolling in professional schools.[3] Physician-surgeons, consequently, received training in physics, chemistry, and biology in high school as well as scientific and clinical specialties in medical school, including histology, physiology, medical chemistry, ophthalmology, bacteriology, gynecology, and mental diseases. Increasingly, instruction emphasized practical experiences in the lab, in the hospital, and at the bedside. Medicine was the largest program at the medical school, though it also offered programs in obstetrics, pharmacy, dentistry, and nursing.

The reforms of the mid-nineteenth century created a legal tension for the practice of medicine. While a liberal constitution established educational and professional freedom, specific regulations unconstitutionally established limits to such liberties. In 1841, the Superior Board of Health [Consejo Superior de Salubridad] substituted the Protomedicato and assumed its licensing functions. Licensing procedures were similar to the ones of the colonial period, though legislation eliminated birthright requirements and adopted Spanish as the official language of instruction and examination. The Board paid particular attention to the licensing of foreign doctors, though ruling governments frequently challenged the Board's decisions. The constitution of 1857 granted Mexicans the freedom to pursue the education and occupation they desired. Degrees and certifications, in principle, did not prevent anyone from practicing medicine. Yet, the 1867 Law of Instruction of Mexico City established the curriculum of the National School of Medicine and provided general guidelines to organize instruction and issue professional degrees. The Board lost control over examination requirements and curricular content, but it kept control over licensing. The Liberal government's rationale to issue regulations that contravened the constitution was that only academically trained physicians possessed adequate knowledge to treat disease and bring people back to health. Medical degrees, then, became legal documents that gave their holders authority over personal and public health, while governments gained a means to control the provision of medicine. It is important to emphasize, however, that this authority and control was very limited, due to legal tensions and the challenges of reaching the rural countryside. The liberalism of the nineteenth century created a profound legal paradox for professional education and practice that took a century to remediate.

Although the hierarchy of physician-surgeons, healing occupations, and healers retained in the nineteenth century essentially the same configuration as in the colonial period, some changes challenged this order (Carrillo 1998). The union of medicine with surgery, for example, made these two independent categories disappear from the hierarchy, while the figure of physician-surgeon, also called medical doctors or just doctors, emerged. While changes in medical theories made bloodletting less frequent, regulations authorizing bloodletters to pull teeth gave rise to dentistry. At the top of the hierarchy and with control of the medical school, doctors controlled the training of dentists, pharmacists, and midwives. Traditional gender roles in nineteenth-century Mexican society and the gendered spaces of medicine made women's access to academic training in medicine and obstetrics difficult (Carrillo 1998), though their experiential knowledge made them qualified midwives in high demand (Jaffary 2016). The clergy and *curanderos* continued competing with medical elites and being disqualified by them, but a new group of practitioners emerged: the empirics. These individuals offered medical treatments unsupported by contemporary medical science, but ratified by a great number of patients. With popular support, empirics raised the suspicion and harsh criticism of medical elites. Some examples of these empirics were Ulises de Seguier, who claimed to have the royal healing touch and toured Mexico City in 1869, the *Médico Santo* [Holy Medic], who treated diseases with saliva in 1870, and Rafael de J. Meraulyock, who dazzled the masses with his panaceas in 1865 (Agostoni 2000). Homeopaths became a group at the margin of professional regulation (Hernández Berrones 2017). Despite the diversification of healers and healing occupations in this period, most of the population relied on homemade remedies described in domestic medical manuals or learned through oral tradition to treat everyday ailments.

During the Porfiriato (1876–1911), the country enjoyed unprecedented stability that was reflected in medical and public health institutions. Given the importance of public health to economic development, the government led by Porfirio Díaz made doctors essential agents of modernization in Mexico (Agostoni 2003). It employed doctors in medical schools, research institutes, public health offices, jails, hospitals, and other government institutions. Doctors shaped these institutions following their own academic, scientific, and market interests, developing a sense of identity and autonomy and gaining a larger control over the provision of health to the population. The power of doctors, however, resulted from the privileged position they were granted by the Porfirian administration. Political ideologies and legal frameworks opposed the monopoly of doctors over medicine. For instance, prevailing liberalism favored freedom of education and occupation, limiting the intended effects of medical licensing regulations promoted by doctors. Similarly, the federalist system led to a decentralized medical apparatus that restricted doctors' regulatory plans to the municipal jurisdiction, leaving to each political entity the liberty to legislate in response to their own situation and needs. If public health policies and institutions remained local during the Porfiriato, they also became the foundation of a national health system after the Revolution.

## The Medical Profession after the Revolution

The Porfirian regime brought social order and economic progress at the cost of increasing socioeconomic inequalities and political repression of dissident voices. The Revolution of 1910 sought to correct the socioeconomic and political consequences of thirty years of dictatorship. Seven years of armed struggle ended with the formulation of a new constitution and the challenge of building a new nation. In terms of medicine and public health, the decades that followed the Revolution were a period of institutional reorganization. The constitution of 1917 made health a right of all Mexicans, sanitation a responsibility of the executive, and sanitary policies mandatory all over the country. Scholars, politicians, public health officers, and authorities linked disease and health to the socioeconomic conditions of the Mexican population and targeted rural and working-class communities as subjects of sanitary intervention. The Department of Public Health [currently, Secretaría de Salud] was created in 1917 to design sanitary interventions to prevent and contain the spread of epidemic disease in the national territory. In the following years, the department expanded its scope to the organization and regulation of healthcare. In this process, public health authorities increasingly associated health conditions with poor urbanization, low socioeconomic status, and Indigenous background. Consequently, public health programs such as vaccination campaigns, sanitation of public and private spaces, distribution of hygienic propaganda, inspection of drugs and food, and special training of medical staff, among others, were frequently imbued with redemptive undertones that aligned with the values of the national medical community and international funding agencies (Birn 2006).

Social medicine, however, conflicted with liberal medicine. The National School of Medicine was one of the founding institutions of the re-established National University [Universidad Nacional Autónoma de México] (UNAM) in 1910, where it continued its development. This school privileged the study of the new sciences of Bacteriology and Physiology and promoted clinical practice and medical specialization. This approach to medical education emphasized the physical, natural, or biological nature of disease, disregarding or minimizing its social and cultural component. If graduates agreed on public health interventions to control disease and even worked for the department in these efforts, they resisted any state intervention that threatened the academic autonomy of medical education and the freedom of graduates to practice medicine where they found fitting. Public health authorities sought to familiarize new generations of physicians with the social determinants of health and promoted their mobilization from urban centers to rural areas. In other words, they aimed to socialize medicine. Supported by the Rockefeller Foundation, they sought to train specialists in public health at the Johns Hopkins School of Public Health in the United States; these specialists would occupy leadership positions on their return (Solórzano 1996). Later, Mexican public health authorities created programs and institutions to train a new generation of socially and public health oriented medical practitioners: a public health program at the newly created School of Public Health in Mexico (1922), a social service program which required medical students to spend a semester in rural communities, as a pre-requisite for graduation at the National School of Medicine (1936), and a program in rural medicine to train students from rural populations at the recently founded National Polytechnic Institute [Instituto Politécnico Nacional] (IPN) in 1938 (Agostoni 2013; Soto Laveaga 2013).

Professional hierarchies and licensing regulations from the nineteenth century continued after the Revolution. While some women graduated in medicine at the turn of the century, men still dominated the healing professions in the mid-twentieth century. This situation began to change in the 1970s (Penyak 2003). As medical schools increasingly offered post-graduate opportunities in the second half of the twentieth century, professional medical researchers began to staff schools, hospitals, and research centers. The National University created professional schools of dentistry in 1914 and pharmacy in 1919, and these professionals earned their own prestige (Godínez Reséndiz and Aceves Pastrana 2014). The National School of Medicine created a nursing program in 1912 in order to train the increasing number of women who worked at public and private hospitals to aid predominantly male doctors. Nursing remained a profession of women controlled by men. In 1936, the Polytechnic Institute assumed the administration of a school of homeopathy, originally created in 1896, to train working-class students who were expected to practice in rural and working-class communities (Francois Flores 2007). Centralizing efforts of postrevolutionary governments limited efforts to establish private medical schools [*escuelas libres*]. The limitations of health programs in rural communities allowed the prevalence of Indigenous medicine all over the country. Anthropologists at the National Institute of Indigenous People [Instituto Nacional Indigenista] (INI) did extensive ethnographies to document these traditions (Mellado Campos and Carrillo Farga 1994) and designed programs to improve the health of Indigenous communities (Aguirre Beltran 1955; Campos-Navarro 2010).

In the 1930s and 1940s, the Department of Public Health approached licensing of the healing occupations as a sanitary campaign. The office required healing practitioners to register their degrees, but it only recognized the ones issued by schools with government oversight. With this, the Department dismissed practitioners without formal academic training. In coordination with the National University and the Secretariat of Public Education [Secretaría de Educación Pública] (SEP), the department unified regulations that established specific academic and licensing requirements all over the nation. As these offices refined their policies, sanitary codes centralized oversight, increasing the privileges of licensed practitioners and marginalizing other healers. Public and private institutions used licenses to certify health professionals' suitability to be expert witnesses, issue death certificates, prescribe narcotics, and offer professional services. The department's office for licensing had agents all over the country who verified practitioners' licensing requirements, reported violations, and fined transgressors.

Licensing regulations contravened the freedom of professional practice granted by the constitution of 1917. Consequently, numerous practitioners sued the department with partial success. Courts supporting the sanitary policy toward licensing originally ruled based on the right of Mexicans to receive proper medical treatment by licensed practitioners. Later, courts sided with the constitution, ruling in favor of individual rights of practitioners. The 1945 Law of Professions ended the legal contradictions between the constitution and sanitary legislation, and normalized state control over training and licensing.

Postrevolutionary governments used public health programs as a tool for modernization. The sanitary campaigns of the 1920s and 1930s sought to transform the culture of health of Mexicans, yet health practitioners discovered socioeconomic realities of both rural and urban populations that prevented Mexicans from attaining the ideal model of healthy and strong citizens of the modern Mexican nation. In the following three decades, governments refined existing institutions and created new ones to bring healthcare to all Mexicans. In 1937, the Department of Public Health turned into the Secretariat of Public Health and Social Welfare [Secretaría de Salubridad y Asistencia Pública], a transition that pointed out the government's realization of the socioeconomic determinants of health. The Mexican Institute of Social Security [Instituto Mexicano del Seguro Social] (IMSS) was founded in 1943 and the Institute for Social Security and Services for State Workers [Instituto de Seguridad y Servicios Sociales para Trabajadores del Estado] (ISSSTE), in 1959, to provide comprehensive healthcare to workers (Frenk 1994). Both institutions became the most important providers of jobs for medical graduates. Anthropologists housed at the National School of Anthropology and History [Escuela Nacional de Antropología e Historia] (ENAH), founded in 1938, and at the National Institute for Indigenous People, founded in 1948, described the health and healing among Indigenous populations and the relationship of these communities' beliefs with academic medicine and public health interventions. With these institutions and programs, postrevolutionary governments established a national health system aimed at controlling medical education, certification, licensing, research, and labor, as well as the provision of services by health professionals, with the caveat of limited reach into Indigenous communities.

## Healing Occupations in the Neoliberal Period

The trend to implement social medicine in Mexico reverted in the last decades of the twentieth century when economic pressures pushed governments to implement neoliberal policies aimed at decentralizing the provision of health and making it more efficient and cost-effective. The goal remained the same—to provide health services to the most vulnerable elements of society—but it now faced the challenge of an unprecedented population growth coupled with decreased state resources. The first indicator of the limits of health provision by state institutions was a strike in November 1964 of medical residents at Mexico City's November 20 Hospital that reached national visibility and support (Soto Laveaga 2011). Residents reacted to unfulfilled government commitments related to the provision of labor stability and adequate remuneration to medical students. The strike represented the limits of social medicine in Mexico, something the national census of 1970 corroborated (Frenk et al. 1995). In spite of the programs to socialize doctors during the 1930s, the distribution of doctors by state in the nation remained uneven in the last three decades of the twentieth century, the majority concentrated in urban areas. This trend contrasted with the increasing number of graduates in medicine during this period in response to the efforts of local states to establish their own medical schools and the growing number of private medical schools (de la Fuente 1993; Frenk-Mora et al. 1990). The labor market encouraged medical specialization since it became a determinant for attaining a position suitable to their skills; however, less than half of the medical graduates were able to pursue such a path. Doctors without a specialty were more likely to be unemployed or underemployed in the 1980s. The gender ratio of medical graduates shifted in the 1990s when more than half of medical students were women. These changes demanded a new relationship between medical schools and institutions that provided jobs to graduating physicians. Medical sociologists and public health scholars have pointed out the need for increased state oversight to match the demands of new health systems with the supply of medical staff (Nigenda et al. 2013).

The overspecialization of healing occupations increased during the second half of the century to such an extent that each one of them required an individual section to examine its own developments. Nurses, pharmacists, dentists, sanitary officers, public health administrators, as well as many medical specialties including pediatrics, obstetrics, internal medicine, neurosurgeons, psychiatrists, psychologists, immunologists, and pathologists among many others created programs, academic societies, schools, and clinics to train human resources, regulate curricula, and provide health services to the population. If the professionalization of the healing occupations began in the late-nineteenth century, it consolidated during the twentieth. Even disciplines undermined and marginalized by academic medicine such as homeopathy, osteopathy, Indigenous medicine, and midwifery adopted practices and forms of organization that their practitioners borrowed from their academic peers, though these practices and forms of organization were facilitated to a certain extent by new legislation and incentivized by specific government initiatives. For instance, with the institutional support of the National Polytechnic Institute, homeopaths diversified and specialized their profession in ways similar to the rest of the medical profession, creating graduate programs, organizing academic societies, regulating the homeopathic pharmacopeia, and expanding the industry of homeopathic medicines (Francois Flores 2007).

Similarly, the government resumed former efforts by biologists, chemists and pharmacists to understand the medicinal properties of plants from Indigenous medical traditions and created the Mexican Institute for the Study of Medicinal Plants [Instituto Mexicano para el Estudio de las Plantas Medicinales] in 1976 (Montiel Reyes 2000). Other institutions embraced this project in the following decades, creating a research and clinical network among private and public institutions. If bioprospecting efforts mined the knowledge of Indigenous communities, other state programs such as IMSS General Coordination of the National Plan for Depressed Zones and Marginalized Groups [Coordinación General del Plan Nacional de Zonas Deprimidas y Grupos Marginados] (COPLAMAR) promoted the participation of local communities with their own intellectual and material resources in development projects to increase health services. The neoliberal political framework in general and this program in particular opened the doors for the incorporation of traditional medical knowledges into institutional efforts that used academic medical and sanitary knowledges (Lozoya L. et al. 1988).

Another example is midwifery, a discipline that was considered parallel to or part of the practice of nursing even when their training programs in the first half of the twentieth century functioned separately. In 1945, the National School of Nursing and Obstetrics unified their programs to one single institution. Traditional midwives continued acquiring practical knowledge in their communities, but neoliberal policies allowed advocates of traditional midwifery to create training programs with official certification and linked certified traditional midwives with state and private institutions of primary care (Freyermuth et al. 2018).

The neoliberal period brought a new balance between the occupations in charge of delivering health services and the state institutions in charge of regulating the training and practice of these occupations. On one hand, this balance expanded the state's preference for one medical system—academic medicine or biomedicine—over other systems of medicine. On the other hand, this expansion reiterated the control of Mexican governments and the national state over the organization, regulation, and administration of the healing occupations. For instance, practitioners of Indigenous or unorthodox medical systems saw limited incorporation into medical institutions, but with a license, they could widely offer their services in the private sector. This dynamic undermined the relative power achieved by the national medical profession during the first half of the twentieth century and offered a legal space for medical pluralism in twenty-first century Mexico.

## Conclusions

What are the healing occupations in Mexico and what is their history? In this overview, I have used knowledge about disease and health, transmission of such knowledge, public certification of possession of this knowledge, entitlement to practice medicine, social hierarchy of health practitioners, and regulation of provision of health services as analytical categories to explain the historical changes in the organization of healers and healing in the course of Mexican history. These categories are the ones that sociologists typically associate with the medical profession. Yet, I argue that even if health practitioners had a model at any point in time in Mexico, it was not homogenous among them and state authorities were responsible to implement it. A history of medical professionalization should emphasize that there is no abstract perfect model toward which these analytical categories move. I have shown that what constitutes the medical profession in Mexico changed rapidly over time and that if large historical periodizations suggest trends, they also fail to capture slow transitions. Furthermore, I have emphasized that in Mexico, as in other countries of Latin America, medical pluralism prevailed in spite of efforts by doctors and governments to privilege a singular model of medicine during specific historical periods. I have also emphasized that after 1519 state institutions have always played an important role in the way healing occupations fulfill their role in society. This five-hundred-year tradition of central government institutions in Mexico makes the use of analytical categories for the medical profession relevant for the historical study of healing occupations in Mexico. However, historians should emphasize the continuous presence of non-academic healing systems in the country in order to identify the continuities and changes in the constant tensions and negotiations among the multiple actors involved in the provision of healthcare and avoid the recurring teleological narratives of the medical profession.

## Notes

1. Precolonial sources of Indigenous medicine are abundant. Alchon (2003) and López Austin (1988) offer perhaps the best guides to this literature. Among the most widely used sources are the *Florentine Codex* and its Spanish translation; *General History of the Things of New Spain* by Bernardino de Sahagún; the *Codex de la Cruz-Badiano*, Hernando Ruiz de Alarcón's *Treatise on the Heathen Superstitions that Today Live among the Indians Native to this New Spain*; and the works of Francisco Hernández.

2. For the concept of purity of blood, see María Elena Martínez's 2008 book: *Genealogical Fictions: Limpieza de Sangre, Religion, and Gender in Colonial Mexico*.

3. Positivism is a philosophical system proposed by the French philosopher Auguste Comte. It proposes that all reliable knowledge comes from sensorial experience, interpreted by reason and systematized through logic. The model of this type of knowledge is physics and, by extension, the remaining natural sciences. For a detailed study of the introduction of positivism in Mexico see Hale's 1989 book *The Transformation of Liberalism in Late Nineteenth-Century Mexico*.

## References

Agostoni, Claudia. 2000. "Médicos científicos y médicos ilícitos en la ciudad de México durante el Porfiriato." *Estudios de Historia Moderna y Contemporánea de México* 19: 13–31.

———. 2003. *Monuments of Progress: Modernization and Public Health in Mexico City, 1876–1910, Latin American and Caribbean Series*. Boulder; Calgary, Alberta; Mexico: University Press of Colorado; University of Calgary Press; Instituto de Investigaciones Históricas, UNAM.

———. 2013. "Médicos rurales y medicina social en el México posrevolucionario (1920–1940)." *Historia Mexicana* 63 (2): 745–801.

Aguirre Beltrán, Gonzálo. 1955. *Programas de salud en la situación intercultural*. Mexico City: Instituto Nacional Indigenista.

———. 1963. *Medicina y magia. El proceso de la aculturación en la estructura colonial*. Mexico City: Instituto Nacional Indigenista.

Alchon, Suzanne Austin. 2003. "Amerindians and Disease before 1492." In *A Pest in the Land: New World Epidemics in a Global Perspective*, 32–59. Albuquerque: University of New Mexico Press.

Andalón González, Mónica Guadalupe. 2016. "El tícitl en la cultura náhuatl del Posclásico." *Cuicuilco Revista de Ciencias Antropológicas* 67: 181–202.

Arce Gurza, Francisco, Anne Staples, Dorothy Tanck de Estrada, Josefina Zoraida Vázquez. 1982. *Historia de las profesiones en México*. Mexico City: SEP, Colegio de México.

Armus, Diego. 2003. *Disease in the History of Modern Latin America: From Malaria to AIDS*. Durham: Duke University Press.

Birn, Anne-Emanuelle. 2006. *Marriage of Convenience: Rockefeller International Health and Revolutionary Mexico*. Rochester, NY: University of Rochester Press.

Burnham, John C. 1998. *How the Idea of Profession Changed the Writing of Medical History.* London: Wellcome Institute for the History of Medicine.

Campos-Navarro, Roberto. 2010. "La enseñanza de la Antropología médica y la salud intercultural en México: Del indigenismo culturalista del siglo XX a la interculturalidad en salud del siglo XXI." *Revista peruana de medicina experimental y salud pública* 27 (1): 114–22.

Carrillo, Ana María. 1998. "Profesiones sanitarias y lucha de poderes en el México del siglo XIX." *Asclepio* 50 (2): 149–68.

Carrillo, Ana María, and Juan José Saldaña. 2005. "La enseñanza de la medicina en la Escuela Nacional durante el Porfiriato." In *La casa de Salomón en México. Estudios sobre la institucionalización de la docencia y la investigación científica,* edited by Juan José Saldaña, 257–82. Mexico City: UNAM.

Castañeda López, Gabriela, and Ana Cecilia Rodríguez de Romo. 2007. "Henry Sigerist y José Joaquín Izquierdo: Dos actitudes frente a la historia de la medicine en el siglo XX." *Historia Mexicana* 57 (1): 139–91.

Cleaves, Peter S. 1985. *Las profesiones y el estado: El caso de México.* Mexico City: Colegio de México, Centro de Estudios Sociológicos.

Cruz, Martín de la. 1964. *Libellus de medicinalibus indorum herbis: Manuscrito azteca de 1552 según traducción latina de Juan Badiano.* Mexico: Instituto Mexicano del Seguro Social.

Cueto, Marcos, and Steven Paul Palmer. 2015. *Medicine and Public Health in Latin America: A History.* New York, NY: Cambridge University Press.

de la Fuente, Juan Ramón. 1993. "Medical Education in Mexico." *Mexican Studies/Estudios Mexicanos* 9 (2): 295–302.

De Vos, Paula S. 2021. "Galenic Pharmacy and the Materia Medica of the Nahuas." In *Compound Remedies: Galenic Pharmacy from the Ancient Mediterranean to New Spain,* edited by Paula S. De Vos, 149–82. Pittsburgh: University of Pittsburgh Press.

Fee, Elizabeth, and Theodore M. Brown. 2004. "Using Medical History to Shape a Profession." In *Locating Medical History: The Stories and Their Meanings,* edited by Frank Huisman and John Harley Warner, 139–64. Baltimore: The Johns Hopkins University Press.

Foster, George M. 1987. "On the Origin of Humoral Medicine in Latin America." *Medical Anthropology Quarterly* 1 (4): 355–93.

Francois Flores, Fernando Darío. 2007. *Historia de la homeopatía en México.* Mexico City: Biblioteca de Homeopatía de México, A. C.

Freidson, Eliot. 1970. *Profession of Medicine: A Study of the Sociology of Applied Knowledge.* New York: Dodd, Mead.

Frenk, Julio, ed. 1994. *Médicos, educación y empleo.* Guadalajara: Universidad de Guadalajara.

Frenk, Julio, Luis Durán-Arenas, Alonso Vázquez-Segovia, Carlos García, and Domingo Vázquez. 1995. "Los médicos en México, 1970–1990." *Salud Pública de México* 37 (1): 19–30.

Frenk-Mora, Julio, Cecilia Robledo-Vera, Gustavo Nigenda-López, Catalina Ramírez-Cuadra, Oscar Galván-Martínez, and Julio Ramírez-Ávila. 1990. "Políticas de formación y empleo de médicos en México, 1917–1988." *Salud Pública de México* 32 (4): 440–48.

Freyermuth, Graciela, Marisol Vega, Aline Tinoco, and Gabriela Gil. 2018. *Los caminos para parir en México en el siglo XXI: Experiencias de investigación, vinculación, formación y comunicación*. México: Centro de Investigaciones y Estudios Superiores en Antropología Social.

Gimmel, Millie. 2008. "Reading Medicine in the Codex De La Cruz Badiano," *Journal of the History of Ideas* 69 (2): 169–92.

Godínez Reséndiz, Rogelio Trinidad, and Patricia Aceves Pastrana. 2014. *Proyectos, realidades y utopías. La transformación de la farmacia en México (1919–1940)*. Mexico City: UNAM.

Hafferty, Fredric W., and John B. McKinlay. 1993. *The Changing Medical Profession: An International Perspective*. New York: Oxford University Press.

Hale, Charles A. 1989. *The Transformation of Liberalism in Late Nineteenth-Century Mexico*. Princeton, NJ: Princeton University Press

Hernández Berrones, Jethro. 2017. "Homeopathy 'for Mexicans': Medical Popularisation, Commercial Endeavours, and Patients' Choice in the Mexican Medical Marketplace, 1853–1872." *Medical History* 61 (4): 568–89.

Hernández Sáenz, Luz María. 1997. *Learning to Heal: The Medical Profession in Colonial Mexico, 1767–1831*. New York: Peter Lang.

———. 2018. *Carving a Niche: The Medical Profession in Mexico, 1800–1870*. Montreal; Chicago: McGill-Queen's University Press.

Hippocrates. 1950. "The Nature of Man." In *The Medical Works of Hippocrates*, compiled and translated by John Chadwick and W. N. Mann. Springfield, IL: Charles C. Thomas.

Huber, Brad R, and Alan R Sandstrom. 2010. *Mesoamerican Healers*. Austin: University of Texas Press.

Jaffary, Nora E. 2016. *Reproduction and its Discontents in Mexico: Childbirth and Contraception from 1750 to 1905*. Chapel Hill: University of North Carolina Press.

Lanning, John Tate. 1967. "Legitimacy and Limpieza De Sangre in the Practice of Medicine in the Spanish Empire." *Jahrbuch Für Geschichte von Staat, Wirtschaft und Gesellschaft Lateinamerikas* 4 (1): 37–60.

Lanning, John Tate, and John Jay TePaske. 1985. *The Royal Protomedicato: The Regulation of the Medical Professions in the Spanish Empire*. Durham: Duke University Press.

López Austin, Alfredo. 1967. "Cuarenta clases de magos del mundo náhuatl," *Estudios de Cultura Náhuatl* 7: 87–117.

———. 1988. *The Human Body and Ideology: Concepts of the Ancient Nahuas*. 2 volumes. Salt Lake City: University of Utah Press.

———. 2017. "The Human Body in the Mexica Worldview." In *The Oxford Handbook of the Aztecs*, edited by Deborah L Nichols and Rodríguez-Alegría Enrique, 399–409. New York: Oxford University Press.

Lozoya L., Xavier. 1986. *La medicina invisible: Introducción al estudio de la medicina tradicional en México*. Colección el hombre y su salud. Mexico City: Folios ediciones.

Lozoya L, Xavier, Georgina Velázquez Díaz, Ángel Flores Alvarado, and Programa IMSS-COPLAMAR. 1988. *La Medicina Tradicional en México: Experiencia del Programa IMSS-COPLAMAR*. Mexico City: Instituto Mexicano del Seguro Social.

Lozoya L., Xavier. 1994. *Plantas, medicina y poder: Breve historia de la herbolaria mexicana*. Colección los libros del consumidor. Mexico City: Procuraduría Federal del Consumidor.

Martínez, María Elena. 2008. *Genealogical Fictions: Limpieza de Sangre, Religion, and Gender in Colonial Mexico*. Stanford: Stanford University Press.

Márquez Morfín, Lourdes, and Patricia Hernández Espinosa, coordinators. 2006. *Salud y sociedad en el México prehispánico y colonial*. México: ENAH.

Martínez Barbosa, Xóchitl. 2011. "Inicios de la historia de la medicina en México: Influencias y relaciones con el extranjero (1935–1960)." *Boletín Mexicano de Historia y Filosofía de la Medicina* 14 (1): 17–22.

Mellado Campos, Virginia, and María del Carmen Carrillo Farga, eds. 1994. *La medicina tradicional de los pueblos indígenas de México*, edited by Carlos Zolla. 3 volumes. Mexico City: Instituto Nacional Indigenista.

Montiel Reyes, Diana. 2000. "Red de investigación científica y tecnológica de plantas medicinales mexicanas." *Revista Mexicana de Sociología* 62 (3): 69–78.

Nigenda, Gustavo, Laura Magaña-Valladares, and Doris Verónica Ortega-Altamirano. 2013. "Recursos humanos para la salud en el contexto de la reforma sanitaria en México: Formación profesional y mercado laboral." *Gaceta Médica de México* 149: 555–61.

Penyak, Lee M. 2003. "Obstetrics and the Emergence of Women in Mexico's Medical Establishment." *The Americas* 60 (1): 59–85.

Polanco, Edward. 2019. "Tiçiyotl and Titiçih: Late Postclassic and Early Colonial Nahua Healing, Diagnosis, and Prognosis." *Oxford Research Encyclopedia of Latin American History* (October) http://dx.doi.org/10.1093/acrefore/9780199366439.013.792

Quesada, Noemí. 1989. *Enfermedad y maleficio. El curandero en el México colonial*. Mexico City: UNAM.

Ruiz de Alarcón, Hernando. 1984. *Treatise on the Heathen Superstitions that Today live among the Indians Native to this New Spain, 1629*. Translated by J. Richard Andrews and Ross Hassig. Norman: University of Oklahoma Press.

Sahagún, Fray Bernardino de. 1905. *Historia general de las cosas de Nueva España*. Translated by Francisco del Paso y Troncoso. Madrid: Fototipia de Hauser y Menet.

———. 2009. *Florentine Codex*. Tempe: Bilingual Review Press.

Solórzano, Armando. 1996. "La influencia de la Fundación Rockefeller en la conformación de la profesión médica mexicana, 1921–1949." *Revista Mexicana de Sociología* 58 (1): 173–203.

Soto Laveaga, Gabriela. 2011. "Doctors, Hospitals and Intelligence Agencies: The Mexican Medical Movement (1964–1965) as seen from Intelligence Reports." *Salud Colectiva* 7 (1): 87–97.

———. 2013. "Bringing the Revolution to Medical Schools: Social Service and Rural Health Emphasis in 1930s Mexico." *Mexican Studies/Estudios Mexicanos* 29 (2): 397–427.

Starr, Paul. 1982. *The Social Transformation of American Medicine*. New York: Basic Books.

Viesca Treviño, Carlos. 1990. *Medicina prehispánica en México. El conocimiento médico de los nahuas*. Mexico City: Panorama Editorial.

Zolla, Carlos, coordinator. 2015. *Obras completes de Francisco Hernández*. Mexico: UNAM.

# 2

# A Systematic Approach to Health and Development in Mexico over the Last Century

KATHERINE E. BLISS

Strengthening the health system to stimulate economic development and improve the population's well being has been a public policy priority in Mexico since the end of the Mexican Revolution (1910–1917). The Constitution of 1917 anticipated health as a key driver of national economic progress and set the groundwork for new institutions and disease eradication campaigns to improve the public's well being. Since 1920, the health situation in Mexico has changed dramatically, with the top causes of death shifting from pneumonia, diarrhea, and malaria in 1922 to non-communicable diseases such as cardiovascular disease, kidney failure, and Type II diabetes in the early twenty-first century (Institute for Health Metrics and Evaluation 2019). Over the same period, life expectancy has more than doubled, from 33 years in 1930 (Bustamante et al. 1982) to 75 years in 2019 (World Bank 2021). But even as Mexico has successfully addressed long-standing health challenges such as communicable disease and high rates of infant and maternal mortality—including by implementing specialized domestic programs to improve the health status of the nation's most vulnerable populations—the country of more than 130 million people has faced new risks to health, including HIV/AIDS, drug-resistant tuberculosis, Zika virus, and dengue virus, with people in the lowest income quintiles being the likeliest to be the most affected. The violence associated with the production and trafficking of illicit drugs from and through Mexico over recent decades also affects health outcomes, with homicide becoming the number one cause of premature death in 2017 (Institute for Health Metrics and Evaluation 2019).

## Building a Revolutionary Healthcare System

The Mexican Revolution—during which peasants fought for recognition of traditional land rights while laborers struggled for better working conditions and the middle class sought a greater share of political power–was one of the deadliest conflicts of the twentieth century. The country's population declined from 15.1 million people in 1910 to 14.3 million in 1921, thanks to violence, food insecurity, emigration, and the spread of infectious disease, including the global influenza pandemic of 1918 (Cabrera 1994, 106–07; Ochoa 2000, 28–29). Through public agencies intended to carry out Revolutionary mandates, officials sought to use reorganized state institutions to eradicate cultural practices they perceived as unhealthy, and to encourage new behaviors they viewed as ways to renew the ravaged agricultural sector and stimulate industrial growth in the precarious postwar economy.

The Department of Public Health [Departamento de Salubridad] (DSP), founded in 1917, was Mexico's first national-level social welfare institution. In the early years, the Department's primary responsibilities were port sanitation and border health, outbreak response, the provision of vaccines, and food and drug safety. The institution both built on and expanded the responsibilities of the older nineteenth century Superior Council for Health [Consejo Superior de Salubridad] which, until 1917, dealt primarily with outbreaks such as smallpox, yellow fever, and malaria, and had limited jurisdiction outside the capital (Bustamante et al. 1982, 40–41). To guide planning efforts and train the next generation of specialists, in 1922 Mexico also established the nation's first school of public health during a period when such schools were being established across the hemisphere (Bustamante et al. 1982).

The high rate of infant mortality during the early postrevolutionary period, particularly in urban areas, was especially concerning to public officials. In Mexico City, for example, each year between 1920 and 1925 roughly 171 children per 1,000 under the age of one year died, primarily from such complications as acute respiratory infections or diarrheal disease (Departamento de Salubridad Pública 1930, 9, 14). Three years later, the Department established the Infant Hygiene Service [Servicio de Higiene Infantil] to deliver prenatal care to Mexico City's women and improve the health of newborns. Clinics were situated in underserved barrios where mothers-to-be were least likely to access medical services prior to giving birth (Departamento de Salubridad Pública 1930, 3). Efforts to improve birth outcomes and protect newborn health also led to the deployment of visiting nurses to impoverished urban neighborhoods (Agostoni 2007, 90) and the engagement of first ladies and other influential women to improve the public perception of motherhood and generate a national dialogue regarding positive child rearing practices (Rodríguez and Martínez Báez 1934, iii). These programs were slow to get off the ground; by 1932, the infant death rate in the city had decreased slightly to 157.2 per 1,000, but health officials worried it was still too high. They also lamented the city's high rate of stillbirths associated with maternal infection with syphilis and other sexually transmitted diseases (Departamento de Salubridad Pública 1933, 9), and they worried about the health conditions of migrants from rural areas who arrived in the city each day. Recognizing the importance of improving health conditions in the countryside, the Department began to expand its activities to rural areas in the 1930s, establishing the rule that graduates of the nation's medical, dental, and nursing programs would be required to perform between six months and two years of social service in the countryside before obtaining their licenses (Homedes and Ugalde 2006, 47). To encourage a high birth rate, the 1936 Population Law [Ley de Población] established an Advisory Council, which promoted population growth by featuring images of large families in textbooks and popular publications, establishing awards for large families, offering prizes to prolific mothers, and outlawing the manufacture and dissemination of contraceptive devices. In some states, pronatalist incentives were especially stringent. For example, in the northeastern state of Tamaulipas, the state legislature penalized childless families and unmarried people over the age of twenty-five with an additional 20 percent tax on household income (Cabrera 1994, 109).

While Mexican health officials in the immediate postrevolutionary era primarily focused on domestic challenges, they shared their experiences with colleagues from other countries and drew inspiration from research presented at international meetings by specialists from the United States, Europe, and Latin America. Since the mid-nineteenth century Mexican health officials had interacted with their peers throughout the hemisphere, forging bilateral and regional agreements on maritime health and migration issues. Mexico was a founding member of the International Sanitary Bureau, which was created in 1902 to formalize inter-American cooperation on health matters, and played a leading role in encouraging other countries to participate in the organization during its early years. Mexico's engagement on health programs with foreign institutions grew in the 1920s and 1930s (Cueto 2004, 67). The International Health Division of the US-based Rockefeller Foundation provided funding for the public health school and advised Mexican officials on how to control yellow fever and hookworm (Birn

2006). And in the mid-1930s, Mexico hosted several international health conferences, including the Seventh Pan American Child Congress, inviting doctors, nurses, social workers, and welfare experts from the Americas to Mexico City to exchange ideas regarding modern approaches to pediatric medicine and child rearing (Sanders 2011, 1).

## Midcentury Expansion of Federal Health Programs

The period between 1940 and the late 1970s saw an unprecedented expansion of federally managed health programs in Mexico. As early as the 1930s, the Department of Public Health began incorporating social assistance programs, such as public dining halls, day care centers, shelters, and food distribution into its responsibilities. In 1943, the Department was elevated within the federal bureaucracy and renamed the Secretariat of Health and Assistance [Secretaría de Salubridad y Asistencia] (SSA). That same year, President Manuel Ávila Camacho launched the Mexican Institute of Social Security [Instituto Mexicano del Seguro Social] (IMSS), which built on older, voluntary social security programs organized at the state level and guaranteed healthcare to people formally employed in the private sector, along with their families (Homedes and Ugalde 2006, 51). In the 1940s, the IMSS headquarters, as well as a series of IMSS–managed clinics and hospitals around the country, were constructed to meet the health needs of private sector employees (Méndez-Vigatá 1997, 81–82), while new public institutions such as the National Institute of Cardiology [Instituto Nacional de Cardiología] and Children's Hospital [Hospital Infantil] provided specialized services in the capital (Homedes and Ugalde 2006, 51). A revised Population Law passed in 1947 reinforced the nation's pronatalist outlook, with Article 5 specifying methods for stimulating population growth (Diario Official 1947), even as new research suggested that soil erosion, reduced water tables, and food scarcity would be the inevitable consequences of continued demographic growth. Into the 1950s, officials continued to encourage high fertility rates, resolving that Mexico would redouble its efforts to reduce poverty and malnutrition rather than limit family size (Gill 1951). This policy stance accompanied a period of focus on boosting agricultural production and led to massive federally funded reclamation projects, such as the damming of the Papaloapan River in the southern states of Oaxaca, Veracruz, and Puebla to make land in the vast watershed arable and capable of supplying food for Mexico's growing population (Poleman 1964, 89–90). As Mexico encouraged population growth and sought to address the core challenge of food security, health officials launched several campaigns to reduce the burden of infectious diseases. Programs such as health service by the Papaloapan Commission [Comisión del Papaloapan] and the National Commission to Eradicate Malaria [Comisión Nacional para la Erradicación del Paludismo] (CNEP) served as platforms to extend immunization programs and improve access to water and sanitation in targeted regions of the country (Bliss 2020; Cueto 2007).

With the expansion of the federal government and the rise of a large class of government employees after the 1950s, Mexico created a new set of social insurance programs for civil servants, employees of the national oil company and the national electric company, and the armed forces, providing healthcare for beneficiaries and their families. For example, the State Employees' Institute for Social Security and Services for State Workers [Instituto de Seguridad y Servicios Sociales de los Trabajadores del Estado] (ISSSTE) was launched in 1959. Following the lead of the World Health Organization's Expanded Program on Immunization, Mexico launched its National Immunization Program [Campaña Nacional de Vacunación] in the early 1970s, enhancing existing efforts to provide vaccines to all citizens at low cost or free of charge (Trumbo et al. 2018). In 1979, recognizing that a large sector of the population that was self-employed or working informally was not covered by insurance, President José López Portillo inaugurated the IMSS-COPLAMAR initiative (an agreement between the IMSS and the Office of the President's General Coordination of the National Plan for Depressed Zones and Marginalized Groups [Coordinación General del Plan Nacional de Zonas Deprimidas y Grupos Marginados de la Presidencia de la República]) granting the unemployed and uninsured—particularly those living in rural areas—access to health services similar to programs accessed by people working in the private sector. Like other insurance programs such as IMSS or ISSSTE, IMSS-COPLAMAR managed its own set of rural health posts, clinics, and hospitals, where subscribers could seek health consultations and benefit from health services (*Proceso* 1981).

As health conditions in midcentury Mexico improved, fertility increased, and mortality fell, some demographers began to worry that Mexico might have a population of more than one billion people by 2000. At the height of Cold War tensions between the United States and the Soviet Union, US officials became concerned that social conditions south of the border could make Soviet-style communism attractive to Mexico's poorest and most vulnerable populations. By the 1960s, when the average number of children born to each woman in Mexico had reached a high of seven, foreign assistance from bilateral donors, as well as private foundations, flooded into the country (Brambila 1998, 157–89). Beginning in 1966, the US-based Ford

Foundation supported Mexico's IMSS in undertaking national surveys regarding attitudes toward family planning and resesarching post-abortion birth control approaches at the IMSS-operated Mexico City Hospital (Harkavay, Sauncers and Southam 1968, 551). By 1967, the United States Agency for International Development (USAID) supported two groups in Mexico: the Association for Family Well-being [Asociación para el Bienestar de la Familia Mexicana] and the Foundation for Population Studies [Fundación para Estudios de la Población] (FEPAC). After promoting population growth domestically (although supporting family planning at some international meetings), by the 1970s Mexican officials, themselves, became convinced that unchecked population growth threatened the nation's economic prospects. A new Population Law in 1974 authorized voluntary family planning for the first time (Gallegos et al. 1977, 197) and established a National Population Council [Consejo Nacional de Población] (CONAPO) charged with implementing the new policies (Cabrera 1994, 114).

## Reducing Costs while Trying to Improve Healthcare Access for the Poor

The collapse of global oil prices in 1980 and a high level of debt to foreign creditors led to the Mexican government's efforts to reduce federal-level responsibilities for health programs which had historically been funded through budget transfers from national energy accounts. In this context, the national government also sought to place greater responsibility for the provision of healthcare at the state and local levels. First, in 1983 the Congress amended Article 4 of the Mexican Constitution to guarantee all Mexicans the right to health protection (Homedes and Ugalde 2006, 55). Second, the government embarked upon a process of decentralizing health services, in which health program financing, infrastructure, and management were transferred to the states (Homedes and Ugalde 2006, 51–53). In 1984, the popular IMSS-COPLAMAR program for the poor and uninsured was brought under the SSA for oversight. But with much of the core funding for health services remaining within the federal bureaucracy, states were hard-pressed to improve health conditions, and in some of the most impoverished regions, the quality of services was low. Following Mexico's accession to the North American Free Trade Agreement (NAFTA) with the United States and Canada in 1994, the uprising in the southern state of Chiapas led by the Zapatista National Liberation Army [Ejército Zapatista de Liberación National] (EZLN) called attention to the deplorable health conditions experienced by the state's Indigenous peoples, among whom "poverty-related diseases, preventable through vaccination and sanitary measures—such as intestinal and respiratory infections, tuberculosis, malaria, and river blindness—[were] the main causes of illness and death" (Katzenberger 1995, 34).

When Vicente Fox, the National Action Party's [Partido de Acción Nacional] candiate, was elected as president in 2000, it was the first time since the early twentieth century that a candidate from a party other than the Institutional Revolutionary Party [Partido Revolucionario Institucional] (PRI)—or its predecessor, the National Revolutionary Party [Partido Nacional Revolucionario] (PNR)—had reached the country's highest office. Under Fox, Mexico renewed its commitment to promoting greater health equity and access to health services for the poorest populations. Recognizing the limits of past efforts to ensure healthcare for the poor and those working in the informal sector, in 2003 the Mexican Congress passed laws authorizing the System for Social Protection in Health, known as Seguro Popular, that focused on equitable access to quality and affordable health services. At the time, 40 percent of the population was covered by IMSS, 7 percent by ISSSTE, and 2–3 percent by private insurance, leaving roughly half of the people in the country forced to pay out of pocket for health services (Knaul and Frenk 2005). In 2012, following a multi-year effort to expand access to public health clinics and use conditional cash transfer programs to incentivize families to ensure their children received required vaccinations and regular checkups, Mexico was lauded for having achieved universal health coverage (UHC). According to the editors at *The Lancet* (2012), "Central to Mexico's progress is an ideological shift: health insurance is no longer seen as an employment benefit but a right of citizenship" (622).

Yet in advancing toward UHC, Mexico maintained the older health insurance programs such as IMSS, ISSSTE, and others, while adding a new program for uninsured, informal sector workers known colloquially as Seguro Popular. Seguro Popular, which included a fund to prevent catastrophic expenditures for specialty procedures, also administered by the Ministry of Health, enabled Mexico to reach an additional 50 million uninsured men, women, and children with basic services and protection against medical impoverishment. But there were some notable limitations to the initiative (Pearson et al. 2016). For example, the government continued to allow each agency to administer its own network of hospitals, clinics, pharmacies, and providers, with limited portability, making it difficult or impossible for a person to access services or programs administered by different agencies among the diverse institutions (Manatt Jones 2015). As a result, people seeking healthcare today can confront a confusing patchwork of programs and benefits. Moreover, services covered under the various programs are not equivalent. Seguro Popular, for example, does not pay for the healthcare costs associated with having a heart attack over the age of 60, strokes, dialysis after renal failure, multiple sclerosis, and lung cancer (Aggarwal et al. 2015).

## Sharing Mexico's Experience Internationally

Even as Mexico has focused on improving domestic health programs over the past century, it has embraced opportunities to share its experience with other countries. Mexico has continued to play an important role in the Pan American Health Organization (PAHO)—the regional arm of the World Health Organization—and has hosted numerous high-level international gatherings related to such global health issues as HIV/AIDS, water security, and maternal and newborn health. A middle-income country and member of the Organization for Economic Cooperation and Development (OECD), Mexico has also joined the circle of global health donors, having established an agency for international cooperation under its Ministry of Foreign Affairs [Secretaría de Relaciones Exteriores] (SRE) in September of 2011.

The Mexican International Cooperation Agency [Agencia Mexicana de Cooperación Internacional de Desarrollo] (AMEXCID) coordinates Mexico's external assistance efforts and focuses program outreach in Latin America and the Caribbean. Health is a substantial focus, along with environment and energy issues (SRE 2011). The government of Mexico sees its provision of technical assistance in the area of global health as a natural outgrowth of the country's own experience benefiting from international support. As such, it articulates its role as one of a "natural bridge of interlocution between countries in different states of development, such as its interaction with countries in the North and South and through triangular cooperation initiatives" (SRE 2011).

One signature effort has been the US$150 million Mesoamerican Health Initiative (Salud Mesoamérica 2015), a private-public partnership involving the Inter-American Development Bank, the Carlos Slim Foundation, the Government of Spain, and the Bill & Melinda Gates Foundation, along with the Mexican and Central American country health ministries, as organizing partners (Inter-American Development Bank 2010). Mexico played a leading role in setting the initiative's agenda and has shared lessons learned from its own experience addressing disparities in health outcomes in the southern state of Chiapas.

Mexico also engages with multilateral and public–private partnerships to promote global health security. As the first country to report unusually virulent influenza activity to the World Health Organization (WHO) in April 2009, Mexico became a focus of international efforts to address the global H1N1 influenza pandemic over the course of that year (CDC 2009). During the 2015–2016 Zika virus outbreak in the Americas, Mexican officials coordinated closely with counterparts in United States border states and neighboring countries in Central America to disseminate public health messages and assess the risks to pregnant women for being infected with Zika (Grajales-Muñiz et al. 2019). And in 2016, Mexico became the first country in the world to roll out the new vaccine against dengue virus.

## Conclusion

By tracing the evolution of the health system in Mexico and considering the extent to which health indicators have changed and improved over time, this essay shows that approaches to health in Mexico over the last century reflect a consistent emphasis on health services as an engine of economic development and a source of popular political support. With employment-based insurance schemes in place since the 1940s, officials' focus on non-insured groups has expanded from the urban poor and rural populations to include marginalized migrant and Indigenous groups. In 2012, Mexico celebrated reaching the goal of universal health coverage by providing 52 million previously uninsured citizens with publicly financed healthcare through the Seguro Popular Program, but considerable gaps in terms of access to quality and affordable services remain (The Lancet 2012). In 2018, President Andrés Manuel López Obrador announced plans to eliminate Seguro Popular (Frenk, Gómez-Dantés, and Knaul 2019, 301), and the new Institute of Health for Wellbeing [Instituto de Salud para el Bienestar], established in 2020, envisions access to primary healthcare free of charge for all Mexicans who do not currently have access to insurance. As Mexico balances the competing priorities of security, economic development, and regional diplomacy, ensuring sustainable financing for and equitable access to health programs at all social levels remains critical.

## References

Aggarwal, Ajay, Karla Unger-Saldana, Grant Lewison, and Richard Sullivan. 2015. "The Challenge of Cancer in Middle-income Countries with an Ageing Population: Mexico as a Case Study." *Ecancer Medical Science* 9: 536 http://doi.org/10.3332/ecancer.2015.536.

Agostoni, Claudia. 2007. "Las mensajeras de la salud: Enfermeras visitadoras en la Ciudad de México durante la década de los 1920." *Estudios de Historia Moderna y Contemporánea de México* 33: 89–120.

Birn, Anne-Emanuelle. 2006. *Marriage of Convenience: Rockefeller International Health and Revolutionary Mexico.* Rochester, NY: Rochester University Press.

Bliss, Katherine E. 2020. "Under Surveillance: Public Health, the FBI, and Exile in Cold War Mexico." In *Peripheral Nerve: Health and Medicine in Cold War Latin America*, edited by Anne-Emanuelle Birn and Raúl Necochea López, 31–54. Durham, NC: Duke University Press.

Brambila, Carlos. 1998. "Mexico's Population Policy and Demographic Dynamics: The Record of Three Decades." In *Do Population Policies Matter? Fertility and Politics in Egypt, India, Kenya, and Mexico*, edited by Anrudh Jain, 157–89. New York: Population Council.

Bustamante, Miguel E., Carlos Viesca Treviño, Federico Villaseñor C., Alfredo Vargas Flores, Roberto Castañon, and Xochitl Martínez B. 1982. *La salud pública en México, 1959–1982*. Mexico City: Secretaría de Salubridad y Asistencia.

Cabrera, Gustavo. 1994. "Demographic Dynamics and Development: The Role of Population Policy in Mexico." *Population and Development Review* 20: 105–20.

Centers for Disease Control and Prevention (CDC). 2009. "Outbreak of Swine-Origin Influenza A (H1N1) Virus Infection—Mexico, March–April 2009." *Morbidity and Mortality Weekly Report* 58 (17): 467–70. https://www.cdc.gov/mmwr/preview/mmwrhtml/mm58d0430a2.htm.

Cueto, Marcos 2004. *The Value of Health: A History of the Pan American Health Organization* Washington, DC: Pan American Health Organization.

———. 2007. *Cold War, Deadly Fevers: Malaria Eradication in Mexico, 1955–1975*. Baltimore: Johns Hopkins University Press.

Departamento de Salubridad Pública. 1930. *Servicio de Higiene Infantil, Colaboración al VI Congreso Panamericano del Niño en la Ciudad de Lima, Perú*. Mexico City: Departamento de Salubridad Pública.

———. 1933. *La mortalidad en la Ciudad de México*, Folleto que dedica el Departamento de Salubridad Pública de México al XXI Congreso Internacional de Estadística. Mexico City: Departamento de Salubridad Pública.

———. 1947. Diario Oficial, "Ley General de Población," December 27, 1947, 3–4.

Frenk, Julio, Octavio Gómez-Dantés, and Felicia Marie Knaul. 2019. "A Dark Day for Universal Coverage." *The Lancet* 393: 301–03. https://www.thelancet.com/action/showPdf?pii=S0140-6736%2819%2930118-7.

Gallegos, Alfredo, Jorge García Peña, Jose Antonio Solís, and Alan Keller. 1977. "Recent Trends in Contraceptive Use in Mexico." *Studies in Family Planning* 8 (8): 197–204.

Gill, Tom. 1951. *Land Hunger in Mexico*. Washington, DC: The Charles Lathrop Pack Forestry Foundation.

Grajales-Muñiz, Concepción, Victor Hugo Borja-Aburto, David Alejandro Cabrerra-Gaytán, Teresita Rojas-Mendoza, Lumumba Arriaga-Nieto, and Alfonso Vallejos-Parás. 2019. "Zika Virus: Epidemiological Surveillance of the Mexican Institute of Social Security." *PLoS One* 14 (2). https://doi.org/10.1371/journal.pone.0212114.

Harkavay, Oscar, Lyle Sauncers, and Anna L. Southam. 1968. "An Overview of the Ford Foundation's Strategy for Population Work." *Demography* 5 (2): 541–52.

Homedes, Núria, and Antonio Ugalde. 2006. "Decentralization of Health Services in Mexico: A Historical Review." In *Decentralization of Health Services in Mexico: A Case*

*Study in State Reform*, edited by Núria Homedes and Antonio Ugalde, 45–94. La Jolla, CA: UCSD Center for US-Mexican Studies.

Institute for Health Metrics and Evaluation (IHME). 2019. "Mexico." Institute for Health Metrics and Evaluation. http://www.healthdata.org/mexico.

Inter-American Development Bank. 2010. "Uniting to Closing the Gap in Access to Life-saving Health in Mesoamerica." Inter-American Development Bank. June 14, 2010. https://www.iadb.org/en/news/uniting-closing-gap-access-life-saving-health-mesoamerica.

Katzengerger, Elaine, ed. 1995. *First World, Ha Ha Ha! The Zapatista Challenge*. San Francisco: City Lights Books.

Knaul, Felicia Marie, and Julio Frenk. 2005. "Health Insurance in Mexico: Achieving Universal Coverage Through Structural Reform." *Health Affairs* 24 (6): 1467–76.

Lancet, The. 2012. "Mexico: Celebrating Universal Health Coverage," Editorial. *The Lancet*, August 18, 2012. 380.

Manatt Jones Global Strategies. 2015. "Mexican Healthcare System: Challenges and Opportunities." *Wilson Center*. https://www.wilsoncenter.org/sites/default/files/mexican_healthcare_system_challenges_and_opportunities.pdf.

Méndez-Vigatá, Antonio E. 1997. "Politics and Architectural Language: Post-Revolutionary Regimes in Mexico and Their Influence on Mexican Public Architecture, 1920–1952." In *Modernity and the Architecture of Mexico*, edited by Edward R. Burian, 61–89. Austin: University of Texas Press.

Ochoa, Enrique C. 2000. *Feeding Mexico: The Political Uses of Food since 1900*. Wilmington, DE: Scholarly Resources.

Pearson, Mark, Francesca Colombo, Yuki Murakami, and Chris James. 2016. *Universal Health Coverage and Health Outcomes, Final Report*. Paris: OECD. http://www.oecd.org/els/health-systems/Universal-Health-Coverage-and-Health-Outcomes-OECD-G7-Health-Ministerial-2016.pdf.

Poleman, Thomas. 1964. *The Papaloapan Project: Agricultural Development in the Mexican Tropics*. Stanford: Stanford University Press.

Proceso Editorial Board. 1981. "La filosofia del programa IMSS-COPLAMAR, en riesgo de perderse reconoce el coordinador." *Proceso*, May 9, 1981.

Rodríguez, Aída S. de, and Manuel Martínez Báez. 1934. *Libro para la madre mexicana*. Mexico City: Tall. Linotipográficos de la Beneficencia Pública Centro Industrial Rafael Dondé.

Sanders, Nichole. 2011. *Gender and Welfare in Mexico: The Consolidation of a Postrevolutionary State*. University Park: Pennsylvania State University Press.

Secretaría de Relaciones Exteriores (SRE). 2011. *Informe Annual de Cooperación Internacional para el Desarrollo*. Agencia Mexicana de Cooperación Internacional para el Desarrollo (AMEXCID).

Trumbo, Silas R., Marcela Contreras, Ana Gabriela Félix García, Fabio Alberto Escobar Díaz, Misael Gómez, Verónica Carrión, Karim Jaqueline Pardo Ruiz, Renee Aquije, M. Carolina Danovaro-Holliday, and Martha Velandia-González. 2018. "Improving Immunization Data Quality in Peru and Mexico: Two Case Studies Highlighting Challenges and Lessons Learned." *Vaccine* 36 (50): 7674–81.

World Bank Group. 2021. "Life Expectancy at Birth, Total (years)." *World Bank Data*. https://data.worldbank.org/indicator/SP.DYN.LE00.IN?locations=MX.

# 3

# Health after Internal Migration within Mexico

The Role of Age at Migration, Motivations, and Place of Origin and Destination

Gabriela León-Pérez

Internal migration in Mexico is six times larger than international migration (Romo Viramontes, Téllez Vázquez, and Ramírez López 2013, 84), yet it is underrepresented in the academic literature (Canales and Montiel 2007). Most of the existing research on Mexican internal migration examines four broad areas: the volume of migration, origin–destination flows, the sociodemographic characteristics of migrants, and postmigration employment and earnings. Comparatively less attention has been given to the health of internal migrants. Knowing about the health of people who move in and out of a community can help adapt the healthcare system to better serve the population and respond to changes in the demand for services. This is especially important in a country where approximately half a million individuals migrate internally every year (Sobrino 2010, 64).

This chapter contributes to our understanding of the health of Mexican internal migrants once they have settled in their new destination. Using longitudinal (that is, pre and postmigration) quantitative data from the Mexican Family Life Survey (MxFLS; Rubalcava and Teruel 2006a, 2006b, 2013), I examine changes in the health of male and female migrants and evaluate whether health varies depending on the characteristics of the migratory trip. Specifically, I investigate the role played by age at migration as well as migration motivations, and the place of origin and destination in shaping postmigration physical and mental health. I study the health of men and women separately because the nature and patterns of Mexican internal migration vary substantially across gender (Curran and Rivero-Fuentes 2003; INEGI 2015; Sobrino 2010). Thus, it is possible for postmigration health to differ by gender as well.

## Background

### Who Are Mexico's Internal Migrants?

Early internal migration in Mexico was facilitated by the construction of more than 12,000 miles of railways during the period of the Porfiriato (1876–1911). The expansion of the railroad boosted the domestic economy, created many jobs, and enabled internal mobility. Rural–urban moves dominated Mexican internal migration flows during the first half of the twentieth century as a result of the deterioration of economic and social conditions in rural areas and the fast urbanization and industrialization of the country (Sobrino 2010). During this time, large numbers of people moved at record rates from less to more developed areas—mostly from *el campo* [the countryside] to the three largest metropolitan areas—as the manufacturing, construction, and service sectors grew and as the demand for labor increased (Canales and Montiel 2007; Sobrino 2014). Over the decades, the rapid urbanization of the country and Mexico's growing role in the global economy has led to the diversification of internal migration flows.

One important change in recent years has been a shift in origins and destinations. Since 2000, urban–urban moves have surpassed rural–urban movements and have become the dominant internal migration flow. In 2015, urban–urban moves constituted 67 percent of migration flows and rural–urban moves, 16 percent (Sobrino 2016, 61). Urban–rural moves are also on the rise, going from 5 percent in 2000 to 13 percent in 2015 (Sobrino 2016, 62). This flow includes individuals returning to their communities of origin and others attracted by economic development as capital moves to rural areas with lower costs of production (Pérez-Campuzano and Santos-Cerquera 2013). Rural–rural migration represents a small but consistent share of migration flows within Mexico, making up 4 percent of all moves in 2000 and 2015 (Pérez-Campuzano and Santos-Cerquera 2013, 67).

While men have historically dominated migration from Mexico to the United States (Donato, Wagner, and Patterson 2008), women have had a long-standing presence in migration flows within Mexico (Sobrino 2014). Female participation in internal migration spiked in the 1940s, and women have dominated domestic migration flows since the 1980s (Curran and Rivero-Fuentes 2003). Today, both rural–urban and urban–urban migration streams are predominantly female (Sobrino 2016). Women's internal migration tends to be characterized by long-duration moves and steady employment; men, on the other hand, tend to move to destinations closer to and smaller than their places of origin (Curran and Rivero-Fuentes 2003; Sobrino 2014). These gender differences in migration experiences result in different networks and resources for prospective migrants and may similarly result in different health outcomes.

Internal migration flows in other countries are usually dominated by young people, but in Mexico migrants tend to be dispersed across the age spectrum (Bernard, Bell, and Charles-Edwards 2014). In fact, Bernard, Bell, and Charles-Edwards's (2014) cross-national research revealed that the age at which migration peaks in Mexico is one of the oldest in the world. Still, internal migration happens relatively early in an individual's work trajectory given that the search for better job opportunities is one of the main drivers of domestic relocations in Mexico (Sobrino 2014; 2016).

In terms of education, Mexican internal migrants tend to have more schooling than migrants to the United States. Individuals with higher levels of education usually favor internal over international migration because their credentials and qualifications may not be adequately rewarded by jobs available to them in the United States (Quinn and Rubb 2005, 156). College-educated men and women are the most likely to relocate domestically (Romo Viramontes, Téllez Vázquez, and López Ramírez 2013), but there is also an important presence of low-skilled individuals (Pérez-Campuzano and Santos-Cerquera 2013). Overall, there is a regional educational selectivity whereby individuals with college degrees or more qualifications dominate urban–urban migration streams and those with low educational attainment dominate rural–urban streams (Pérez-Campuzano and Santos-Cerquera 2013; Sobrino 2014), a pattern that Sobrino (2016) calls the "territorial redistribution of human capital" (63). The educational level of migrants directly affects the types of jobs they can perform. Almost 50 percent are employed in the service sector (which includes transportation, communication, professional, financial, and government jobs); the rest work in the trade (21 percent), manufacturing (17 percent), construction (8 percent), and agricultural (5 percent) sectors (Téllez Velázquez, López Ramírez, and Romo Viramontes 2014, 18).

## The Health of Internal Migrants

While existing research provides a clear profile of who Mexican internal migrants are, we know significantly less about their physical and mental health. There is evidence that migration to the United States negatively impacts health and that, in many cases, migrants' health trajectories become different from those of their counterparts who stayed in Mexico (see, for example, Goldman et al. 2014; Ullmann, Goldman, and Massey 2011; Wong and Gonzalez-Gonzalez 2010). In the case of internal migration, there are few (if any) differences in postmigration health between internal migrants and non-migrants. For example, studies of older Mexican adults have found no differences between internal migrants and non-migrants in the prevalence of chronic conditions (Wheaton and Crimmins 2013; Wong and Gonzalez-Gonzalez 2010).

Even if there are no observed health differences in the overall internal migrant versus non-migrant populations, it is possible that migrants differ from one another based on the conditions in which their migration occurred. Some individuals may exhibit poor postmigration health due to work, family, and interpersonal stress, or to the stress of adjusting to city life. Emotional well being may also be impacted by separation from family and friends and the social isolation that results from migration. Indeed, prior studies have found that the disruption of social ties and networks after migration is related to increased risk of psychological distress (Lu 2010a).

However, migration does not necessarily have to be detrimental to health. It is possible for migrants to experience health improvements if the living conditions and access to healthcare in the destination community are better than in the origin one. Migrating from less to more developed areas may improve socioeconomic and life circumstances thanks to educational and employment opportunities that would be unavailable in the place of origin (Canales and Montiel 2007). In addition, improved health may result from having more autonomy and freedom from social and cultural norms that exist in the origin community (Nauman et al. 2015).

## Characteristics of Migration Trip as Predictors of Postmigration Health

The characteristics of the migration trip could potentially capture sources of selection, as well as explain observed differences in postmigration health. For example, age is related to premigration health and may also play an important role in shaping health outcomes after migration. Because health deteriorates as individuals age, those who migrate at younger ages usually have better postmigration health than those who migrate at relatively older ages (Angel et al. 2010). In terms of gender, women tend to be less mobile during childbearing years due to social norms and household responsibilities, potentially leading to gender differences in postmigration health.

It is also important to consider the motivation that drives the decision to migrate. There is evidence that family migration motivations shape immigrant children's academic trajectories. For example, Hagelskamp, Su, and Hughes (2010) found that when families migrated to the United States for educational opportunites, their children had a higher Grade Point Average (GPA) in high school. On the other hand, migrating for work prospects was related to a faster decline in children's GPA throughout the high school years. A similar phenomenon might be occurring in terms of health, whereby the reason for migration is associated with postmigration health. Indeed, research on Chinese internal migrants suggests that economic migrants (especially low-skilled ones) are usually healthier than those who migrate for family reasons (Lu 2008). Over time, however, migrating for family reasons might be protective for migrants' well-being given that family members can serve as a source of social support (Lu 2010a, 2010b). In Mexico, the top two reasons for internal migration are work (especially for men) and family (especially for women) (Sobrino 2014). Migration for education is also prevalent among men and women (Canales and Montiel 2007; Sobrino 2010). In addition, recent national data reveal an increase in migration motivated by the rising insecurity in many regions of Mexico (INEGI 2015).

The level of urbanization of the places of origin and destination could also play a role in shaping postmigration health. Urban areas potentially offer opportunities for health improvements such as access to higher levels of household consumption and standards of living that might be unattainable in the origin region (International Organization for Migration [IOM] 2015; Lu 2010b). At the same time, urbanization is related to less physical activity, poorer health behaviors, and more non-communicable diseases (IOM 2015). Research on the mental health consequences of urban migration is limited and mixed, with some finding positive effects (Nauman et al. 2015) and others negative ones (Chen 2011). In terms of gender, prior studies have found that urban migration has a negative impact on men's health (Wheaton and Crimmins 2013) and is protective for women (Wong and Gonzalez-Gonzalez 2010).

## Methods

### Data Source

Data come from the Mexican Family Life Survey (MxFLS; Rubalcava and Teruel 2006a, 2006b, 2013), a longitudinal survey of the well being of individuals and families in Mexico. The survey was developed and is managed by Mexican researchers at Universidad Iberoamericana and Centro de

Investigación y Docencia Económicas (CIDE) in collaboration with Duke University researchers (see Rubalcava and Teruel 2006a for more details about the survey methodology). The MxFLS fielded three surveys over a period of ten years and collected social, economic, demographic, and health data, as well as information on internal and international migration trips done between interviews. The baseline survey was collected in 2002 using a probabilistic, stratified, and multi-staged cluster design. It included interviews with 19,800 individuals from 8,400 households in 150 urban and rural communities throughout Mexico (Rubalcava and Teruel 2006a). The second and third surveys were fielded during 2005–2006 and 2009–2012, and achieved a 90 percent and 85 percent re-contact rate at the household level, respectively (Rubalcava and Teruel 2006b, 2013).

The present study focuses on survey participants who migrated within Mexico at any time during the study period (2002–2012). At each follow-up interview, respondents were asked: "Since [year of last interview] have you moved for a year or longer outside of the locality/neighborhood where you used to live?" If they answered "yes," respondents were then asked to list all the places where they lived, both within the country and internationally. Using this information, I identified individuals who relocated domestically between interviews (respondents who stayed in their communities at all times and those who migrated internationally were excluded from the analyses). The analytical sample includes data on 1,338 internal migrants (505 men and 833 women) ages fifteen to fifty, who had complete migration histories, and complete data in all study variables.

**Dependent Variables**

The two health outcomes of interest were self-rated health and depressive symptoms. In this study, health is measured at two time points: before migration (when respondents were still in their origin community, measured at the first interview) and after migration (after they have migrated and settled in their destination, measured at the last interview). Including baseline health in the statistical models makes it possible to account for any health differences that existed before individuals migrated.

Self-rated health is a robust indicator of morbidity, subsequent disability, and mortality (Idler and Benyamini 1997). It is especially useful when studying populations that do not have widespread access to healthcare services, such as many rural areas in Mexico.[1] In the MxFLS, respondents were asked: "Currently, could you say that your health is very good, good, regular, bad, or very bad?" Responses range from 1 to 5, with higher scores indicating better health. This outcome has been used in many studies of internal migration and health (for example, Anglewicz et al. 2017; Lu 2010b; Malmusi, Borrell, and Benach 2010). It has also been widely used to assess the health of Mexicans, including men and women, those with and without migration experience, rural versus urban, and elderly populations (Goldman et al. 2014; Ullmann, Goldman, and Massey 2011).

In terms of mental health, the survey includes a module with twenty-one questions that capture a variety of depressive symptoms. The first twenty questions comprise a scale drawn from the Clinical Questionnaire for the Diagnosis of Depressive Syndrome [*Cuestionario Clínico para el Diagnóstico del Síndrome Depresivo*] (CCDSD). The CCDSD was developed by the Mexican Institute of Psychiatry (Calderón Narváez 1997) and its items are similar to those in the Center for Epidemiologic Studies Depression (CES-D) scale. The questions capture symptoms such as feelings of sadness, anxiety, fear, trouble sleeping, and poor appetite. For each item, respondents reported how often they experienced symptoms in the last four weeks, ranging from 1 = never to 4 = all the time. Respondents' answers to each of the twenty questions were summed, yielding an overall score that ranges from 20 to 80 with higher scores indicating more depressive symptoms. Summed scores were log-transformed in the statistical models to correct for the skewed distribution.

**Independent Variables**

The predictors of interest capture the characteristics of the migration trip. Most respondents migrated only once between interviews (77 percent of men and 78 percent of women). For those who migrated more times, I used the characteristics of the last migration trip they undertook.

Age at migration is operationalized into categories to account for potential curvilinear effects: 15–24 (reference), 25–34, 35–44, and 45–50 years. Motivation captures the main reason that prompted the move and was coded into six categories: family (for example, to be closer to family, marriage/union, pregnancy, death of spouse/partner); work/education (work or education/training of respondent or other household member); independence (to become independent of family or move to own house); health (of respondent, spouse, or other person); safety (insecurity, political instability, or natural disasters); and other reasons. Origin/destination measures include two dichotomous variables that identify the type of community that respondents originated from and to where they migrated. Following the definition used by the Mexican National Institute of Statistics and Geography (INEGI), rural origin was coded as 1 if the origin community had a population of less than 2,500; otherwise it was coded as 0. Urban destination was coded as 1 if they migrated to a city and 0 if they migrated to a ranch, town, ejido, or other community.

**Control Variables**

Control variables account for participant characteristics that could independently influence the outcomes. Education was coded into four categories following the Mexican educational system: elementary school or less (0–6 years), middle school (7–9 years), high school (10–12 years), and college or more (13 years or more). Because postmigration conditions may have independent effects on observed health outcomes, models also include dichotomous variables that capture respondents' characteristics at the time of the last interview (postmigration): employment status (1 = employed; 0 = not employed), marital status (1 = married or living with partner; 0 = else), and whether there were any children ages 0–14 living in the household (1 = yes; 0 = no). Self-rated health models control for postmigration depressive symptoms to adjust for potential psychosomatic effects on respondents' perceived health. Similarly, depressive symptoms models control for postmigration self-rated health to account for the relationship between somatic symptoms and mental health.

**Analytic Strategy**

First, I calculated descriptive statistics and estimated chi-square tests to examine if male and female migrants differed in the characteristics of their migration trip, educational attainment, and postmigration conditions. Next, I estimated lagged dependent variable (LDV) models using ordinary least-squares (OLS) regressions to predict postmigration self-rated health and a separate set of models to predict postmigration depressive symptoms. The LDV regressions estimate postmigration health (measured at the last interview) as a function of age at migration, migration motivations, and place of origin and destination, while accounting for premigration health (measured at the first interview) and other covariates. By including the baseline measurement of the dependent variable (in this case, health status before migration), LDV models address possible selection bias by adjusting for prior health and unmeasured characteristics (Wooldridge 2002). Therefore, they allow for more stringent tests than cross-sectional models. All analyses are estimated using robust standard errors to correct for the clustering of multiple individuals within the same household. Analyses were stratified by gender because Mexican internal migration patterns, and migration in general, vary for men and women. Distinct processes, motivations, and social norms influence and shape men and women's migration outcomes; thus, the internal migration–health relationship may differ by gender.

## Results

### Descriptive Differences between Male and Female Migrants

Table 3.1 presents descriptive statistics for all study variables by gender. The last column indicates if the percentage distributions for men and women are significantly different. Both male and female migration were concentrated within the 15–34 years age range, with women being overall younger than men. Over one-third of both groups migrated for family reasons; the other top migration motivations were work/education (men 30 percent; women 25 percent) and independence (men 23 percent; women 25 percent). Approximately 3 percent of both samples migrated due to health-related reasons, 2–3 percent due to safety concerns, and the rest for other reasons. There were no significant differences between men and women in terms of their origins and destinations—more than one-third of both samples originated in rural communities and over half migrated to cities. There were, however, significant gender differences in educational attainment and postmigration conditions. Male migrants had significantly higher levels of education, postmigration employment, and marriage than their female counterparts. Women had higher rates of living in households with children.

### Do the Characteristics of the Migration Trip Shape Postmigration Self-Rated Health?

Next, I present results on the relationship between postmigration self-rated health and the characteristics of the migration trip. Table 3.2 shows unstandardized coefficients from LDV regressions for men and women. Positive and significant coefficients indicate that a variable is related to better health after migration, whereas negative and significant coefficients indicate that the variable is associated with worse health after migration. Overall, these regression models are a better fit for men than women: they explain 26 percent of the variance in postmigration self-rated health for men and 20 percent of the variance for women.

We begin with the results for male migrants. As would be expected, prior health is a positive and significant predictor, such that better premigration health is associated with better postmigration health. Variables that capture the characteristics of the last migration were important predictors of men's

Table 3.1. Characteristics of Mexican male and female internal migrants (Mexican Family Life Survey, 2002–2012)

|  | Men (N=505) percent | Women (N=833) percent | Sig. |
|---|---|---|---|
| **CHARACTERISTICS OF THE MIGRATION TRIP** | | | |
| *Age at migration* | | | |
| 15–24 years | 23.0 | 28.8 | * |
| 25–34 years | 41.0 | 35.5 | * |
| 35–44 years | 19.6 | 21.8 | |
| 45–50 years | 16.4 | 13.8 | |
| *Motivation* | | | |
| Family | 33.7 | 33.9 | |
| Work/Education | 30.3 | 25.2 | * |
| Independence | 23.2 | 25.1 | |
| Health | 3.0 | 3.4 | |
| Safety | 1.8 | 2.8 | |
| Other | 8.1 | 9.7 | |
| *Origin/Destination* | | | |
| Rural community of origin | 36.8 | 36.5 | |
| Urban destination | 55.1 | 58.3 | |
| **EDUCATIONAL ATTAINMENT** | | | |
| Elementary school or less | 28.7 | 36.6 | ** |
| Middle school | 38.8 | 32.7 | * |
| High school | 16.6 | 19.2 | |
| College or more | 15.8 | 11.5 | * |
| **POSTMIGRATION CHARACTERISTICS** | | | |
| Employed | 92.3 | 49.9 | *** |
| Married | 74.7 | 70.5 | † |
| Children living in household | 45.5 | 60.0 | *** |

*Note:* Asterisks denote significant differences between men and women where †p < 0.10; *p < 0.05; **p < 0.01; ***p < 0.001.

Table 3.2. Regression models predicting self-rated health after internal migration by gender (Mexican Family Life Survey, 2002–2012)

|  | Men | | Women | |
| --- | --- | --- | --- | --- |
|  | B | SE | B | SE |
| Premigration self-rated health | 0.321*** | (0.050) | 0.264*** | (0.040) |
| **CHARACTERISTICS OF MIGRATION TRIP** | | | | |
| *Age at migration* (ref=15–24) | | | | |
| 25–34 years | -0.173* | (0.087) | -0.057 | (0.062) |
| 35–44 years | -0.293** | (0.096) | -0.097 | (0.078) |
| 45 years or older | -0.460*** | (0.113) | -0.171* | (0.086) |
| *Motivation* (ref=family) | | | | |
| Work/Education | -0.146† | (0.084) | -0.052 | (0.066) |
| Independence | -0.114 | (0.089) | -0.085 | (0.069) |
| Health | 0.052 | (0.168) | -0.217* | (0.107) |
| Safety | 0.463* | (0.200) | -0.082 | (0.143) |
| Other | -0.267* | (0.122) | -0.087 | (0.086) |
| *Origin/Destination* | | | | |
| Rural origin | -0.055 | (0.077) | 0.082 | (0.057) |
| Urban destination | 0.193** | (0.073) | 0.044 | (0.052) |
| **EDUCATION (REF=ELEMENTARY OR LESS)** | | | | |
| Middle school | 0.042 | (0.085) | 0.147* | (0.058) |
| High school | 0.031 | (0.101) | 0.241** | (0.075) |
| College or more | 0.228* | (0.105) | 0.286** | (0.093) |
| **POSTMIGRATION CHARACTERISTICS** | | | | |
| Employed (ref=unemployed) | 0.344** | (0.115) | 0.061 | (0.052) |
| Married (ref=not married) | 0.072 | (0.080) | 0.002 | (0.054) |
| Children in household (ref=no children) | -0.114 | (0.077) | 0.039 | (0.056) |
| Depressive symptoms | -0.023*** | (0.005) | -0.019*** | (0.003) |
| Constant | 2.891*** | (0.302) | 2.986*** | (0.190) |
| R-square | 0.26 | | 0.20 | |
| N | 505 | | 833 | |

*Note*: †p < 0.10; *p < 0.05; **p < 0.01; ***p < 0.001.

postmigration health. Age at migration was negatively related to health and the relationship was linear, such that individuals who migrated at older ages reported worse postmigration health than those who migrated at younger ages. Men who migrated for work/education and other reasons reported significantly worse postmigration health than those who migrated for family reasons, but men who migrated due to safety concerns reported better health. There were no significant differences between rural vs. urban migrants, but those who migrated to a city reported better postmigration health than those who moved to non-urban destinations. In terms of education, the only significant variable was college or more, suggesting that college-educated migrants reported better health than those with elementary education or less. In terms of postmigration characteristics, being employed was related to better health and those who reported more depressive symptoms experienced worse health. Marital status and children in the household were not significant predictors.

Women's postmigration self-rated health is shaped by different factors than men's. Again, premigration health was a significant and positive predictor of postmigration health. In contrast to men, women's self-rated health did not vary significantly across age groups (except the oldest group) or by origin/destination. There were no statistically significant differences in postmigration health between women who migrated for family reasons and those who migrated for work/education, safety, or other reasons. Health-related motivations were not significant for men, but they were significant and negative for women, indicating that migration for health reasons was related to worse health after migration compared to migrating for family motives. Education had a positive and significant effect such that having higher levels of education positively impacted female postmigration self-rated health. Similar to men, depressive symptoms were negatively related to women's health.

### Do the Characteristics of the Migration Trip Shape Postmigration Depressive Symptoms?

Table 3.3 presents the results from analyses exploring the relationship between the characteristics of the migration trip and postmigration mental health. A positive coefficient suggests that a variable is related to an increase in depressive symptoms (that is, worse mental health) and a negative coefficient indicates that a variable is related to a decrease in symptoms (that is, better mental health). In terms of model fit, these regressions explain 15 percent of the variance in postmigration depressive symptoms for men and 18 percent of the variance for women.

Table 3.3. Regression models predicting depressive symptoms after internal migration by gender (Mexican Family Life Survey, 2002–2012)

|  | Men | | Women | |
|---|---|---|---|---|
|  | B | SE | B | SE |
| Premigration depressive symptoms | 0.239*** | (0.060) | 0.253*** | (0.041) |
| **CHARACTERISTICS OF MIGRATION TRIP** | | | | |
| *Age at migration* (ref=15–24) | | | | |
| 25–34 years | -0.008 | (0.027) | 0.025 | (0.023) |
| 35–44 years | -0.025 | (0.030) | -0.005 | (0.029) |
| 45 years or older | -0.057† | (0.033) | 0.005 | (0.032) |
| *Motivation* (ref=family) | | | | |
| Work/Education | -0.039 | (0.024) | -0.054* | (0.023) |
| Independence | -0.023 | (0.027) | -0.054* | (0.025) |
| Health | -0.007 | (0.043) | 0.019 | (0.055) |
| Safety | 0.011 | (0.064) | -0.013 | (0.078) |
| Other | -0.040 | (0.037) | 0.021 | (0.036) |
| *Origin/Destination* | | | | |
| Rural origin | -0.052** | (0.020) | -0.008 | (0.021) |
| Urban destination | 0.004 | (0.019) | 0.012 | (0.020) |
| **EDUCATION (REF=ELEMENTARY OR LESS)** | | | | |
| Middle school | -0.045† | (0.024) | -0.043† | (0.023) |
| High school | -0.062* | (0.028) | -0.055* | (0.027) |
| College or more | -0.022 | (0.030) | -0.115*** | (0.027) |
| **POSTMIGRATION CHARACTERISTICS** | | | | |
| Employed (ref=unemployed) | -0.009 | (0.041) | 0.028 | (0.018) |
| Married (ref=not married) | -0.016 | (0.022) | -0.012 | (0.019) |
| Children in household (ref=no children) | 0.018 | (0.021) | 0.027 | (0.022) |
| Self-rated health | -0.067*** | (0.012) | -0.086*** | (0.012) |
| Constant | 2.763*** | (0.205) | 2.781*** | (0.155) |
| R-square | 0.15 | | 0.18 | |
| N | 505 | | 833 | |

Note: †p < 0.10; *p < 0.05; **p < 0.01; ***p < 0.001.

Among men, migrants in the oldest age group present less depressive symptoms than the youngest migrants. In contrast to the self-rated health findings, migration motivations were not associated with men's mental health. In terms of origin/destination, men from rural communities reported less depressive symptoms but there were no significant differences by type of destination. Different patterns emerged among female migrants. Women's postmigration depressive symptoms did not vary significantly across age, origin, or destination. Interestingly, women who migrated for work/education and those who migrated for independence reported significantly less depressive symptoms than those who migrated for family reasons. Depressive symptoms decreased among men and women with higher levels of education and those with better self-rated health. Employment status, marital status, and children in the household were not related to postmigration mental health.

## Discussion

The purpose of this research was to examine if the characteristics of the migration trip are related to postmigration health among Mexican internal migrants. I used longitudinal data from the Mexican Family Life Survey to explore if age at migration, migration motivations, and the places to and from which a person migrated were associated with postmigration self-rated health and depressive symptoms. Results from lagged dependent variable regressions revealed that the characteristics of the migration trip were indeed related to postmigration health, but the effects varied across gender and outcomes.

Age at migration is a key variable used to understand the health outcomes of international migrants (Angel et al. 2010), yet it has been seldom examined in studies of internal migration. The results presented here provide initial evidence that age at migration is not an important predictor of Mexican internal migrants' health—that is, there are few differences in postmigration health across age groups. The only exception was found in models of men's self-rated health, where results indicated that men who migrated at older ages perceived their health to be worse after migration.

There were interesting gendered patterns in the health effects of migration motivations. Compared to migrating for family reasons, migrating for work/education was detrimental for men's self-rated health but beneficial for women's mental health. These findings highlight the vast research that confirms that family support, especially from spouses, is more important for men's health than for women given that men's networks are more reduced and less intensive, whereas women draw support from multiple sources and larger networks (Belle 1987). Thus, for men, migrating for family reasons may be a protective health factor, whereas migrating for work/education may be detrimental due to family separation and reduced social support. Another explanation could be that migration due to work and education may lead to increased stress compared to migrating for family and, consequently, result in poorer health. On the other hand, the finding that women who migrate for work/education and for independence exhibit less depressive symptoms than those who migrate for family reasons may suggest that internal migration could be a vehicle for female empowerment. This may be especially true in the context of a patriarchal society like Mexico which has greatly limited women's migration to the United States (Donato, Wagner, and Patterson 2008).[2] Thus, leaving the origin community for employment, education, or simply for independence may lead to more autonomy and freedom for women and, consequently, better mental health outcomes.

Prior research suggests that the distinct social and economic contexts in the origin and destination communities may result in different postmigration health profiles (Malmusi, Borrell, and Benach 2010). This was only evident among male migrants: men who originated in rural communities reported fewer postmigration depressive symptoms than their urban counterparts; however, migrating to a city was associated with better self-rated health. The latter finding could be related to greater access to household consumption and healthcare services, as well as better living conditions in Mexican cities compared to less developed areas.

A few limitations need to be acknowledged. First, I did not account for any socioeconomic and behavioral changes that occurred after migration and which could potentially impact postmigration health. There is evidence that internal migrants usually experience gains in socioeconomic standing after migration (Lu 2010a; Parrado and Gutierrez 2016). At the same time, health behaviors tend to change after migration, both positively and negatively. For instance, internal migration is related to declines in physical activity, increased weight gain, and improvements in diet (IOM 2015). Future research should explore whether socioeconomic and behavioral mechanisms mediate the association between internal migration and health.

Notwithstanding these limitations, this research makes several contributions. Scholarship on the internal migration–health relationship has predominantly focused on moves within countries in East and Southeast Asia (see, for example, Chen 2011; Lu 2008, 2010b; Nauman et al. 2015) and Africa (see, for example, Anglewicz et al. 2017). The present study contributes to this literature by investigating the health of Mexican internal migrants and the factors that shape it. In addition, the stratified gender analyses contribute to our understanding of the gender-migration-health relationship. Few studies have explicitly assessed gender differences in the health effects of internal migration (see, for example, Malmusi, Borrell, and Benach 2010; Wheaton and Crimmins 2013; Wong and Gonzalez-Gonzalez 2010). My findings reveal that migration motivations, age at migration, and type of origin and destination shape the health of Mexican male and female migrants differently.

## Notes

1. Rural populations are largely dependent on public healthcare services offered by the Mexican Institute of Social Security (IMSS) and by state-run hospitals and clinics. However, these rural health institutions, especially those that serve Indigenous populations, tend to be difficult to access, under-funded, oversaturated, and under-staffed (Montero Mendoza 2011).

2. See, for example, Lilia Soto's (2018) qualitative account of how young Mexican women's migration is discouraged and often blocked by their fathers.

## References

Angel, Ronald J., Jacqueline L. Angel, Carlos Díaz Venegas, and Claude Bonazzo. 2010. "Shorter Stay, Longer Life: Age at Migration and Mortality among the Older Mexican-Origin Population." *Journal of Aging and Health* 22 (7): 914–31.
Anglewicz, Philip, Mark Vanlandingham, Lucinda Manda-Taylor, and Hans-Peter Kohler. 2017. "Cohort Profile: The Migration and Health in Malawi (MHM) Study." *PSC Working Paper Series* 7: e014799.
Belle, Deborah. 1987. "Gender Differences in the Social Moderators of Stress." In *Gender and Stress,* edited by B. Rosalind, L. Biener, and G. Baruch, 257–77. New York: Free Press.
Bernard, Aude, Martin Bell, and Elin Charles-Edwards. 2014. "Life-Course Transitions and the Age Profile of Internal Migration." *Population and Development Review* 40 (2): 213–39.
Calderón Narváez, Guillermo. 1997. "Un cuestionario para simplificar el diagnóstico del síndrome depresivo." *Revista de Neuro-Psiquiatría* 60: 127–35.
Canales, Alejandro, and Israel Montiel. 2007. "De la migración interna a la internacional. En búsqueda del eslabón perdido." In *Taller Nacional sobre "Migración interna y desarrollo en México: Diagnóstico, perspectivas y políticas."* Mexico City: Universidad de Guadalajara. https://www.cepal.org/sites/default/files/courses/files/acanales.pdf
Chen, Juan. 2011. "Internal Migration and Health: Re-Examining the Healthy Migrant Phenomenon in China." *Social Science & Medicine* 72 (8): 1294–301.
Curran, Sara R, and Estela Rivero-Fuentes. 2003. "Engendering Migrant Networks: The Case of Mexican Migration." *Demography* 40 (2): 289–307.

Donato, Katharine M., Brandon Wagner, and Evelyn Patterson. 2008. "The Cat and Mouse Game at the Mexico-U.S. Border: Gendered Patterns and Recent Shifts." *The International Migration Review* 42 (2): 330–59.
Goldman, Noreen, Anne R. Pebley, Mathew J. Creighton, Graciela M. Teruel, Luis N. Rubalcava, and Chang Chung. 2014. "The Consequences of Migration to the United States for Short-Term Changes in the Health of Mexican Immigrants." *Demography* 51 (4): 1159–73.
Hagelskamp, Carolin, Carola Su, and Diane Hughes. 2010. "Migrating to Opportunities : How Family Migration Motivations Shape Academic Trajectories among Newcomer Immigrant Youth." *Journal of Social Issues* 66 (4): 717–39.
Idler, Ellen L., and Yael Benyamini. 1997. "Self-Rated Health and Mortality: A Review of Twenty-Seven Community Studies." *Journal of Health and Social Behavior* 38 (1): 21–37.
Instituto National de Estadística y Geografía (INEGI). 2015. "Estadísticas a propósito del Día Internacional del Migrante (18 de diciembre)," 1–9.
International Organization for Migration (IOM). 2015. "World Migration Report 2015–Migrants and Cities: New Partnerships to Manage Mobility." Geneva, Switzerland.
Lu, Yao. 2008. "Test of the 'Healthy Migrant Hypothesis': A Longitudinal Analysis of Health Selectivity of Internal Migration in Indonesia." *Social Science & Medicine* 67 (8): 1331–39.
———. 2010a. "Mental Health and Risk Behaviours of Rural–Urban Migrants: Longitudinal Evidence from Indonesia." *Population Studies* 64(2): 147–63.
———. 2010b. "Rural-Urban Migration and Health: Evidence from Longitudinal Data in Indonesia." *Social Science & Medicine* 70 (3): 412–19.
Malmusi, Davide, Carme Borrell, and Joan Benach. 2010. "Migration-Related Health Inequalities: Showing the Complex Interactions between Gender, Social Class and Place of Origin." *Social Science & Medicine* 71 (9): 1610–19.
Montero Mendoza, Elda. 2011. "Percepción de los habitantes indígenas de áreas rurales respecto al primer nivel de atención médica. El caso del sureste de Veracruz, México." *Salud Colectiva* 71 (1):73–86.
Nauman, Elizabeth, Mark VanLandingham, Philip Anglewicz, Umaporn Patthavanit, and Sureeporn Punpuing. 2015. "Rural-to-Urban Migration and Changes in Health among Young Adults in Thailand." *Demography* 52 (1): 233–57.
Parrado, Emilio A., and Edith Y. Gutierrez. 2016. "The Changing Nature of Return Migration to Mexico, 1990–2010: Implications for Labor Market Incorporation and Development." *Sociology of Development* 2 (2): 93–118.
Pérez-Campuzano, Enrique, and Clemencia Santos-Cerquera. 2013. "Tendencias recientes de la migración interna en México." *Papeles de Poblacion* 19 (76): 53–88.
Quinn, Michael A., and Stephen Rubb. 2005. "The Importance of Education-Occupation Matching in Migration Decisions." *Demography* 42 (1): 153–67.
Romo Viramontes, Raúl, Yolanda Téllez Vázquez, and Jorge López Ramírez. 2013. "Tendencias de la migración interna en México en el periodo reciente." In *La situación demográfica de México 2013*, 83–106. Mexico City: Consejo Nacional de Población.
Rubalcava, Luis, and Graciela Teruel. 2006a. "User's Guide for the Mexican Family Life Survey, First Wave."

———. 2006b. "User's Guide for the Mexican Family Life Survey, Second Round."
———. 2013. "User's Guide for the Mexican Family Life Survey, Third Round."
Sobrino, Jaime. 2010. *Migración interna en México durante el siglo XX*. Mexico City: Consejo Nacional de Población.
———. 2014. "Migración interna y tamaño de localidad en México." *Estudios Demográficos y Urbanos* 29 (3[87]): 443–79.
———. 2016. "Migración interna en México, 1995–2015." *Coyuntura Demográfica* 10: 57–65.
Soto, Lilia. 2018. *Girlhood in the Borderlands: Mexican Teens Caught in the Crossroads of Migration*. New York: New York University Press.
Téllez Velázquez, Yolanda, Jorge López Ramírez, and Raúl Romo Viramontes. 2014. *Prontuario de migración interna*. Consejo Nacional de Población.
Ullmann, S. Heidi, Noreen Goldman, and Douglas S. Massey. 2011. "Healthier before They Migrate, Less Healthy when They Return? The Health of Returned Migrants in Mexico." *Social Science & Medicine* 73 (3): 421–28.
Wheaton, Felicia V., and Eileen M. Crimmins. 2013. "In Hindsight: Urban Exposure Explains the Association between Prior Migration and Current Health of Older Adults in Mexico." *Journal of Aging and Health* 25 (3): 422–38.
Wong, Rebeca, and Cesar Gonzalez-Gonzalez. 2010. "Old-Age Disability and Wealth among Return Mexican Migrants from the United States." *Journal of Aging and Health* 22 (7): 932–54.
Wooldridge, Jeffrey M. 2002. *Econometric Analysis of Cross Section and Panel Data*. Cambridge, MA: MIT Press.

# 4

## Practicing Medicine in Post-Revolution Mexico

The Case of John Steinbeck and Emilio Fernández

Douglas J. Weatherford

In 1940, American Pulitzer Prize–winning author and future Nobel laureate John Steinbeck met the still fairly unknown but soon-to-be iconic Mexican director Emilio "El Indio" Fernández. Although the details of that meeting are not well known, that first encounter would blossom into a productive transnational relationship that would mark the artistic careers of both men. Steinbeck was in Mexico to film the semi-documentary *The Forgotten Village*, but it was not his first time south of the Rio Grande.[1] Indeed, Steinbeck, who was fluent in Spanish, had traveled through much of central Mexico and would continue to return to the country (especially to Mexico City, Puebla, Oaxaca, and Cuernavaca), often staying for weeks at a time (Bercini 2013, 73). The California-bred author was, of course, quite familiar with, and sympathetic to, the presence of Mexican and Mexican American laborers in his own community and he often included individuals of Hispanic descent in his fiction, giving his work what Charles L. Etheridge Jr. (2007) has called a "Mexican sensibility" (226). In 1940, however, Steinbeck was not looking simply to flavor his fiction with Hispanic characters; rather, he was attracted by the possibility of creating something that would be truly Mexican. As it turns out, Steinbeck's encounter with Fernández would culminate in his writing the short novel, *The Pearl* in 1945. This novel was adapted by Fernández for the big screen, first in the Spanish as *La perla*, released in Mexico in 1947, and then in the English as *The Pearl*, released in the United States in 1948. These versions of the film cemented the American author's place in Mexican film history and that of Mexico in his own artistic oeuvre. At the heart of Steinbeck's fascination with his southern neighbor is a quartet of texts that were created almost entirely in Mexico and that are set fully in that country: *Sea of Cortez: A Leisurely Journal of Travel and Research* (1941), *The Forgotten Village* (1941), *The Pearl* (1947), and *Viva, Zapata!* ([1952] 1993).

Fernández's direct participation in this grouping is limited to *The Pearl*, and I will return to that work at the end of this study. And yet, a comparison of the Mexican vision of Steinbeck and Fernández might be found just as productively in an examination of the semi-documentary film *The Forgotten Village* that the California native was working on when he met the future director of many of Mexico's most cherished movies. That piece shares an important connection to *Río Escondido* [Hidden River] (1947), a feature-length film that Fernández directed a half-decade after *The Forgotten Village* and that became one of the most important additions to the so-called Golden Age of Mexican Film.[2] Both Fernández in *Río Escondido* and Steinbeck in *The Forgotten Village* examine the national condition in the decades following the Mexican Revolution of 1910[3] and commend the central government's efforts to send assistance to the farthest corners to cure what they considered to be two of the nation's lingering maladies: disease and ignorance. Along the way, both artists created didactic works whose reach—like that of the *maestros rurales* and *médicos rurales* [rural teachers and doctors] that they honor—is intended to extend far and wide.[4] Indeed, Steinbeck and Fernández create what Marijane Osborn (2013) has called participatory parables in an effort to make an impact on the viewing public. This meta-cinematic instructional imperative is reflected in both works through the obsessive creation of on-screen learning environments where the movie-going public on this side of the big screen observes another audience projected in black and white absorbing a lesson (be it about health or history) that each socially committed artist hoped would change lives on both sides of the so-called fourth wall. A lot has been said already about the presence of medicine and medical practitioners in Steinbeck and Fernández's work.[5] My research complements those earlier investigations by illuminating both individuals' interest in the possibilities of art to influence national film audiences who might recognize themselves in the faces of on-screen learners. At the same time, I show that John Steinbeck, acclaimed chronicler of the North American experience in a healthcare-based cinematic endeavor, fits well within the social and artistic environment of midcentury Mexico.[6]

## John Steinbeck, Emilio Fernández, and the Visualization of Mexico

John Steinbeck's interest in his southern neighbor was not new when filming began on *The Forgotten Village*. Nor was it insincere or fleeting. The author had a strong grounding in that country's history and culture, and he cultivated relationships with Mexican intellectuals, including Miguel Covarrubias and Diego Rivera (see Etheridge 2007). In many ways, Steinbeck was not unlike many other artists (including the Soviet Sergei Eisenstein, the Italian Tina Modotti, the North American Paul Strand, the Spaniard Luis Buñuel, and the German Walter Reuter, to name just a few) who were drawn to Mexico during the first half of the twentieth century for artistic and political reasons. The nation's social and artistic rebirth in the decades following the Revolution, especially as it was spearheaded by the muralist movement, proved irresistible to many, while others came in search of a safe harbor from the violence of European conflict in the 1930s (the Spanish Civil War) and the 1940s (World War II). Although Steinbeck's wanderings through Mexico—both literal and figurative—were never a retreat from his home country, the author expressed enthusiasm for working on *The Forgotten Village,* a project that was significantly grounded in a Mexican rather than an American film environment.[7] He would show the same eagerness a few years later about the film, *La perla/The Pearl.* In January 1945, he wrote in a letter to a friend that he and Emilio Fernández had decided "to make [that film] straight without any concessions to Hollywood" (qtd. in Benson 1984, 565). Steinbeck wrote *The Forgotten Village* together with Herbert Kline in Mexico City during the spring of 1940 (Schultz and Li 2005, 86). It was filmed in the fall on location in the states of Puebla and Tlaxcala, included numerous Mexican crew and cast members, and relied fully upon non-professional actors who, as Steinbeck believed, needed merely to reprise scenes from their own lives.[8] And yet Steinbeck was not interested only in the art, but also in the cause, and he believed that by crossing the border to shoot a documentary about health and education, he could improve lives in both Mexico and the United States while also building bridges between the two nations. The future Nobel laureate would place his creative destiny even more securely in foreign hands when he wrote *The Pearl* specifically for Emilio Fernández, who, ironically like Steinbeck, had moved back to his home country only a few years earlier to participate in a Mexican film industry showing new promise.

Fernández had begun an accidental career in film years earlier when he arrived in Hollywood in the mid-1920s after working at a number of odd jobs throughout the United States. It was while he was in Hollywood that he learned of the newly flourishing environment for film in his home country, and the expatriate decided that his future in cinema lay not in Hollywood but in Mexico. Although Steinbeck first met Fernández as the cineaste was transitioning from acting to directing, the pair would join forces to film *La perla/The Pearl* in the very moment—the mid-1940s—in which the cineaste known affectionately as "El Indio" [the Indian] would reach the height of his directorial career. Steinbeck, who was attracted to Fernández's personality and his potential as a filmmaker, described his collaborator in January 1945 as "an ex-cowboy actor, ex-revolutionary leader [who] started directing pictures." Steinbeck continues, "I think Indio [Fernández] will emerge as one of the great directors of the world" (qtd. in Benson 1984, 565).

It is not surprising that Emilio Fernández and John Steinbeck would find common ground. Indeed, crossing the United States' southern border to participate in the prospering Mexican cinema is only one characteristic that the two have in common. Both men lived large while being attracted artistically and politically to the vulnerable members of their nations' populace. And both men have been accused of creating an ambivalent body of work that vacillates between faith and fear in the modern world. That fluctuation can be seen clearly in *La perla/The Pearl* that the two made together and also in separate ventures that, although produced apart, seem in many ways to be two versions of the same project: *The Forgotten Village* and *Río Escondido*. Each of these three movies considers Mexico's postrevolutionary condition through the lens of modern medicine and universal education, and each creates parables that ask audiences to act on behalf of the nation's vulnerable. *The Forgotten Village* and *Río Escondido* do so with optimism, while the skepticism of *La perla*, as we shall see later, offers a cautionary tale.

## Seeing Is Believing: *The Forgotten Village* and *Río Escondido* as Participatory Parables

*The Forgotten Village* is, of course, a cooperative creation and Steinbeck is only one of several individuals who contributed to its production. Although a number of filmmakers and technicians appear on the film's credits, the primary co-creators were Herbert Kline, who directed and produced the initiative, and Alexander Hammid (listed as Alexander Hackensmid) who co-directed and was responsible for the photography. Both individuals were essential to the production and must be seen as equally responsible for the work's emphasis on medicine as metaphor. Nonetheless, it would be difficult to overstate Steinbeck's role in *The Forgotten Village*. Although credited only for the film's "story and screenplay," the novelist's presence is far deeper than simply having put pen to paper. He participated in many aspects of pre- and post-production and was a major figure on set during the film's shooting. And, in many ways, the project was a response to the writer's very personal attraction to his southern neighbor.[9]

Steinbeck was full of optimism when he headed to Mexico to film *The Forgotten Village*. In his mind, the venture was practical and socially responsible. "Literature was not promulgated," as the author would assert in his 1962 Nobel lecture, "by a pale and emasculated critical priesthood singing their litanies in empty churches—nor is it a game for the cloistered elect. . . ." *The Forgotten Village* is the ideal reflection of the author's model of committed art and, based on this didactic raison d'être, Marijane Osborn (2013) has labeled the film, along with *The Pearl*, as "participatory parables" (241–42).[10] Both works, it might be said, seek more than a simple understanding of social injustice from their readers and viewers—they demand action. Steinbeck implies this instructional imperative largely through the recurrent depiction of learning environments in which trainees, whether young or old, are taught principles of history and medicine. In the present study that seeks to find common ground between Steinbeck and Fernández, it goes without saying that *Río Escondido* shares the same obsession for pedagogy as *The Forgotten Village*.

Of course, Steinbeck and Fernández were not the first artists to refer in their work to the field of medicine as practiced in Mexico. Providing effective medical care had been, after all, a major concern during the 1910 uprising and would be one of the first imperatives of the postrevolutionary government. The very practical need to care for soldier and citizen would appear in a variety of creative texts. And yet this interest in doctoring was not limited to the real as novelists, muralists, and filmmakers during and, especially after, the Revolution looked to the metaphoric potential of medicine as a reflection of the national condition.[11] To be sure, as early as 1915 the doctor-turned-novelist Mariano Azuela (1873–1952) sought to diagnose the national character in *Los de abajo* [The Underdogs] in part through medical discourse. "We could say" [*podríamos decir*], Luis Leal (1962) would explain, "that Azuela sees reality, in all of its facets, with the eyes of a doctor. . . . His novelistic production, like his profession, is guided by a well-defined purpose that is never lost from sight: improving the health of Mexico, of that Mexico that pained him so deeply and that he knew so well how to capture in his work" [*que Azuela ve la realidad, en todos sus aspectos, con ojos de médico. . . . Su obra novelística, como su profesión, se encamina hacia una meta bien definida y que nunca pierde de vista: mejorar la salud de su México, de ese México que tanto le dolía y que tan bien supo captar en su obra*] (303).[12] Azuela fictionalized his inclination to see the nation with the "eyes of a doctor" through Luis Cervantes. And although this character with the imposing literary name—an allusion to Miguel de Cervantes—is quickly exposed as an opportunist, Azuela never calls into question his abilities as a medical practitioner. As David Laraway (1999) has shown, Azuela singles out Cervantes's dedication to empirical thought as the appropriate way to understand the Republic. Yet Azuela never suggests that such understanding should be limited to a few. In one illustrative scene, for example, the novelist emphasizes the process of learning through observation when Cervantes, while treating his own wound, teaches Camila about microbes. The girl's persistent questions, as Laraway (1999) points out, "reveal crucial details about modern medical thought and its foreign, exotic quality in the *eyes* of the physician's provincial audience" (55; emphasis mine). She asks: "Listen, and who taught ya to cure like that?" Her interrogation continues: "And whatcha boil the water for? [ . . . ] Is that really alcohol? Well, what d'ya know, I thought alcohol was only good for colic! [ . . . ] Little tiny animals livin' in the water if you don't boil the water! Phooey! I sure don't see nothin' when I look at it!" (Azuela [1915] 1960, 28–29).[13]

"Such questions," as Laraway (1999) suggests, "should not be regarded as signals of either simple ignorance or inattentiveness on Camila's part" (55). Rather, they are an indication that Camila had "not been initiated into a world in which [microbes] are both meaningful and discernible . . ." (56–57). The scene is a tribute to the power of observation to treat illness and, more generally, to improve lives. But by fictionalizing the process of learning in which the reader *sees* a protagonist *see* an observable but previously unknown medical truth, Azuela suggests that all Mexicans, when taught what to look for, are capable of understanding and perhaps curing the national malady. Obviously, such a positive analysis belies the cynicism of Azuela's novel. But it does prefigure an optimism that will define the postrevolutionary government's decision to send doctors—the famous *médicos rurales*—flooding into the countryside. And it points to the later tendency of socially committed artists (painters, filmmakers, authors) to envision the teaching of medical principles as a metaphor for growth and progress.[14] Both *The Forgotten Village* and *Río Escondido* adopt this pedagogical trope and—through the meta-cinematic representation of one audience watching another audience learn (with medicine and history being the primary attractions)—both films hope to extend their influence beyond the silver screen.

The importance of the medical field is obvious throughout *The Forgotten Village* as the film highlights instruments of that profession: stethoscopes, microscopes, glass slides, syringes, flasks, beakers, and others. It is not surprising, of course, to see such items represented in a medical documentary. And yet their presence as a visual motif underscores a faith in modern technology that is at the heart of the film, especially when these progressive

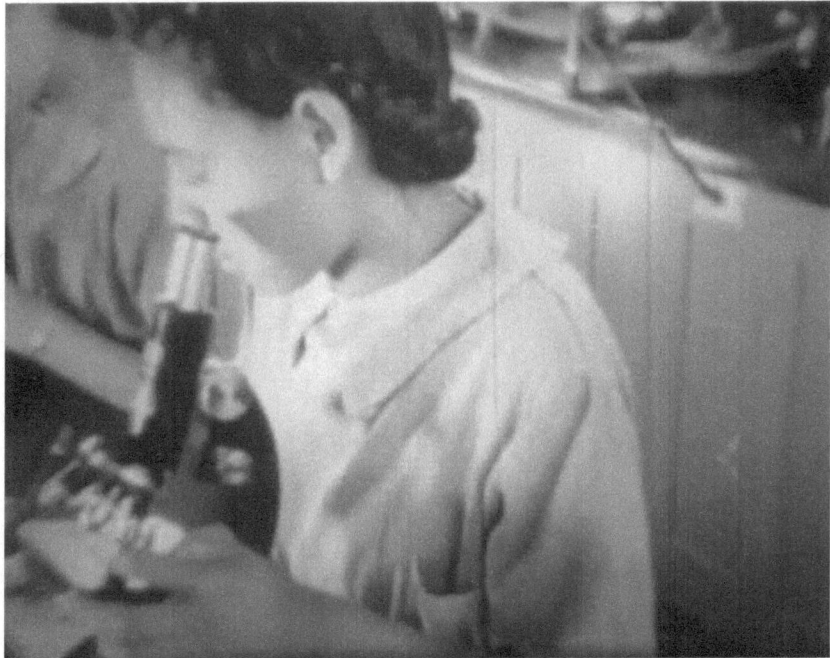

Figure 4.1. In this still from *The Forgotten Village* (1941) a female student looks through a microscope in a school in Mexico City.

tools of the trade are compared to the snakeskin and incense of the hapless *curandera* (or healer, referred to in the film as the "wise woman").[15] But these medical supplies are not placed in the hands of a trained elite whose learning lifts them above the uneducated. Instead, the film emphasizes a technology that is accessible to all through education. The doctors of *The Forgotten Village* do not simply practice medicine; they teach principles that will cure beyond a single patient. To be sure, each time a medical instrument is shown in the film—whether in the small town of Santiago or in the schools of Mexico City—it is connected in some way to an individual who is being taught. In one of the most iconic images of the documentary, for example, a young female student is photographed next to a microscope, a juxtaposition that is hardly insignificant for audiences on both sides of the Río Grande that might not yet be comfortable with women studying to be physicians and for an audience in the United States that might be unaccustomed to seeing Mexico represented as a progressive nation (see fig. 4.1).

*The Forgotten Village* overflows with images of learning environments as the camera focuses on individuals—young and old—who gather to be instructed (see fig. 4.2). Although a struggle between new and old lies at the

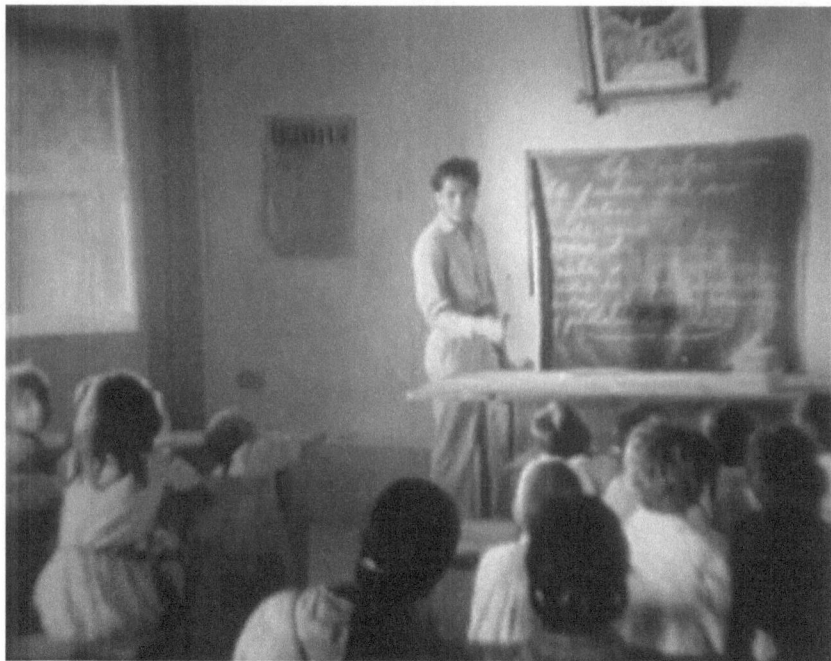

Figure 4.2. *The Forgotten Village* (1941), based on a text by John Steinbeck, overflows with images of learning environments.

heart of the semi-documentary and the village residents initially reject the remedies that they are offered, the film projects a faith that knowledge will overcome fear. The locus of that optimism is a capital city and the institutions that it houses that are shown, in the postwar years, to be modernizing, well-ordered, and caring. "The streets [of Mexico City] were quiet," Burgess Meredith, the off-screen narrator, explains, "for order was restored and the day of fighting was over." *The Forgotten Village* concludes as Juan Diego, the young villager who initially sought assistance for his community, sets off once more for the capital. It is this young man—and many others like him, one assumes—who will gain an education before returning home. Additionally, as his pious name seems to suggest, an homage to the Chichimec believer who saw the Virgin of Guadalupe in 1531 on a hill north of Mexico City, Juan Diego will redeem his people.[16]

It is difficult in this collaborative project to know who played what role in *The Forgotten Village*'s visual and thematic insistence on the metaphoric quality of learning environments. It is likely, of course, that Steinbeck was an essential—if not the dominant—voice in that creative process. As biographer Jackson J. Benson (1984) writes, Steinbeck "seemed to operate during most of his life in two modes—writer or learner. A series of still photographs taken throughout his life might very well show that his most characteristic posture was that of a man, sitting or standing, near a campfire, at the counter of a coffee shop, aboard a ship, or hunched over in a chair in someone's living room—listening" (237). Furthermore, the novelist, as already mentioned, was familiar with Mexican history and was appreciative of the efforts by Mexico's postrevolutionary government—especially in the creation of the *médicos* and *maestros rurales*—to improve the nation through education and modern medicine. It is also likely that the Californian was aware that the artistic representation of learning as a national value was already taking hold among committed Mexican intellectuals (like José Vasconcelos), authors (like Mariano Azuela), and muralists (like Diego Rivera).[17]

*The Forgotten Village*'s exploration of a nation's attempt to extend medical care and learning to the farthest reaches of the nation is just one example of how Steinbeck, acclaimed chronicler of the North American experience, fits comfortably within the social and artistic environment of midcentury Mexico. Nowhere is such a statement seen more clearly than in *Río Escondido*, one of the most recognizable efforts by postrevolutionary artists to reflect upon (and, in Fernández's case, to praise) the doctors and teachers sent to change the nation.

Shot in 1947 and released the following year, *Río Escondido* was immediately popular among audiences at home and abroad. The film is now considered a classic of Golden Age Mexican cinema and a witness to the talent of many of that country's most iconic cineastes at the height of their careers. Working alongside Emilio Fernández, to name just a few examples, were Gabriel Figueroa, one of Mexico's most celebrated cinematographers; Mauricio Magdaleno, a talented and prolific screenwriter; and María Félix, among the nation's most popular female actors of any generation. Set in the mid-1940s, *Río Escondido* follows Rosaura, a dedicated *maestra rural* who, hiding a heart condition that should keep her home, is sent by the president of the Republic to open a school in the northern provincial village of Río Escondido. Far from the civilizing reaches of Mexico City, the town is dominated by a local cacique, or boss, Don Regino, who initially frustrates Rosaura's efforts. Things change, however, when a contagion spreading through town infects Don Regino. The strongman calls for the *médico rural*, Felipe, who arrived with Rosaura and lives in a nearby town. In exchange for his own treatment, Don Regino allows the entire village to be vaccinated and the school to be opened.

The similarities between *The Forgotten Village* and *Río Escondido* are striking, especially in both films' juxtaposition of education and medicine.

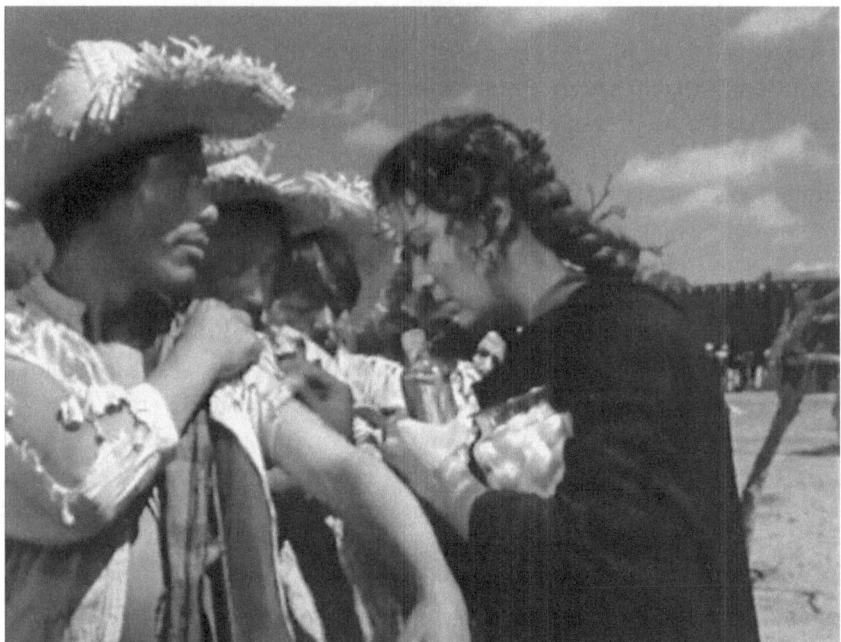

Figure 4.3. In the Mexican film *Río Escondido* (1947), Rosaura prepares a long line of patients for inoculation.

To be sure, it is through the combined efforts of Felipe (as a *médico rural*) and Rosaura (as a *maestra rural*) that the progressive forces of the postrevolutionary Republic are able to reach the national periphery and tap the potential (the hidden river of the film's title) of all of its citizens. But the similarities extend further. In a metaphoric flourish not uncommon in Emilio Fernández's films, Rosaura is presented as a Marian figure, seen most clearly when the unmarried, sexually innocent woman takes on the maternal responsibilities (a figural virgin birth) of caring for three recently orphaned children.[18] The symbolism of Rosaura's saving power extends to the children, especially the youngest, who is described in perhaps all-too-obvious ways at the end of the film as the future of the nation ("*Este niño es México*" [This child is Mexico]) by a Rosaura who, on her deathbed, has literally and figuratively given her life for her country. Rosaura, in other words, is as closely associated with the Virgin of Guadalupe as a foundational myth of the Mexican nation as is Juan Diego. Yet, the Marianist/Messianic quality of Rosaura is just one of many connections that *Río Escondido* shares with *The Forgotten Village*. She, like Juan Diego in the earlier film, for example, travels between the capital and the periphery in a symbolic pilgrimage that, despite its pious underpinnings, is meant to expand the reaches of an apparently

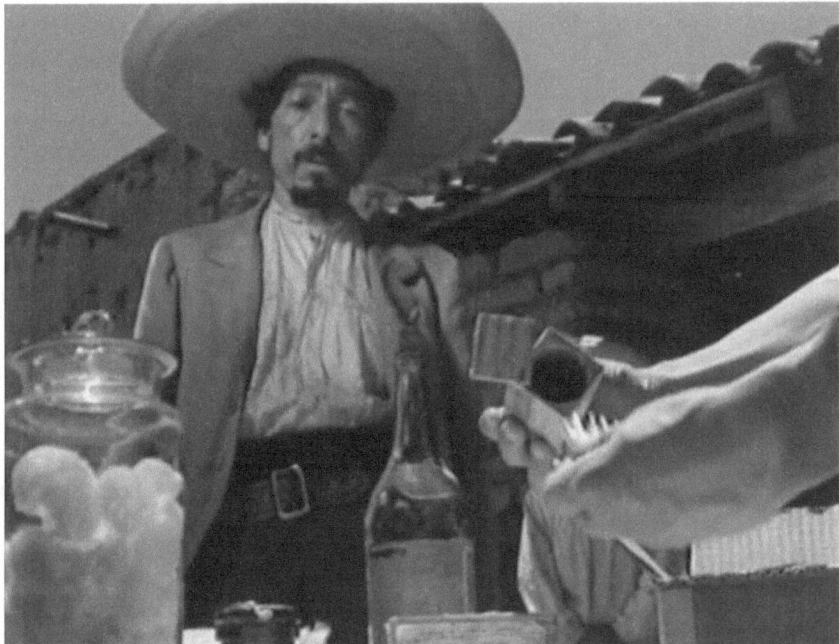

Figure 4.4. The doctor's tools of trade are laid out with almost religious admiration in Emilio Fernández's *Río Escondido* (1947).

benevolent, secular government through pedagogy and science. Ultimately, one of the more striking parallels between Steinbeck and Fernández is the obsessive need each artist felt to create visual and thematic motifs that highlight medical discourse and learning environments.

In one of *Río Escondido*'s most memorable scenes, the villagers have lined up to receive a vaccination. The black and white cinematography of Gabriel Figueroa is interested as much in aesthetics as pragmatics, and it highlights an artistic mise-en-scène, eye-catching contrasts, and vertical lines. The scene is also designed, however, as an homage to modern medicine. The doctor, Felipe, and the teacher, Rosaura, who assists him, are held in reverence by their placement on-screen and by the long line of patients who await their inoculation (see fig. 4.3). The pair, representing twin pillars of progress, are the episode's dominant (primary focus) throughout several shots. Also important, however, are the healthcare workers' tools of trade—vials of medicine, syringes, cotton swabs, alcohol for sterilization, and a doctor's bag—shown admiringly on the table at the head of the line (see fig. 4.4). The scene feels like religious devotion, and in one long shot a cross in the background hovers above the setting, suggesting that the intermingling of reason and faith is not accidental. Nor is it pure artistry. Instead, *Río Escondido* is a

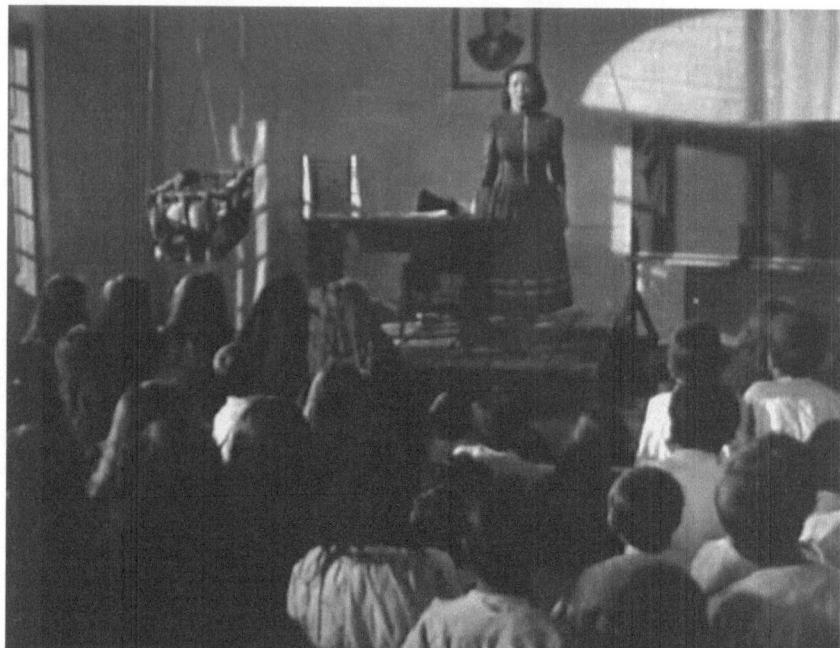

Figure 4.5. In *Río Escondido* (1947), Rosaura stands at the front of the class in the newly opened school. The painting above her is of Benito Juárez, Mexico's first Indigenous president.

highly didactic film that appropriates a wide range of symbols that uphold the efforts of the postrevolutionary state and promote modern healthcare practices. The latter motivation is seen particularly well in another important scene. A gathering of women, clad in black shawls wait in line for their turn to collect water from the town's only public well. The hieratic stillness of the image again reflects Figueroa's tendency toward the aesthetic. Felipe is positioned by and above the women and, in a scene reminiscent of the already mentioned conversation in *Los de abajo* between Cervantes and Camila, the doctor explains: "And above all, don't forget what I've just recommended: always boil your water and that way you won't get sick." [*Y sobre todo, no se les olvide lo que acabo de recomendarles: hiervan siempre el agua y así no se enfermarán.*] This is, of course, a repetition of the learning environments so present in *The Forgotten Village*. And like that earlier film, *Río Escondido* slowly reveals itself as another metafictional "participatory parable" where the filmgoing audience is asked to witness the learning of another audience on-screen.

*The Forgotten Village* privileges medical instruction over the learning of national history. Nonetheless, the semi-documentary understands that medical advances are integral to, not separate from, Mexico's unique historical arc. This fact is seen in the film's frequent allusions to the Virgin of Guadalupe and in a respectful fascination with Indigenous characters as the camera, in medium and close-up shots, often lingers on the faces of villagers, especially in a scene that shows Juan Diego reading to his family about Benito Juárez, Mexico's first Indigenous president. *Río Escondido*, however, inverts the hierarchy and chooses Rosaura, the *maestra rural*, rather than Felipe, the *médico rural*, as the film's primary protagonist. To be sure, with the townsfolk inoculated, healthcare gives way to pedagogy, when, in the very next scene, Rosaura stands in front of a large class of children eagerly awaiting instruction in their newly opened school (see fig. 4.5). The film returns often to learning environments (especially, but not limited to, the classroom) where Rosaura teaches the alphabet, Mexican history (again through the biography of Benito Juárez), personal responsibility (by rejecting Don Regino's advances), and national ethics (by explaining the difference between *malos mexicanos* [bad Mexicans] and *buenos mexicanos* [good Mexicans]). And it is through these lessons that Rosaura will help the villagers and, by extension, the national audience that watches her story on the big screen, to take a step toward regional and national progress.

### *La Perla /The Pearl:* A Cautionary Tale

It might be difficult for a modern audience to watch *The Forgotten Village* and *Río Escondido* and not recognize immediately some of the concerns that Steinbeck and Fernández's progressive optimism disregard. Both works are paternalistic and imagine a world in which centralized institutions are wise and benevolent, and where assimilation is key for marginalized and vulnerable communities. Despite Steinbeck's sympathetic eye for Mexico, some might see in *The Forgotten Village*, as Reyes Bercini (2013) has, "some of the stereotypes that foreigners have regarding Mexicans" [*algunos estereotipos que tiene el extranjero con respecto al mexicano*] (62). Despite the confidence in the future that *The Forgotten Village* and *Río Escondido* exhibit, neither Steinbeck nor Fernández was unaware of the costs of progress and both artists vacillated in their view of modernity across their literary and filmic oeuvres. The novelist's call for intervention in Indigenous communities in *The Forgotten Village* so aggravated his good friend, Ed Ricketts, who traveled to Mexico with him and collaborated on *Sea of Cortez: A Leisurely Journal of Travel and Research*, that he proposed writing an anti-script to oppose the film's premise. Ricketts did not need to write that challenge, however, as Marijane Osborn (2013) has suggested, since Steinbeck did it himself when he penned *The Pearl* in 1945, which he later adapted for the big screen and filmed side-by-side with Emilio Fernández—both the English and the Spanish versions.[19]

Based on a story that Steinbeck heard while traveling by boat along the Baja California peninsula, *The Pearl* turns both *The Forgotten Village* and *Río Escondido* on their heads. "Among other things," Osborn (2013) points out, "the new plot interrogates the basic moral premise in *The Forgotten Village*: that Western medicine has more value than native traditions" (232). Indeed, *La perla/The Pearl*, as shot by Fernández (again with the celebrated photography of Gabriel Figueroa), is a cautionary tale that places much of the weight of its message on the shoulders of a racist doctor who, as a foreigner (likely a Spaniard in the short novel, while seen variously as German or American in Fernández's bilingual renditions), represents the abuse of conquest and oligarchy that comes from afar.[20] In *La perla/The Pearl* outsiders are to be feared, there is no benevolent government, the church is conspiratorial, and medical practitioners are exploitative. And, although *La perla/The Pearl*, like *The Forgotten Village* and *Río Escondido*, emphasizes medical devices and other items (stethoscope, magnifying glass, and pharmaceuticals), these are shown to Kino and Juana, the parents of a son who has been stung by a scorpion, in an attempt to confound rather than instruct and cure (see fig. 4.6). Indeed, the one scene that duplicates the learning environments of the other films is an overwrought vision of a happy future for his son, Coyotito, that Kino sees reflected in the giant pearl that he has found: "My son will know how to read and he'll know what a book is. And my son will learn how to write. That will make him free. He'll have knowledge and through him we'll also come to know." [*Mi hijo sabrá leer y sabrá lo que es un libro. Y mi hijo aprenderá a escribir. Es[o] nos [hará] libres. Él tendrá saber y por él nosotros también llegaremos a saber.*][21] The episode, followed by Coyotito's death, creates an obvious paradox: Is this story a positive call to education or a reminder that "progress" does not always improve one's life? Either way, *La perla* returns to the practice of medicine in rural Mexico and, in the process, offers a cautionary tale that the optimism of *The Forgotten Village* and *Río Escondido* might be misguided, or at least incomplete.[22]

## Conclusion: Practicing Medicine in Postrevolutionary Mexico

In the 1940s, two of North America's most iconic artists explored medicine as metaphor to speak to the national condition in the years following the 1910 Revolution. Despite their ambivalence, *The Forgotten Village, Río*

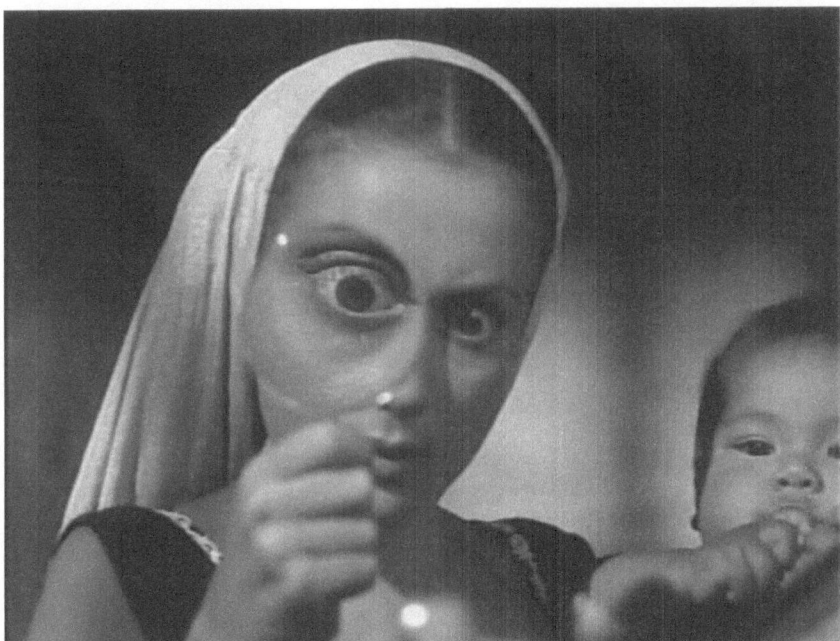

Figure 4.6. In *La perla* (1947), an adaptation of John Steinbeck's short novel by the same title (*The Pearl*), medical instruments and medical practitioners are used to confuse and deceive rather than instruct.

*Escondido,* and *La perla/The Pearl* are participatory parables that hope to influence a generation of moviegoers to see, to understand, and to act for the betterment of society. *La perla* and *Río Escondido* enjoyed critical and popular success and continue to be shown and discussed widely. Sadly, *The Forgotten Village,* a film obsessed with spectators who see and thus understand, never received a commercial release, and has never found a significant audience. And while the English-language version of *The Pearl* became the first full-length Mexican film to earn wide release in the United States, it has not enjoyed the place it deserves in the annals of this country's film history. Indeed, Steinbeck's cross-border conversation about medicine might be interpreted—as Steinbeck biographer Jackson J. Benson (1984) has defined *The Forgotten Village*—as essays "on perception." Benson explains: "A boy, a family, a village have a choice—to deal with the world on the basis of superstition or to deal with it on the basis of scientific *observation*. If they wish, the people can *look* into the microscope and *see* the animals in their water that are killing them" (457; emphases mine). Ultimately, John Steinbeck and Emilio Fernández offer films that are participatory parables that ask us to look, along with its characters, into the microscope or the magnifying glass and to see Mexico—the good and the bad—and to work for that nation's betterment. All three films also want us to see Mexico seeing, a reaction shot that offers a positive face of the nation: inquisitive, strong, and learning.

### Notes

1. *The Forgotten Village* was released in the fall of 1941 along with a companion book by the same title that included Steinbeck's narration from the film and 136 photographs taken by Rosa Harvan Kline and Alexander Hackensmid. *The Forgotten Village* is considered a semi-documentary, that is, a film based on nonprofessional players acting in scenes that, although imagined, are related to their actual lives.

2. The Golden Age of Mexican film lasted from about 1936 to 1956 and represents a period of intense production—in both quantity and quality—of Mexican film. Emilio Fernández is one of the most celebrated directors of this period.

3. The Mexican Revolution began in November 1910 and ended in 1917 (others suggest 1920). It was a complex movement that had at its heart an attempt to improve the conditions of Mexico's largely lower-class population. In the decades that followed, the postrevolutionary government attempted—with varying degrees of commitment and success—to implement the ideals of the 1910 uprising.

4. The programs that sent *médicos rurales* and *maestros rurales* into the Mexican countryside began in the early 1920s. Although not without problems, this postrevolutionary initiative is often celebrated as a positive result of the Mexican Revolution. "By 1936," as Thomas Benjamin (2000) notes, "there were more than 11,000 rural schools, with 14,000 teachers giving instruction to more than 700,000 children" (480).

5. Reyes Bercini (2013), David S. Dalton (2018), and Adela Pineda Franco (2018) are three critics, among others, who consider the role of medicine in Steinbeck and Fernández's work. Pineda Franco's monograph, titled *Steinbeck y México: Una mirada cinematográfica en la era de la hegemonía estadounidense,* is of particular interest and may be consulted by those interested in an expanded discussion of Steinbeck's presence in Mexico.

6. Although I emphasize the Mexican origins of Steinbeck's interest in the story of *The Forgotten Village,* it is also true that the film owes a significant debt to his work on a medical documentary set in Chicago: *The Fight for Life* (1940). This film, commissioned by the Roosevelt administration in advance of health legislation proposals, highlighted ongoing efforts to combat high infant mortality rates. Although uncredited, Steinbeck worked with director/producer Pare Lorentz on the project and wrote the narrative portions of the film (Schultz and Li 2005, 83).

7. Adela Pineda Franco (2018), as mentioned earlier, offers a wide-ranging view of Steinbeck's relationship to Mexico for readers wanting to learn more about this topic. The critic sees a progression in Steinbeck that, according to her, "begins with the image of a progressive writer, defender of the Cardenista State in the 1930s and culminates with that of a staunch defender of US policy as it competes with communism in Mexico in the 1960s" ["*inicia con la imagen de un escritor progresista, defensor del Estado cardenista en*

*los años treinta, y culmina con la de un acérrimo defensor de la política estadounidense de contención en contra del comunismo en* México *durante los años sesenta"*] (23).

8. In his preface to the published version of *The Forgotten Village* (1941) Steinbeck described the process as follows: "The working method was very simple, and yet required great patience. A very elastic story was written. Then the crew moved into the village, made friends, talked, and listened. [ . . . ] To tell this story we had only to have people re-enact what had happened to them. Our *curandera* was a real 'wise woman,' one who practiced herbology and magic in the village; our teacher was a real teacher in the government school; our doctors real doctors; our mother a real mother who had lost a number of children. If they moved through scenes with sureness and authority it was because they had been through them many times before when no cameras were there" (5–6).

9. Jackson J. Benson (1984) has suggested that the original idea for *The Forgotten Village* belonged to Kline, with Steinbeck making significant alterations: "Its genesis had come months earlier when producer-director of documentaries Herbert Kline approached Steinbeck with an idea to do a film about a poor Mexican family caught up in the turmoil of revolution. The writer liked the focus on a peasant family but suggested, in line with his concern with science, that instead of revolution the conflict come out of the attempt to bring modern medicine to a backward area. This was a theme that had been in his mind for some time, ever since his encounters with the problems faced by public health nurses in attempting to deal with the prejudices of Okie and Mexican migrant workers, and it had been stimulated further by his work on [the medical documentary] *The Fight for Life.* . . ." (452–53).

10. Osborn also includes *Viva Zapata!* in the category of participatory parables. Readers of Osborn's study will find that she and I do not use the term "participatory parable" (242) in exactly the same way. They will also find, however, that this critic's insightful reading of Steinbeck's Mexican canon is an important influence on my own approach, and I owe her my gratitude. For his part, Steinbeck would define *The Pearl* in the following way in a letter he wrote in late January 1945: "A folk tale I hope. A black-white story like a parable" (qtd. in Benson 1984, 564).

11. Readers wanting to investigate this topic more might examine, as only one of many examples, David S. Dalton's (2018) *Mestizo Modernity: Race, Technology, and the Body in Postrevolutionary Mexico* (see chapter 3 in particular).

12. All translations are mine, unless otherwise indicated.

13. All quotes from *Los de abajo* come from Sergio Waisman's (2008) translation titled *The Underdogs*. For simplicity, I chose to not include the original Spanish of this long and fragmented quote.

14. I will point simply to Diego Rivera as one of many individuals who see medicine as metaphor. See, for example, this artist's mural "Historia de la medicina en México: El pueblo en demanda de la salud" [The History of Medicine in Mexico: The People Demand Better Health]. Completed in 1953 and located in the Hospital Centro Médico La Raza in Mexico City, this mural celebrates medical advances in the modern as well as the pre-Colombian world.

15. In this film, and in large measure through the critical representation of the *curandera*, Steinbeck and Hammid privilege modern western medical practices over ancient

and Indigenous ones. A more contemporary sensibility, of course, would likely be less dismissive of alternate approaches. I will return to this concern later when I comment on *La perla*. Ironically, the most controversial scene of the film, depicting an Indigenous woman giving birth from a standing position, is also the one that most clearly attempts to show non-traditional medical practices from a respectful perspective.

16. The idea of redemption as a national value in post-Revolution Mexico is not unique to Steinbeck. Instead, the California native is taking part in a dialogue among Mexican intellectuals that includes the writings, among others, of Manuel Gamio (*Forjando patria*, 1916) and José Vasconcelos (*La raza cósmica*, 1925).

17. One of the primary ideals of the Mexican muralist movement was, of course, the didactic responsibility of art, placed in large public spaces, to instruct the population—whether literate or not—in national traditions and values. The aspiration of the muralist movement to teach its viewers is often reflected in scenes depicted within the artwork itself. That is certainly the case in many of Diego Rivera's murals, including *La maestra rural* [*The Rural Schoolteacher*] (1932) and *El hombre controlador del universo* [Man, Controller of the Universe] (1934). See Charles L. Etheridge (2007) for more information on possible connections between Steinbeck's own artistic worldview and that of Mexican muralism.

18. Dalton (2018) goes as far as classifying Rosaura as a cyborg Virgin because of the intersection of her Marian nature and the fact that she, unlike the town's inhabitants, has received an immunization for smallpox (107–27).

19. Steinbeck adapted *The Pearl* along with Fernández and Jack Wagner, and filming began in 1946. Upon its release in the United States, as Joseph R. Millichap (1983) has explained, *The Pearl* (English-language version) became "the first Mexican-made film to win general release in American theaters" (96). *The Pearl* was adapted again in 2001, in English, by Mexican director Alfredo Zacarías.

20. See Fernando Fabio Sánchez (2009) and Dolores Tierney (2010) as examples of two critics who consider the nationality of the doctors across the various literary and film versions of *The Pearl*.

21. It is curious to note that Fernández was developing *Río Escondido* (filmed in 1947) almost in the same moment that he was working on *La perla* (shot in 1946), and the two films, with two very different tones, appear side-by-side in chronological listings of Fernández's directorial oeuvre.

22. The ambivalence of *La perla* offers another point of contact between Steinbeck and the Mexican cultural scene. The optimistic, pro-government tenor of *The Forgotten Village* fits comfortably into a post-Revolution artistic context that often wanted to laud the advances of the nation and that frequently—especially in the case of muralism and cinema—was supported financially by state institutions that encouraged positive representations. There were those, however, who used their art to question the narrative of the Revolution as an idealistic endeavor followed by progressive governance. Mariano Azuela, in the already mentioned *Los de abajo* (1915), belongs to that grouping, as do the filmmaker Luis Buñuel (e.g. *Los olvidados* [The Forgotten Ones], 1950), the photographer Nacho López, and the authors Juan Rulfo (e.g. *Pedro Páramo*, 1955) and Rosario Castellanos (e.g. *Oficio de tinieblas* [The Book of Lamentations], 1962).

# References

Azuela, Mariano. (1915) 1960. *Los de abajo*. Mexico City: Fondo de Cultura Económica.
———. *The Underdogs*. 2008. Translated by Sergio Waisman. New York: Penguin Classics.
Benjamin, Thomas. 2000. "Rebuilding the Nation." In *The Oxford History of Mexico*, edited by Michael C. Meyer and William H. Beezley, 467–502. New York: Oxford University Press.
Benson, Jackson J. 1984. *The True Adventures of John Steinbeck, Writer*. New York: The Viking Press.
Bercini, Reyes. 2013. *Poética del instinto: La perla de John Steinbeck y Emilio Fernández*. Mexico City: Universidad Nacional Autónoma de México.
Buñuel, Luis, director. 1950. *Los olvidados*. Ultramar Films.
Castellanos, Rosario. 1957. *Balún Canán*. Mexico City: Fondo de Cultura Económica.
Dalton, David S. 2018. *Mestizo Modernity: Race, Technology, and the Body in Postrevolutionary Mexico*. Gainsville, FL: University of Florida Press.
Etheridge, Charles L., Jr. 2007. "Steinbeck, Rivera, and Mexican Modernism." In *John Steinbeck and His Contemporaries*, edited by Stephen K. George and Barbara A. Heavilin, 221–303. Lanham, MD: Scarecrow Press.
Fernández, Emilio, director. *La perla*. 1947. Argument by John Steinbeck.
———. *Río Escondido*. 1947. CLASA Films.
Gamio, Manuel. 1916. *Forjando Patria: Pro Nacionalismo*. Mexico City: Porrúa Hermanos.
Kline, Herbert, and Alexander Hackensmid, directors. 1941. *The Forgotten Village*. Pan-American Films Inc.
Laraway, David. 1999. "Doctoring the Revolution: Medical Discourse and Interpretation in *Los de abajo* and *El águila y la serpiente*." *Hispanófila* 127 (Sept): 53–65.
Leal, Luis. 1962. "Mariano Azuela, novelista médico." *Revista Hispánica Moderna* 28 (2/4): 295–303.
Lorentz, Pare, director. 1940. *The Fight for Life*. Columbia Pictures.
Millichap, Joseph R. 1983. *Steinbeck and Film*. New York: Frederick Ungar Publishing.
Osborn, Marijane. 2013. "Participatory Parables: Cinema, Social Action, and Steinbeck's Mexican Dilemma." In *A Political Companion to John Steinbeck*, edited by Cyrus Ernesto Zirakzadeh and Simon Stow, 227–46. Lexington: University Press of Kentucky.
Pineda Franco, Adela. 2018. *Steinbeck y México: Una mirada cinematográfica en la era de la hegemonía estadounidense*. México: Bonilla Artigas.
Rulfo, Juan. 1955. *Pedro Páramo*. Mexico City: Fondo de Cultura Económica.
Sánchez, Fernando Fabio. 2009. "From the Silver Screen to the Countryside: Confronting the United States and Hollywood in 'El Indio' Fernández's *The Pearl*." In *Mexico Reading the United States*, edited by Linda Egan and Mary K. Long, 78–95. Nashville: Vanderbilt University Press.
Schultz, Jeffrey, and Luchen Li. 2005. *Critical Companion to John Steinbeck: A Literary Reference to His Life and Work*. New York: Checkmark Books.
Steinbeck, John, and Edward F. Ricketts. 1941. *Sea of Cortez: A Leisurely Journal of Travel and Research*. New York: The Viking Press.

———. 1941. *The Forgotten Village with 136 Photographs from the Film of the Same Name*. Photographs by Rosa Harvan Kline and Alexander Hackensmid. New York: The Viking Press.
———. 1947. *The Pearl*. New York: The Viking Press.
———. (1952) 1993. *Viva, Zapata!* In *Zapata* by John Steinbeck, edited by Robert E. Morsberger, 224–330. New York: Penguin Books.
———. 1962. "Nobel Lecture." NobelPrize.org.
Tierney, Dolores. 2010. "Emilio Fernández 'in Hollywood': Mexico's Postwar Inter-American Cinema, *La perla/The Pearl* (1946) and *The Fugitive* (1948)." *Studies in Hispanic Cinemas* 7 (2): 81–100.
Vasconcelos, José. 1925. *La raza cósmica*. Madrid: Agencia Mundial de Librería.

# PART II

## Healthcare in United States Latino/a/x Communities

# 5

# Colonial Care

## Medicalizing Latino/a Bodies in the United States, 1894–1970s

Benny J. Andrés Jr.

The United States absorbed Mexican and Puerto Rican people and the territory through military conquest. After the acquisition of the Southwest from Mexico in 1848, US leaders incorporated and subordinated the far-flung and small Mexican population whom they viewed as "unfit" for democratic governance due to their Indigenous ancestry (González 2004). In 1899, the country acquired Puerto Rico following the Spanish-American War. Both populations quickly became colonized subjects, marginalized politically and economically due to existing racial and cultural dogmas in the United States. Congress granted Puerto Ricans citizenship in 1917, but it refused to convert the territory into a state (Erman 2019). Mexicans and Puerto Ricans differed greatly, and White Americans interacted with them in different ways. Nevertheless, these Latino/as'[1] access to healthcare shared key similarities. US officials stereotyped both as disease carriers who posed biological threats to the nation through deficient hygiene and prolific birth rates (Molina 2006, 46–49; Ramírez de Arellano and Seipp 1983; Trujillo-Pagán 2013a). What is more, US physicians engaged in projects of colonial public health care within both communities to lower rates of infectious disease within (and, significantly, beyond) Latino/a communities and, frequently, to use Latino/a bodies to test innovative new drugs.

Theories and practices of colonial care emerged in US tropical colonies, where military and civilian medical researchers constructed knowledge about bacteriology, parasitology, disease eradication, sanitation, quarantine, and public and private health (Anderson 2006; Hattori 2004). US colonial physicians were an elite corps who professionalized Western medicine (Fairchild 2003, 84–85). They cycled through tours of duty in the Philippines, the Panama Canal, Puerto Rico, Cuba, Hawai'i, and Guam, and shared knowledge of germ eradication programs enacted on racialized subjects. Medics circulated their ideas and experiences in Tropical Medical Schools on both sides of the Atlantic, in scientific journals, medical bulletins, conference talks, letters, reports, public health programs, laboratory research, inventions, public talks, and innumerable conversations (Curtin 1989, 104–129; Farley 1991; Haynes 2001; Palmer 2010; Wilkinson 2000). The central tenet of colonial care was that doctors viewed subaltern bodies both as vectors for disease and as sites for human testing of new treatments. In many cases, US medics carried out sanitation campaigns not as much to protect native populations as to ensure the continued health of the colonizers (Anderson 2006; Stern 2006).[2] Douglas Haynes (2001), an historian of imperial medicine, notes: "The wide swaths of the tropics, ranging from Africa to South America to China, designated as the 'white man's grave' testified to stubbornly high levels of mortality and morbidity among European imperial servants" (3). Colonial public health reflected the West's scientific paradigms of the day. While Europe and the United States engaged in imperialism, a parallel universe of scientific, biological, and behavioral discourse emanated from the Western world justifying colonialism. This included casting subjugated persons as "polluted" and disease prone (Ahuja 2016; Palmer 2010), which, in turn, led to the popularization of eugenics—the scientific theory of human betterment (Kevles 1985).

Eugenics encompassed a wide variety of theories about human development (Turda 2010, 63). The two main lines of thinking were neo-Lamarckian and Mendelian genetics. The neo-Lamarckian approach leaned on ideas about environmental factors influencing heredity and was known as positive or soft eugenics. Followers of positive eugenics believed that developing public health, sanitation, and education provided a holistic life experience for improving racial health. This viewpoint was most commonly held in Latin America and the Middle East (Rosemblatt 2018, 29–87; Schell 2010; Stepan 1991, 67–70, 73–95; Stern 2005, 14–15). Proponents of Mendelian (also called Spencerian or neo-Malthusian) genetics, in contrast, focused primarily on heredity fixed at birth to explain intelligence, physique, and behavioral characteristics (Kevles 1985). Since genes determined everything according to Mendelian genetics, the theory was called negative or hard eugenics. Hereditarians ascribed negative and positive traits to genetics. As the elite of Western society, Mendelians believed they had achieved a eugenic ideal; because racialized human traits were fixed and innate, Mendelians thought interracial mixing diluted the genetic line of superior races (Stepan

1991, 24–26, 75, 95–100, 102–134; Stern 2005, 14–17; Turda 2010). Rather than engage in the improvement of supposedly unfit groups through medicine and charity, Mendelian eugenicists preferred to let dysgenic bodies die off and leave natural resources for superior specimens (Stepan 1991, 28).

American neo-Mendelians, who trumpeted the harshest version of negative eugenics, constantly worried that immigration and colonialism would result in sexual relations between the elite and the inferior, and cause racial degeneracy (Black 2003, 30–31). They fretted about race degeneration from declining birth rates among White people, coupled with the mushrooming growth of non-White immigrants, as well as prison and asylum inmates (Kevles 1985, 41–128; Klausen and Bashford 2010, 98–100; Kline 2001, 7–12; Largent 2008, 39–63). Determined to address these challenges, they pursued an agenda of racial hygiene to both reflect genetic betterment and disinfect the unfit to remove their offspring from the national gene pool. Racial disinfectant entailed state intervention to curate the population through birth control in any form, including surgical sterilization. The fertility control branch of eugenics was known as neo-Malthusianism (Klausen and Bashford 2010; Kline 2001, 32–94). Neo-Malthusian eugenics reached southwestern Mexican communities and Puerto Rico in the early twentieth century and remained in place until the 1970s.

This chapter begins with Mexican healthcare in the United States–Mexico borderlands. In the decades before and during the Mexican Revolution (1910–1920), an estimated one million Mexicans entered the United States, settling primarily in the Southwest. Drawn to California for its plentiful jobs and mild weather, every year tens of thousands of Mexicans settled or lived seasonally in Los Angeles County (Sánchez 1993). Initially, assimilationist social workers in Los Angeles believed that environmental and social conditions—particularly substandard housing and an inattention to hygiene—caused disease in Mexican settlements. A 1916 typhus epidemic among Mexicans in Los Angeles and across the borderland resulted in a border entry quarantine that remained in effect until World War II. Public health officials replicated colonial medicalization to cleanse diseased Mexican bodies. The stigmatization of Latino/as as vectors for tropical pathogens had a profound impact on how White people viewed and treated them. California's historical violence toward Native Americans and Asian immigrants (Madley 2016; Pfaelzer 2007) set the stage for the continental mainland's most intense sterilization program. Eugenicists claimed that oversexed Mexicans posed a national security threat because their "differential fecundity" would dilute the superior Nordic blood (Stern 1999, 77). Critics articulated these stereotypes to justify Mexican immigration restriction. Congress rejected putting Mexico on the quota list (Montoya 2020), but the cataclysm of the Great Depression offered new opportunities to cast 350,000 Mexican immigrants and naturalized family members out of the nation (Gratton and Merchant 2013, 958–59).

## United States–Mexico Borderlands, 1894–1940

### Los Angeles Public Health, 1916 Typhus Quarantine

Latino/a colonial care began in the continental United States in 1894 when female progressive reformers moved into a settlement house in Sonoratown, the heart of Mexican Los Angeles. Settlement workers developed a range of housekeeping programs emphasizing White, middle-class notions of domestic life, personal hygiene, and sanitation. Reformers also established nursing and basic health outreach and English instruction (Lewthwaite 2009, 19–48). These agents of Americanization believed that Mexicans, like other racial minorities and immigrants were disease carriers (Kraut 1994). In 1913, California created the Commission of Immigration and Housing to prepare immigrants for manual labor jobs and citizenship. It approved an innovative program that sent female teachers and nurses into homes to teach mothers the modern art of nutrition, childrearing, and cleanliness. Mexicans recognized that these Americanizing projects were paternalistic, and they frequently ignored the advice, opting instead to follow their own traditions (Lewthwaite 2009, 103–19).

The era of mass Mexican immigration contributed to the population explosion in Los Angeles. While the region's boosters widely advertised a White metropolis along the Pacific Ocean, local leaders expressed antipathy toward immigrants and people of color, whom they segregated and discriminated against in all aspects of public life (Abel 2007). Promotional literature publicity drew streams of White male itinerant laborers who loitered and sought public relief. Police cracked down on "undesirable" vagrants, arresting, imprisoning, and setting them to work on the chain gang (Hernández 2014). Local officials objected to and stigmatized indigent consumptives (sufferers of tuberculosis) and others with debilitating or contagious diseases. Conservative officials rid the region of non-productive costly medical cases by paying for train tickets and pressuring newcomers to return home (Abel 2007, 31–36). The repression of unwanted visitors—particularly those deemed unfit for assimilation—initiated the reception of Mexicans during both the 1916 typhus and the 1924 bubonic plague epidemics.

To meet the healthcare needs of the working class in the early twentieth century, Los Angeles officials built modest clinics in the sprawling county and began outpatient nursing home care. City and county officials gradually erected a medical infrastructure for migrants and the working poor. Racism and discrimination against minorities guided the establishment of segregated and substantially unequal medical facilities and substandard care, mirroring residential and educational segregation (Abel 2007, 70; Molina 2006, 76–77, 89–91, 97–102). Health officials rooted clinics in the *colonias* to reduce the infant mortality rate, which was two to three times higher for Mexican babies than for White people (Sánchez 1993, 82). Understaffed clinics operated for only a few hours a day, and the facilities had inadequate equipment (Abel 2007, 49–50). In the 1920s, Mexican women began to heed the calls of local officials to give birth in hospitals or to take infants for checkups soon after birth. These services were free or available for a nominal fee (Molina 2006, 100–03).

When a typhus epidemic in Los Angeles County sickened twenty-six railroad workers from June to October 1916, medical authorities instituted a two-week quarantine of *colonias* with armed guards and a brutal sanitation program that mimicked the indiscriminately destructive and humiliating responses in other colonialized settings.[3] Public health officials launched an education and sanitation campaign targeting Mexicans. Because researchers had identified lice as the disease vector for typhus in 1910 (Mckiernan-González 2012, 172), medics inspected and deloused Mexicans by using cyanide gas at one hundred railroad camps and forty *colonias*. Medical staff also invaded schools and homes to delouse Mexican spaces. The health department passed an order making it a public nuisance for anyone to have lice on their body. The quarantine mandated a weekly bathing regime with coal oil and warm water under visual supervision by a health worker. Mexican workers had to bathe in tin tubs because their camps lacked running water. Bedding, clothing, and shoes were deloused in a military-style operation akin to colonial quarantines. Mexicans complied, but they resented the racist and dehumanizing treatment. One group of laborers formally protested to the Mexican consul, stating that they had already endured medical inspections when entering the country and that local officials behaved as if only Mexicans carried pathogens. The petition blamed employers for unsanitary conditions because they only provided railroad boxcars for housing on lots without running water or sewers. During the epidemic, twenty-two Mexicans fell ill and five died of the disease (Molina 2006, 61–68).

## United States–Mexico Border Typhus Quarantine

Eight hundred miles to the east of Los Angeles—and six months earlier—in the border city of El Paso, Texas, a typhus outbreak sparked a half-century of colonial care. The popular belief that Mexicans were diseased produced an unprecedented regime of medicalization and surveillance in Texas and Arizona, surpassing the statutory health requirements of immigrants at Ellis Island near New York City and Angel Island in the harbor of San Francisco (Baynton 2016; Fairchild 2003, 5, 132–59; Kraut 1994). The attention on Mexicans originated in the xenophobic sentiment sweeping the United States in the 1910s. A massive congressional investigation into the impact of immigrants (Benton-Cohen 2018), blamed foreigners for bringing communicable diseases, especially tuberculosis, into the nation. Once contagion breeched the nation's borders; however, health departments and the US Public Health Service (PHS), played a central role in "the most exceptional intrusions of state authority into the privacy of the individual" (Rothman 1993, 291) to enforce health measures, including vaccinations, incarceration, quarantine, and expulsion.

The PHS, stuffed with imperial physicians, rushed to bring health inspections to the United States–Mexico border. In 1913, Dr. Ernest Sweet conducted a study of the interstate migration of persons with tuberculosis in Texas and Arizona. Unsurprisingly, Sweet ignored White consumptives and instead blamed Mexican immigrants for the rising cases (Sweet 1915a, 1915b, 1915c). Published in 1915, Sweet's biased and methodologically flawed report for the PHS focused attention on the non-enforcement of health inspection on the southern border (Sinclair 2016). In El Paso—the main gateway from Mexico into the United States—the tuberculosis study and the diagnosis of three cases of typhus in Laredo, Texas, prompted local officials in December to appeal to the Immigration Service to quarantine the international divide (Pierce 1917, 426). Physicians believed they could sanitize Mexican bodies because of their experiences with tropical pestilence, particularly yellow fever in Cuba and Panama (Espinosa 2009; Pierce 1904; Stern 2006), leprosy in Hawai'i (Ahuja 2016, 29–70; Worboys 2000), the plague in San Francisco and Hawai'i (Shah 2001), and hookworm in Puerto Rico (Trujillo-Pagán 2013a) and the US South (Palmer 2010).

Armed Immigration Service agents and the Public Health Service (organized under a military structure headed by the Surgeon General) flung a medical net across the southern border, taking aggressive steps to wipe out typhus (Fairchild 2003, 153–59). The PHS was intimately familiar with conditions in southern Texas because it had battled smallpox and yellow fever outbreaks since 1891, empowered by a 1905 Supreme Court decision permitting public health officials to quarantine and compel vaccinations to combat transborder pathogens for national defense (Ahuja 2016, 1–3). Reflecting eugenicist ideologies, a PHS doctor intoned: "the mode of living of the Mexicans of the lower class is so contrary to the laws of nature that the wonder is that they live at all" (Mckiernan-González 2012, 171). Physicians isolated contagious patients and administered smallpox immunizations. When residents refused to comply, health officials forcibly disinfected them in their homes. A flabbergasted Cuban-born PHS doctor wrote: "The people endeavor to conceal the fact that any of their family is sick, as they have an antipathy for the American physicians, some of the more ignorant even going so far as to claim that the Americans would give them medicine to poison them" (Mckiernan-González 2012, 125). The PHS succeeded in stamping out contagious outbreaks, but the Immigration Service did not have the resources to implement health inspections at ports of entry on the southern border. Racial and cultural stereotypes of Mexicans had not yet gained enough prominence in the national public consciousness to justify a border patrol (Hernández 2010, 17–33). However, the influx of immigrants during the Mexican Revolution altered the dynamics in favor of the comprehensive medicalization of Mexicans during the 1916 typhus epidemic.

When Claude Pierce, a renowned PHS surgeon experienced in combating scourges in Panama and San Francisco (Pierce 1904; Shah 2001; Stern 2005, 42–48), arrived in El Paso, he designed a quarantine system modeled after seaport immigration stations (Pierce 1916). In 1916, he made architectural plans for a delousing facility. After crossing the Rio Grande bridge from Ciudad Juárez into El Paso, immigrants left their luggage to be steam cleaned. They then walked into gender-segregated rooms to fully disrobe and begin the colonial industrial medical process. Before entering the bathroom, an attendant checked their entire body for lice. Men with lice had their heads shaved; women with lice applied kerosene and vinegar to their hair keeping it under a towel for half an hour. All migrants then walked under a nozzle that sprayed a solution of kerosene, soap, and water. An attendant observed as migrants bathed and proceeded to another room for their clothing and shoes. After multiple steam cleanings with hydrocyanic acid (the deadliest gas at the time), most, if not all, clothing disintegrated and shoes melted. Frequent border crossers received a card permitting them to delouse only once a week. After dressing, everyone received a medical inspection and, if needed, a smallpox vaccination (Pierce 1917; Romo 2017, 235–40).

In the first four months of the quarantine, 871,639 Mexicans in Texas and Arizona endured the border sanitation gauntlet, with 2,830 daily inspections carried out in El Paso. City medical officers and the army patrolled El Paso's barrio, Chihuahuita, and entered homes to forcefully delouse people. Troops cleaned streets, burned refuse, and destroyed shacks, leaving thousands homeless (Mckiernan-González 2012, 181; Romo 2017, 234–35; Stern 1999, 45–48, 56). Race and class were embedded in the inspection enterprise at the United States–Mexico border. While "peons" were compelled to endure chemical baths, fumigation, and degrading full-body visual inspections and surveillance while bathing, well-dressed Mexicans were treated like first-class passenger ship travelers: they were inspected privately and were allowed to skip the delousing baths (Fairchild 2003, 129–31). Colonial medicine at the Mexican border was not required at the Canadian border or at Ellis Island (Fairchild 2003, 63–74, 86–94, 144–50; Kraut 1994, 50–77), though physicians at seaports had the authority to inspect immigrants fully naked, if warranted.[4] This class-based healthcare occurred on the mainland and in Puerto Rico, where paying customers accessed private care.

The government's imperial public health in El Paso spurred massive protest. Incensed by the intrusive germ eradication measures, and furious upon hearing rumors that pictures of naked women adorned local cantinas, Carmelita Torres, a 17-year-old "auburn-haired Amazon" who resided in Ciudad Juárez and worked in El Paso, led an army of several thousand women in a riot on the Rio Grande bridge. They destroyed a streetcar and vehicles crossing into Juárez. With bottles and stones, the women laid low the US immigration inspectors and soldiers, and assaulted the men crossing the bridge. When the feared Mexican cavalry arrived with sabers drawn, the women jeered and forced the troops off the bridge (Mckiernan-González 2012, 183–89; Romo 2017, 225). In 1917, an immigration official noted the anger generated by the degrading quarantine measures: "the lower classes of Mexicans are very resentful of any treatment which would tend to reflect discredit on their habits of personal hygiene, and they not infrequently employ very abusive language" to the inspectors (Fairchild 2003, 156). Although there were only three typhus deaths (all in El Paso) along the entire borderline and there were no significant outbreaks of typhus or smallpox through the 1930s, the PHS refused to lift the quarantine (Mckiernan-González 2012, 240; Stern 1999, 47–49).

Despite the Public Health Service's determination to install Ellis Island-style inspection at every land port on the southern border, budgetary constraints resulted in understaffed gateways and a reliance on part-time local doctors. Outside of El Paso, the border was mostly unpoliced and medical examinations haphazard. After World War I, xenophobic sentiments led many in the United States to bombard federal officials with allegations of lax implementation of immigration law on the US–Mexico line.[5] In November 1923, immigration agents at the southern ports of entry received a memorandum asking if immigration laws, particularly the literacy test and medical inspections, were enforced.[6] Five archived reports from California, Arizona, and Texas present a snapshot of immigration processing. All the respondents claimed full compliance, "as is possible with the limited force [of manpower] available."[7] Three reports from Arizona reveal the inner workings of the machinery. The inspector in Nogales cogently describes the doctor's role in policing the borderlands: "Every alien [while clothed] is inspected from head to foot and special attention is paid to the examination of the eyes" and skin. Physicians probed to detect symptoms of venereal, heart, and lung disease. Medical personnel vaccinated those without a recent smallpox scar and "aliens of the immoral classes" submitted to an examination to detect venereal diseases. The doctors also inspected or treated immigrants at the county jail.[8] Private practice physicians in Douglas served as instruments of empire by following Ellis Island's ritualized procedures, looking for "loathsome or dangerous contagious diseases" for inadmissibility. Examiners, claimed the report's author, observed entrants as they walked and looked "for visible and at times invisible disabilities, defects or diseases" and dispensed smallpox vaccinations.[9]

With the nation's only land quarantine station, El Paso's class-based inspection system epitomized Latino/a colonial care in the twentieth century. El Paso's six-page report reveals how the facility's procedures had evolved since 1916. All first-class (upper-class) train travelers bypassed the quarantine humiliation and received cursory medical inspections onboard. Immigration agents waived the literacy test as a curtesy to avoid delay and disrespect for Mexican professionals and high-ranking officials. Upper-class pedestrians also received expedited processing in the first-class inspection room or the physician's private office. In contrast, second-class (steerage) train travelers disembarked and crossed the bridge with pedestrians into the hands of the PHS. Non-Mexican immigrants were not deloused or fumigated. They proceeded to rooms on the ground floor for inspection, presumably because they did not harbor typhus. Meanwhile, working-class Mexicans entered the quarantine chamber for delousing, fumigation, and vaccines before being physically examined in the basement. Following stereotypes of the era, medical practitioners did not inspect the eyes of Mexicans unless a suspicion arose. Doctors made inquiry of suspected disability in their office. Immigrants also took the literacy test.[10] These five reports demonstrate how eugenicists attempted to replicate Ellis Island–style inspection at the United States–Mexico border, along with typhus quarantine in El Paso solely for Mexicans.

The typhus scare had a lasting impact on the US national consciousness. It implanted the idea that dirty, louse-ridden Mexicans threatened public health. This image was incorporated into eugenicist arguments that defined Mexicans as biologically inferior and culturally unassimilable "Indians." These ideas coalesced into the catch-all term the "Mexican Problem," which referred to low naturalization rates, perceived criminality, feeble-minded and diseased bodies, laziness, refusal to learn English, and unwillingness to Americanize (Abel 2007, 68; González 2004, 71–102, 128–152). The medics at the El Paso port of entry used a variety of insecticides, including Zyklon B, to disinfect bodies and clothing in the building's "gas chamber."[11] The chemicalization of brown, migrant bodies continued during the Bracero Program (1942–1964), when 3.5 million seasonal Mexican male laborers experienced even more sickening fumigation processes than those established in 1916. At ports of entry, gas mask-wearing workers sprayed DDT on long lines of naked braceros, a dehumanizing experience akin to spraying rows of crops. The foul agent made the braceros run away and cough or vomit (Molina 2011, 1027–28; Romo 2017, 223, 237–43). Braceros later recounted the trauma and humiliation of the delousing program (Romo 2017, 237, 240; Stern 1999, 68–69). Despite protests, congressional hearings, and negative publicity, the chemicalization of field workers continues to this day (Nash 2006, 127–208).

### Los Angeles 1924 Plague Quarantine

Because healthcare officials racialized Mexican bodies and associated them with disease and bad parenting, it became especially easy to blame Mexicans for a bubonic plague epidemic in 1924 that killed thirty-one Mexicans, a White priest, and an ambulance driver (Molina 2006, 88). The Los Angeles plague outbreak was the United States' last epidemic of the twentieth century. After an autopsy revealed the black death, alarmed city leaders ordered drastic measures. The city quarantined five Mexican neighborhoods within sight of downtown. For two weeks, four hundred guards watched 2,500 people while doctors and nurses went house to house identifying victims. Lacking a cure, doctors treated the patients with different chemicals to see if anything proved effective. A squadron of rodent killers in military formation went street by street poisoning, trapping, and shooting rats, creating a mountain of rats that was placed on display (Deverell 2004, 176–95). Medical officials dusted off the tropical quarantine playbook from Hawai'i's 1900 bubonic plague eradication, where health officials burned 4,000 homes in Honolulu's Chinatown (Shah 2001, 128). In Los Angeles, the second wave of public health sanitation consisted of fumigating with mercurochrome or tearing down 10,000 structures. After vanquishing the epidemic, officials tagged 2,500 homes as a public nuisance, which permitted the city to burn or tear them down and not provide compensation. The city refused to allow lot owners to rebuild, rendering thousands homeless in a barrio cleansing resembling the one in El Paso during the 1916 typhus quarantine (Deverell 2004, 195–99).

Chastened by the plague epidemic, Los Angeles County conducted health studies. In 1925 and 1926, local reports associated the Mexican population with high incidents of tuberculosis, which required costly treatment; a state report in 1930 upheld these findings (Abel 2003, 823–26, 838). Los Angeles invested heavily in medical infrastructure. Before 1927, the county operated only nine health centers, most of which were located in company towns servicing Mexican workers and their families. After 1927, new health centers treated residents and recently arrived indigents. Outpatient nursing services augmented the medical facilities. Despite the improved healthcare, patients roundly complained about the scarcity of doctors and the underwhelming care (Abel 2007, 50–55, 69). Local newspapers ran stories pathologizing Mexicans as impoverished, ignorant, unclean, and overly fecund. In terms of family health, medical workers pushed a narrative where these women were deficient parents (Molina 2006, 69–71, 77–78).

**Eugenics and Reproductive Sterilization, 1920s–1930s**

In the 1920s, militarized tropical healthcare on the southern borderlands evolved into a neo-Malthusian eugenics movement of population control, which held that only contraception—and particularly compelled sterilization—could ensure that current and future generations would have access to needed natural resources. A prominent neo-Malthusian believed "from the eugenical point of view the sterilization of the woman is more important than" a vasectomy or castration of males (Kline 2001, 71). The campaign of medical biological engineering fit within the contours of invasive medicalization of colonials. According to Alexandra Stern (1999), intrusive medicine was "a far-reaching cultural and scientific formation pivotal to United States imperialism and nation-building in the early twentieth century" (50). Beginning with Indiana in 1907, thirty-two states legalized involuntary medical sterilization in mental institutions, prisons, and hospitals, a practice that resulted in at least 63,841 operations (Largent 2008, 72, 80). California's pursuit of biological fitness made it a national pacesetter in non-elective eugenic sterilization. Its 1909 sterilization law allowed doctors to sterilize more people than any other state; one-third of all US sterilizations occurred there (Stern 2005, 82–114), and the state's Mexican population faced the eugenicist scalpel in greater numbers than their percentage of the overall population. The files also show the ways the patients and their families resisted fertility termination. California's projects of forced sterilization of Mexicans show how eugenics and medicalization were not related to healthcare; rather, they represented a strategic objective of medical population erasure (Lira and Stern 2014). Nationally prominent eugenicists held important public and educational positions in the Golden State (Stern 2005, 82–149). They corresponded with German eugenicists, who passed a eugenics law in 1933 modeled after that of California. Thus, Germany's Final Solution of ridding humanity of "degenerates" and Jews was rooted in California's eugenics law and US inventions of lethal chemical gases (Kline 2001, 103–04).

The eugenics movement shifted American policy from assimilation to immigration restriction by fueling anti-immigration legislation to reduce the proportion of "unfit" foreigners contaminating the nation's genetic pool. After Congress passed the 1924 law setting national immigration quotas, critics began agitating to put Mexico on the quota list (Montoya 2020). The expense of caring for tubercular indigent Mexicans provided additional ammunition to oppose unchecked immigration. David Starr Jordan, a former president and chancellor of Stanford University, was a fervent eugenicist and anti-imperialist who lobbied for immigration restrictions on Mexico. In 1925, Jordan wrote to Charles Davenport, the founder of the Eugenics Records Office in Cold Harbor, New York, and the American Eugenics Society: "The Mexicans have brought with them bubonic plague, small pox, and typhus fever," he fumed. Although Jordan admitted that none of these contagious pathogens had harmed White Californians, he speculated they kept winter tourists from visiting Los Angeles (Stern 1999, 75).

After Congress rejected putting Mexico on the quota list in 1928 (Montoya 2020), California eugenicists expressed outrage. C. M. Goethe (1929), the wealthy founder of the Eugenics Society of Northern California, published "The Influx of Mexican Amerinds" in the national magazine *Eugenics*. He described why Mexican "peons" were unfit and should be excluded from the United States. He disparaged the brown "coolies" who were mostly racial "hybrids," or, worse, full-blooded "Indian" (a racial category used to exclude from naturalization). The eugenicist further alleged that brown, polluted bodies were a sanitation "menace," because they were "contagion carrier[s]" afflicted with typhus fever, pneumonic plague, amoebic dysentery, venereal disease, and alcoholism (6–9). Goethe (1929) finished by proclaiming that Mexicans were addicted to public relief, a frequent critique that foreshadowed the justification for large-scale deportations and coerced repatriations during the Great Depression, when the simple act of accessing public charity for food or medical assistance could get Mexican immigrants—and even their US-born children—deported (Abel 2003, 841–49; Molina 2006, 133–41).

Following the Great Depression, stereotypes of Mexicans as diseased and unhygienic were employed to show that they could not assimilate. School officials used racialized health concerns to justify school segregation (McCormick and Ayala 2007, 22). Grassroots activism and litigation finally succeeded in desegregating schools in the Southwest (Flores 2014, 209–285), but it took more than two decades to compel general compliance (García 2018, 100–161). Clearly, the "Mexican Problem" persisted in the US Southwest; discourses of healthcare and eugenics sat at the heart of these debates. Negative stereotypes about Mexicans provided a context for social scientists and social workers to theorize why Puerto Ricans failed to assimilate. Observers concluded that the "Puerto Rican Problem" was a "culture of poverty" (Whalen 2001, 194–206).

## Puerto Rican Colonial Care and Population Control, 1899–1970s

### Hookworm

Immediately after the United States acquired Puerto Rico, imperial physicians instituted smallpox vaccinations. Despite resistance, in three months, the army inoculated 790,000 residents (Trujillo-Pagán 2013a, 75, 77). The military government discovered anemia was the primary cause of death and doctors speculated that a lack of meat in the diet was responsible. Curious about why patients were chronically lethargic, army surgeon Baily K. Ashford conducted a study and found worms in feces under a microscope. He speculated that these parasites caused hookworm—a common malady in the tropics—when feces came in contact with the skin. His theory sent shock waves through the imperial bureaucracy, challenging racial typologies of subaltern peoples as inherently lazy and diseased (Trujillo-Pagán 2013b). Ashford's parasite field research mimicked European colonial medicine across the globe (Cueto 1996; Farley 1991; Haynes 2001; Palmer 2010; Wilkinson 2000). When Ashford and his Puerto Rican doctor allies advocated for rural sanitation, the military ignored the appeals because anemia did not threaten occupying forces.

Rural health became a priority with the transfer to civilian governance in 1900. Puerto Rican elites were devoted to a scientific program of modernization for economic development, and healthy rural peasants were central to that objective. The insular government funded Ashford's team of American and Puerto Rican physicians to open rural clinics and to train local doctors to detect hookworm. In time, Puerto Rico opened anemia testing centers and built latrines that dramatically reduced hookworm and anemia (Trujillo-Pagán 2013b). Since medical school–trained physicians only practiced in the large towns, the insular government set up the School for Tropical Medicine to train Puerto Rican doctors, who were not educated or certified in an accredited medical school (Trujillo-Pagán 2013a, 63, 69–101). As late as the 1940s, many towns did not have a doctor and only 65 out of 852 physicians had accredited medical school training. In 1949, the government opened a medical school (Córdova 2017, 43–44).

The desire to eradicate hookworm to improve health and economic activity mirrored the actions taken to wipe out bubonic plague in the San Juan slums in 1912. Similar to cases in El Paso and Los Angeles, authorities focused on rat eradication and the destruction of Afro-Puerto Rican homes (Zulawski 2018). The medical modernization of the laboring classes laid the foundation for family planning in the 1920s, which targeted the fertility of mothers, whose perceived excessive fecundity threatened the island's economic well-being. By the 1920s, the island had the basic medical structure to manage its healthcare needs. Urbanites with money accessed private physicians and hospitals, while small towns and rural spaces relied on country doctors and outpatient clinics that focused on hookworm. This medical regime functioned in the same way as the unequal medical care for the working poor and indigent in Los Angeles. In the 1920s and 1930s, healthcare on the island veered in a new direction as socialists, feminists, and the medical profession embraced neo-Malthusian eugenics to curb population growth.

Puerto Rican administrators, doctors, and nurses initially followed the lead of Latin American nations and subscribed to neo-Lamarckian eugenics ideas about preventive medicine, which focused on eliminating environmental factors dangerous to human health. Positive eugenics, however, came under assault by Americans who advocated for racial hygiene as the solution for social and economic ills. US mainland intervention in Puerto Rico viewed Latino/a bodies as dangerous breeding grounds that threatened the health and wealth of the colony. After establishing an international movement to limit population growth, neo-Malthusians joined influential health and population-control foundations such as the Carnegie Institution, the Rockefeller Foundation, the Council on Foreign Relations, and the

Population Council to promote fertility control.[12] Neo-Malthusians published journals and books, and organized international eugenics conferences (Rosemblatt 2018, 60–87; Schell 2010, 479–81; Stepan 1991; Tone 2001, 215). Wealthy fertility reduction activists began birth-control research on poor people around the world as test subjects. Puerto Rican elites embraced an agenda of US-based modernization, falling under the sway of negative eugenics to curb procreation. Population control began in Puerto Rico in the 1920s and gathered steam in the 1930s when the island became a laboratory for temporary and permanent birth-control experiments.

**Contraceptives, 1920s–1930s**

Neo-Malthusian eugenics became a political issue in 1920 when Puerto Rican socialists endorsed birth control to reduce overpopulation, which, they claimed, sapped economic vitality and caused poverty, crime, and disease. Puerto Rican socialists and many elites believed that the working poor were ignorant, oversexed victims of poverty and of a conservativism rooted in patriarchal Catholicism. Socialists demanded decriminalization of contraceptives and elective surgical sterilization as a solution to overbreeding (Briggs 2002, 89–93; Ramírez de Arellano and Seipp 1983, 16–29).

Cultural issues on the mainland strongly influenced Puerto Rico. During the Great Depression, neo-Malthusians branched out from sterilizing the unfit in state institutions to demanding birth control for the unfit in the general population (Klausen and Bashford 2010). At the same time, racial betterment advocates shored up the White, middle-class family with marriage counseling and encouraged procreation (Stern 2005, 150–181). The positive eugenics program for the promotion of better health for fit women and children led to a family planning movement that permitted women to use contraceptives under a doctor's care and sterilization for health reasons. Although society in general opposed artificial birth control, New Deal programs laid the groundwork for government agencies, private industry, and nonprofits to build the medical welfare state. Private care physicians distributed contraceptives to the poor, and health officials established state and county family planning programs (Kline 2001, 124–156). Birth-control leaders such as Margaret Sanger, an unabashed eugenicist (Ordover 2003, 137–58) used poverty and family planning arguments to target poor, undereducated, and marginalized rural women to use non-surgical contraceptives supplied by Sanger's birth-control allies. When the American Eugenics Society, a prominent eugenicist organization, approved Margaret Sanger's agenda in 1933, Puerto Rico became a petri dish for birth-control human trials (Klausen and Bashford 2010, 101–02).

Puerto Rican leaders crafted a program mixing positive and negative eugenics to improve the standard of living. The program implemented neo-Lamarckian public health initiatives: an infant and children milk feeding program, school nurses to combat tuberculosis, dental clinics, and home nursing (Briggs 2002, 101–02). Puerto Rican social workers and nurses, arguing from a feminist nationalist perspective, advocated for birth control to cultivate healthy nuclear families, "to link maternalism, the state, and social advancement" (Briggs 2002, 94). The government sprinkled New Deal funding into a short-term program to open 160 rural birth-control clinics (Briggs 2002, 123; Ramírez de Arellano and Seipp 1983, 37–44).

Sensing an opportunity to expand his birth-control experiments beyond the US mainland, Clarence Gamble, a wealthy graduate of Harvard Medical School, set up shop in Puerto Rico in impoverished and working-class neighborhoods in 1936. Prior to arriving on the island, Gamble worked with pharmaceutical companies to develop inexpensive and easy-to-use contraceptives that he tested on low-income rural women in the US South (Schoen 2005, 21–74).[13] A condescending elitist, Gamble circulated among the imperialist medical school cadre who viewed racialized bodies as biologically inferior test subjects. Among the numerous examples, for instance, physicians tested bubonic plague vaccines on prisoners in India (Shah 2001, 126) and a cholera vaccine on Filipino prisoners where thirteen died (Anderson 2007, 16). In Puerto Rico, for three years, Gamble's staff distributed diaphragms, creams, spermicidal powder, and jellies, but they did not warn the participants of potential side effects. Gamble claimed that, although diaphragms were highly effective, working-class Puerto Rican women lacked the intelligence and commitment to use them correctly. Against the suggestions of his staff, Gamble pushed simple contraceptives, which resulted in many pregnancies (Briggs 2002, 102–04, 107; Ramírez de Arellano and Seipp 1983, 45–48). The unreliability of Gamble's simple contraceptives led public health officials and women to support sterilization; his privately funded medical experiments launched decades of research using female islanders in clinical trials.

### Female Reproductive Sterilization, 1930s–1970s

Island leaders turned Gamble's clinical trials into public health policy, but with a surgical twist. In 1937, the legislature passed three eugenics laws. One permitted the dissemination and use of contraceptives, another authorized maternal health and birth control—including elective sterilization. This sterilization law went further than state laws. It permitted surgeons practicing outside of prisons and asylums to perform asexualization procedures.

As a result, hospitals became centers of on-demand neo-Malthusian eugenics. The third eugenic law permitted involuntary sterilization under the Eugenics Board, which approved forty-eight asexualizations (Briggs 2002, 80–81, 107; Ramírez de Arellano and Seipp 1983, 49–51). Neo-Malthusianism sparked furious opposition. The Puerto Rican Nationalist Party criticized the birth-control experiments, charging that Americans intended to eliminate the island's people within a generation (Briggs 2002, 76). The Catholic Church also opposed artificial birth control. Supporters of the law initiated a test case and a court upheld the legislation in 1939. Funding from the Social Security Act that same year provided funds for birth control on the island. On the continent it was illegal to use public money for birth control, but the insular government maneuvered around this restriction decades before their state-side counterparts (Briggs 2002, 80–81; Ramírez de Arellano and Seipp 1983, 52–55).

By the late 1940s, dire social conditions in Puerto Rico convinced US-based population-control groups to pressure the island's leaders to reduce pregnancies (Briggs 2002, 109–12, 118–121; Mass 1976, 36–40; Ramírez de Arellano and Seipp 1983, 93–104). Most of the population lived in rural settings with limited access to medical care, education, and indoor plumbing. One-third never attended school; one-third did not advance past the fourth grade. Mothers had 6 to 7 children and one-fourth of the children died before reaching their teens. Of these, 40 percent did not have indoor running water; only 11 percent had refrigerators; 20 percent had no latrines, and only 20 percent had a toilet (Córdova 2017, 32). Faced with these challenges, leaders engaged in social and economic reengineering (Briggs 2002, 112–15).

With contraceptives dispensed in clinics and sterilization conducted in hospitals (Briggs 2002, 150; Ramírez de Arellano and Seipp 1983, 134–142), nurses and doctors held tremendous power over undereducated and low income women, whom they encouraged, coerced, or tricked into undergoing sterilization. Puerto Rico was perhaps the only place in the world where surgical sterilization became the primary method of birth control, with 37.4 percent of the female population (mostly voluntarily) undergoing the procedure (Schell 2010, 483–84). The island's women embraced sterilization because it was a permanent method, yet they remained interested in contraceptive clinical trials.

During the 1950s and 1960s, the Puerto Rican elite's modernization program did not result in an economic miracle, but it did facilitate a dramatic improvement in public health. Almost all the islanders had running water, life expectancy rose ten years over the 1940s, and the number of physicians almost tripled. Mortality rates dropped 50 percent. By the early 1970s, 70 percent had toilets (Córdova 2017, 32). While medical standards about human testing on the continent did not apply on the island, it was difficult to find reputable funding sources for contraceptive research. Clinicians thus forged alliances with wealthy population-control patrons and pharmaceutical companies to run large-scale clinical trials (Briggs 2002, 123–125; Mass 1976, 96). These products proved ineffective, but surveys revealed that women's use of contraceptives rose from 34 percent in 1939 to 74 percent in 1968 (Briggs 2002, 122).

## Female Oral Contraceptive Research, 1950s

Once mainland physicians established Puerto Rico as a site for unregulated procreation testing, researchers came calling. In 1956, Gregory Pincus, a reproductive chemist, initiated an unprecedented clinical trial in Puerto Rico to develop a commercial female oral contraceptive. After being denied tenure at Harvard for conducting unethical experiments, Pincus opened a private research laboratory focused on infertility. His research attracted the attention of birth-control activist Margaret Sanger, who encouraged him to develop an oral contraceptive. The birth-control philanthropist Katherine McCormick funded his research and clinical trials. G. D. Searle, a pharmaceutical company, was another of Pincus's early sponsors (Marks 2001, 34–35, 53–57; Ramírez de Arellano and Seipp 1983, 105–113). Sensitive to accusations of engaging in contraceptive research, pharmaceutical companies quietly supplied maverick scientists like Pincus with the needed material for testing. After small studies on the mainland, including a coerced trial on fifteen psychiatric patients in a Massachusetts hospital, Pincus needed a large clinical trial; because he could not conduct large-scale trials in the United States, he turned to colonial care (Marks 1998, 222, 227–33; Tone 2001, 204–20). The medical profession's continued reliance on women of color for human subject research well into the twentieth century reveals how the legacy of eugenics and colonial medicalization shaped the practice and trajectory of Western medicine even after World War II. Researchers did not formulate safety guidelines for human subject experimental drug testing, and clinical efficacy trials remained unregulated until 1962, two years after the pill's approval. The island was the perfect test site. Just off the US coast, it had sixty-seven birth-control clinics with experienced staff, women were in an island "cage," and there were no laws against human contraceptive experiments. Pincus hired two American nursing administrators already working in Puerto Rico to recruit volunteers and oversee the clinical work (Briggs 2002, 129–39; Marks 1998, 233–40; Ramírez de Arellano and Seipp 1983, 108–20; Tone 2001, 220–23).

Desiring reliable, easy, and inexpensive birth control, working-class women enthusiastically volunteered for the trials (Tone 2001, 222–24). The clinicians did not inform participants of potential side effects, which had caused significant limb deformities in the offspring of pregnant women in a different trial (Briggs 2002, 131–32). In the first round of tests, many women reported headaches, dizziness, vomiting, and nausea and the same symptoms plus mid-cycle bleeding in the second round. The side effects were so severe that half the participants withdrew, and Pincus struggled to recruit replacements. The clinicians tabulated the side effects and Pincus adjusted the tablet compound accordingly. Disturbed clinicians expressed deep reservations to Pincus about possible side effects, including the potential for reproductive cancers, but the researcher dismissed their objections. Reports of sickened women elicited outrage in local newspapers and from Catholic priests. The critics forced the on-site director to resign and leave the island (Briggs 2002, 136–39; Ramírez de Arellano and Seipp 1983, 114–20). Pincus's research resulted in the development of a female oral contraceptive, approved by the Federal Drug Administration in 1960. Searle Co. marketed "the pill" as Enovid (Junod and Marks 2002, 124–45; Tone 2001, 225–31).

Pincus's miracle drug turbocharged contraceptive studies in Puerto Rico (Ramírez de Arellano and Seipp 1983, 121–23, 133). In the 1960s, the US federal government embraced neo-Malthusian eugenics when it subsidized sterilization and contraceptives as part of its family planning and anti-poverty programs (Ramírez de Arellano and Seipp 1983, 160–72).

The medical and pharmaceutical industry's reliance on Puerto Rican women for human subject testing reveals how this important medical advancement derived from grotesque violations of subaltern bodies. Beginning in the 1970s, pharmaceutical companies and doctors aggressively pushed dangerous experimental contraceptives on women of color around the world (Ordover 2003, 179–94). This unsavory chapter in contraceptive research—which many laud as a major development in liberating women—must factor into the triumphalist narrative. Puerto Rican leaders encouraged the American clinical trials, and medical researchers ignored or downplayed the collateral damage inflicted on women as an acceptable price for economic vitality and human advancement in the same way imperial physicians implemented colonial medicine along the United States–Mexico borderlands.

The sterilization of Puerto Rican women is complicated by the desire of women for the procedure (Briggs 2002, 153–155; Mass 1976, 94–95, 104). On the mainland in the 1960s and 1970s, however, evidence of widespread coerciveness of asexualization took place in hospitals that routinely sterilized minority women without their knowledge and even when they refused to consent (Nelson 2003, 65–76; Silliman et al. 2004). In New York City, Puerto Ricans were twice as likely to be sterilized as Black women, and seven times more than White people (Nelson 2003, 126). In the late 1960s and 1970s, Puerto Rican, Black, and Native American nationalists rose up against this medieval abuse, facing off against White liberal feminists, doctors, and family planners, eventually forcing an end to the coerced population control in 1978 (Kluchin 2009, 184–213; Nelson 2003, 133–45; O'Sullivan 2016). In 1975, Latinas in Los Angeles who had been sterilized without their permission or were pressured for their consent while in labor filed a class-action suit against hospital administrators (see Dalton's chapter in this book). After Latino/as protested, California legislators put an end to coerced sterilization, but occasional cases of nonconsensual sterilization continued to emerge (Gutiérrez 2008, 35–54, 94–108).

## Conclusion

US colonial tropical medicine had a direct impact on Mexican and Puerto Rican healthcare. Elite physicians departed from the racially and class-segregated mainland to the empire's colonies and returned with new ideas of disease, medical treatment, public health, sanitation, and racial fitness. In the metropole, these experiences meshed with eugenicist theories and fears of overpopulation to discipline colonized bodies. Doctors came to practice colonial medicine on impoverished, poorly educated, marginalized Latino/as. The similarities between Latino/a public health on the mainland and on the island starts with substandard care. Mexican immigrant bodies were violated by abusive inspections and sprayed with delousing poisons, while Puerto Rican women endured mass asexualization and dangerous oral contraceptive clinical trials. US medics were the common denominator in all these instances. The case studies described above reveal how government officials, philanthropists, medical professionals, and social workers enacted public and personal health policies driven by fear of alleged Latino/a working-class cultural and biological deficiencies. Elitists criticized Latino/as for personal hygiene, supposedly unhealthy diets, excessive fertility, poor parenting, and their unsanitary living conditions. These stereotypes, rooted in beliefs of racial, class, and cultural superiority, sought to limit procreation and impose colonial medicine on a population with limited resources.

The convergence of medical science and eugenics found its expression in the cleansing of supposedly germ-carrying Mexican immigrants and Puerto Rican islanders to discipline colonial bodies for industrial labor.

Neo-Malthusian eugenicists used racial hygiene to normalize female sexual reproduction sterilization in Puerto Rico. Medical researchers collaborated with transnational pharmaceutical companies to test birth-control products using healthy Puerto Rican females as human subjects in dangerous and unethical clinical trials that they could not conduct on the mainland (Marks 2001, 89–115). Medical researchers who experimented with subaltern bodies cloaked themselves with the greater-good argument: risking the lives and health of colonials served a higher medical purpose. Scholars who agree with the greater-good argument tend to downplay the invasive nature of the contraceptive clinical trials and coercive asexualization of impoverished and racialized women (Marks 2001, 106–15; May 2010, 7–8, 17–34; Schoen 2005, 30). Although Latino/as resisted colonial care, they frequently had to accept harsh treatment because of their marginalized status. Interpreting Mexican and Puerto Rican healthcare through the prism of medical colonization presents a unique perspective on how the United States incorporated these subjugated populations.

## Notes

1. This essay uses the term Latino/a to refer to all persons of Latin American descent in the United States. The term Mexicans refers to both Mexican citizens and Mexican Americans in the United States.

2. US officials trained subjugated elites to inscribe Western medicine on colonials throughout the empire (Choy 2003).

3. Nayan Shah (2001, 120–157) traces how physicians stigmatized Chinese immigrants as the principal vectors of bubonic plague in San Francisco from 1900 to 1904 despite evidence linking the spread to rats.

4. Asian immigrants at Angel Island experienced quarantine measures on par with their Mexican counterparts (Shah 2001, 179–203).

5. James J. Davis, Memorandum for the Bureau of Immigration, November 17, 1923, file 0614, roll 3, Records Group 85, Records of the Immigration and Naturalization Service Series A, Subject Correspondence Files pt. 2: Mexican Immigration 1906–1930, National Archives and Records Administration (Bethesda, MD: University Publications of America, 1993), hereafter NARA.

6. Assistant Commissioner General to Inspector in Charge, November 30, 1923, file 0611, roll 3, NARA.

7. Inspector in Charge, Los Angeles, Calif., to Commissioner-General of Immigration, December 12, 1923, file 0609–0610, roll 3, NARA. The memorandum from California is the only one that did not describe its procedures.

8. Acting Inspector in Charge, Nogales, Ariz., to The Supervisor, December 12, 1923, file 0599–0601, roll 3, NARA.

9. Inspector in Charge, Douglas, Ariz., to Supervisor, December 8, 1923, file 0593–

0596, roll 3, NARA; see also the report from Naco, Ariz., December 8, 1923, file 0597–0598, roll 3, NARA.

10. Inspector in Charge, El Paso, Texas to Supervisor, December 13, 1923, file 0587–0592, roll 3, NARA.

11. This gas chamber served as inspiration for Nazi Germany in its own projects of border security and, later, in its concentration camps and death camps (Romo 2017, 240–43).

12. Revealing the link between imperial medicalization of Mexican immigrants and birth control, Claude Pierce, the architect of the El Paso quarantine station, and the former medical director of the Public Health Service, left the PHS in 1942 to become the medical director of Margaret Sanger's Planned Parenthood Federation of America. See "Dr. C. C. Pierce Accepts Post," *New York Times*, March 12, 1942.

13. Gamble managed his clinical trials like the Public Health Service's infamous Tuskegee syphilis experiments on African Americans (Jones 1993).

## References

Abel, Emily K. 2007. *Tuberculosis and the Politics of Exclusion: A History of Public Health and Migration to Los Angeles.* New Brunswick: Rutgers University Press.

———. 2003. "From Exclusion to Expulsion: Mexicans and Tuberculosis Control in Los Angeles, 1914–1940." *Bulletin of the History of Medicine* 77 (4): 823–49.

Ahuja, Neel. 2016. *Bioinsecurities: Disease Interventions, Empire, and the Government of Species.* Durham, NC: Duke University Press.

Anderson, Warwick. 2006. *Colonial Pathologies: American Tropical Medicine, Race, and Hygiene in the Philippines.* Durham, NC: Duke University Press.

———. 2007. "Immunization and Hygiene in the Colonial Philippines," *Journal of the History of Medicine and Allied Sciences* 62 (1): 1–20.

Baynton, Douglas C. 2016. *Defectives in the Land: Disability and Immigration in the Age of Eugenics.* Chicago: University of Chicago Press.

Benton-Cohen, Katherine. 2018. *Inventing the Immigration Problem: The Dillingham Commission and Its Legacy.* Cambridge: Harvard University Press.

Black, Edwin. 2003. *War against the Weak: Eugenics and America's Campaign to Create a Master Race.* New York: Four Walls Eight Windows.

Briggs, Laura. 2002. *Reproducing Empire: Race, Sex, Science, and U.S. Imperialism in Puerto Rico.* Berkeley: University of California Press.

Choy, Catherine C. 2003. *Empire of Care: Nursing and Migration in Filipino American History.* Durham, NC: Duke University Press.

Córdova, Isabel M. 2017. *Pushing in Silence: Modernizing Puerto Rico and the Medicalization of Childbirth.* Austin: University of Texas Press.

Cueto, Marcos. 1996. "Tropical Medicine and Bacteriology in Boston and Peru: Studies of Carrión's Disease in the early Twentieth Century." *Medical History* 40: 344–64.

Curtin, Philip D. 1989. *Death by Migration: Europe's Encounter with the Tropical World in the Nineteenth Century.* Cambridge: Cambridge University Press.

Deverell, William. 2004. *Whitewashed Adobe: The Rise of Los Angeles and the Remaking of its Mexican Past*. Berkeley: University of California Press.

"Dr. C. C. Pierce Accepts Post." 1942. *New York Times*, March 12.

Erman, Sam. 2019. *Almost Citizens: Puerto Rico, the U.S. Constitution, and Empire*. Cambridge: Cambridge University Press.

Espinosa, Mariola. 2009. *Epidemic Invasions: Yellow Fever and the Limits of Cuban Independence, 1878–1930*. Chicago: University of Chicago Press.

Fairchild, Amy L. 2003. *Science at the Borders: Immigrant Medical Inspection and the Shaping of the Modern Industrial Labor Force*. Baltimore, MD: Johns Hopkins University Press.

Farley, John. 1991. *Bilharzia: A History of Imperial Tropical Medicine*. Cambridge: Cambridge University Press.

Flores, Ruben. 2014. *Backroads Pragmatists: Mexico's Melting Pot and Civil Rights in the United States*. Philadelphia, PA: University of Pennsylvania Press.

García, David G. 2018. *Strategies of Segregation: Race, Residence, and the Struggle for Educational Equality*. Berkeley: University of California Press.

Goethe, C. M. 1929. "The Influx of Mexican Amerinds." *Eugenics: A Journal of Race Betterment* 2(1): 6–9.

González, Gilbert G. 2004. *Culture of Empire: American Writers, Mexico, and Mexican Immigrants, 1880–1930*. Austin: University of Texas.

Gratton, Brian, and Emily Merchant. 2013. "Immigration, Repatriation, and Deportation: The Mexican-Origin Population in the United States, 1920–1950," *International Migration Review* 47 (4): 944–75.

Gutiérrez, Elena R. 2008. *Fertile Matters: The Politics of Mexican-Origin Women's Reproduction*. Austin: University of Texas Press.

Hattori, Ann P. 2004. *Colonial Dis-Ease: U.S. Navy Health Policies and the Chamorros of Guam, 1898–1941*. Honolulu: University of Hawai'i Press.

Haynes, Douglas M. 2001. *Imperial Medicine: Patrick Manson and the Conquest of Tropical Disease*. Philadelphia: University of Pennsylvania Press.

Hernández, Kelly L. 2014. "Hoboes in Heaven: Race, Incarceration, and the Rise of Los Angeles, 1880–1910." *Pacific Historical Review* 83 (3): 410–47.

———. 2010. *Migra! A History of the U.S. Border Patrol*. Berkeley: University of California Press.

Jones, James H. 1993. *Bad Blood: The Tuskegee Syphilis Experiment*. Revised Edition. New York: The Free Press.

Junod, Suzanne W., and Laura Marks. 2002. "Women's Trials: The Approval of the First Oral Contraceptive Pill in the United States and Great Britain," *Journal of the History of Medicine and Allied Sciences* 57 (2): 117–60.

Kevles, Daniel J. 1985. *In the Name of Eugenics: Genetics and the Uses of Human Heredity*. New York: Alfred A. Knopf.

Klausen, Susanne, and Alison Bashford. 2010. "Fertility Control: Eugenics, Neo-Malthusianism, and Feminism." In *The Oxford Handbook of the History of Eugenics*, edited by Alison Bashford and Philippa Levine, 98–115. Oxford: Oxford University Press.

Kline, Wendy. 2001. *Building a Better Race: Gender, Sexuality, and Eugenics from the Turn of the Century to the Baby Boom*. Berkeley: University of California Press.

Kluchin, Rebecca M. 2009. *Fit to Be Tied: Sterilization and Reproductive Rights in America, 1950–1980*. New Brunswick, NJ: Rutgers University Press.
Kraut, Alan M. 1994. *Silent Travelers: Germs, Genes, and the "Immigrant Menace."* Baltimore: Johns Hopkins University Press.
Largent, Mark A. 2008. *Breeding Contempt: The History of Coerced Sterilization in the United States* New Brunswick, NJ: Rutgers University Press.
Lewthwaite, Stephanie. 2009. *Race, Place, and Reform in Mexican Los Angeles: A Transnational Perspective, 1890–1940*. Tucson: University of Arizona Press.
Lira, Natalie, and Alexandra M. Stern. 2014. "Mexican Americans and Eugenic Sterilization: Resisting Reproductive Injustice in California, 1920–1950." *Aztlán* 39 (2): 9–34.
Madley, Benjamin. 2016. *An American Genocide: The United States and the California Indian Catastrophe, 1846–1873*. New Haven, CT: Yale University Press.
Marks, Lara. 1998. "A 'Cage' of Ovulating Females: The History of the Early Oral Contraceptive Pill Clinical Trials, 1950–1959." In *Molecularizing Biology and Medicine: New Practices and Alliances, 1910s–1970s*, edited by Soraya de Chadarevian and Harmke Kamminga, 221–47. Amsterdam: Harwood Academic Publishers.
Marks, Lara V. 2001. *Sexual Chemistry: A History of the Contraceptive Pill*. New Haven, CT: Yale University Press.
Mass, Bonnie. 1976. *Population Target: The Political Economy of Population Control in Latin America*. Toronto: Latin American Working Group.
May, Elaine T. 2010. *America and the Pill: A History of Promise, Peril, and Liberation*. New York: Basic Books.
McCormick, Jennifer, and César J. Ayala. 2007. "Felícita 'La Prieta' Méndez (1916–1998) and the End of Latino School Segregation in California." *Centro Journal* 19 (2): 12–35.
Mckiernan-González, John. 2012. *Fevered Measures: Public Health and Race at the Texas-Mexico Border, 1848–1942*. Durham, NC: Duke University Press.
Molina, Natalia. 2011. "Borders, Laborers, and Racialized Medicalization: Mexican Immigration and US Public Health Practices in the 20th Century." *American Journal of Public Health* 101 (6): 1024–31.
———. 2006. *Fit to Be Citizens? Public Health and Race in Los Angeles, 1879–1939*. Berkeley: University of California.
Montoya, Benjamin C. 2020. *Risking Immeasurable Harm: Immigration Restriction and US-Mexican Diplomatic Relations, 1924–1932*. Lincoln: University of Nebraska Press.
Nash, Linda. 2006. *Inescapable Ecologies: A History of Environment, Disease, and Knowledge*. Berkeley: University of California Press.
Nelson, Jennifer. 2003. *Women of Color and the Reproductive Rights Movement*. New York: New York University Press.
O'Sullivan, Meg D. 2016. "Informing Red Power and Transforming the Second Wave: Native American Women and the Struggle Against Coerced Sterilization in the 1970s." *Women's History Review* 25 (6): 965–82.
Ordover, Nancy. 2003. *American Eugenics: Race, Queer Anatomy, and the Science of Nationalism*. Minneapolis: University of Minnesota Press.
Palmer, Steven. 2010. *Launching Global Health: The Caribbean Odyssey of the Rockefeller Foundation*. Ann Arbor: University of Michigan Press.

Pfaelzer, Jean. 2007. *Driven Out: The Forgotten War against Chinese Americans.* New York: Random House.
Pierce, C. C. 1917. "Combating Typhus Fever on the Mexican Border." *Public Health Reports* 32 (12): 426–29.
———. 1916. "Typhus Fever: Prevention and Control." *Texas State Journal of Medicine* 12 (4): 182–83.
Pierce, Claude C. 1904. "Sanitary Report of Panama and Vicinity." *Public Health Reports* 19 (8): 273–80.
Ramírez de Arellano, Annette B., and Conrad Seipp. 1983. *Colonialism, Catholicism, and Contraception: A History of Birth Control in Puerto Rico.* Chapel Hill: University of North Carolina Press.
Romo, David D. 2017. *Ringside Seat to a Revolution: An Underground Cultural History of El Paso and Juárez: 1893–1923.* El Paso: Cinco Puntos Press.
Rosemblatt, Karin A. 2018. *The Science and Politics of Race in Mexico and the United States, 1910–1950.* Chapel Hill: University of North Carolina Press.
Rothman, Sheila M. 1993. "Seek and Hide: Public Health Departments and Persons with Tuberculosis, 1890–1940." *The Journal of Law, Medicine & Ethics* 21 (3–4): 289–95.
Sánchez, George J. 1993. *Becoming Mexican American: Ethnicity, Culture, and Identity in Chicano Los Angeles, 1900–1945.* Oxford: Oxford University Press.
Schell, Patience A. 2010. "Eugenics Policy and Practice in Cuba, Puerto Rico, and Mexico." In *The Oxford Handbook of the History of Eugenics,* edited by Alison Bashford and Philippa Levine, 477–92. Oxford: Oxford University Press.
Schoen, Johanna. 2005. *Choice & Coercion: Birth Control, Sterilization, and Abortion in Public Health and Welfare.* Chapel Hill: University of North Carolina Press.
Shah, Nayan. 2001. *Contagious Divides: Epidemics and Race in San Francisco's Chinatown.* Berkeley: University of California Press.
Silliman, Jael, Marlene G. Fried, Loretta Ross, and Elena R. Gutiérrez. 2004. *Undivided Rights: Women of Color Organize for Reproductive Justice.* Cambridge, MA: South End Press.
Sinclair, Heather M. 2016. "White Plague, Mexican Menace: Migration, Race, Class, and Gendered Contagion in El Paso, Texas, 1880–1930." *Pacific Historical Review* 85 (4): 475–505.
Stepan, Nancy L. 1991. *"The Hour of Eugenics": Race, Gender, and Nation in Latin America.* Ithaca, NY: Cornell University Press.
Stern, Alexandra M. 1999. "Buildings, Boundaries, and Blood: Medicalization and Nation-Building on the US-Mexico Border, 1910–1930." *Hispanic American Historical Review* 79 (1): 41–81.
———. 2005. *Eugenic Nation: Faults and Frontiers of Better Breeding in Modern America.* Berkeley: University of California Press.
———. 2006. "Yellow Fever Crusade: US Colonialism, Tropical Medicine, and the International Politics of Mosquito Control, 1900–1920." In *Medicine at the Border: Disease, Globalization and Security, 1850 to the Present,* edited by Alison Bashford, 41–59. London, UK: Palgrave Macmillan.
Sweet, Ernest A. 1915a. "Interstate Migration of Tuberculosis Persons: Its Bearing on the

Public Health, with Special Reference to the States of Texas and New Mexico." *Public Health Reports* 30 (15): 1059–91.

———. 1915b. "Interstate Migration of Tuberculosis Persons: Its Bearing on the Public Health, with Special Reference to the States of Texas and New Mexico." *Public Health Reports* 30 (16): 1147–73.

———. 1915c. "Interstate Migration of Tuberculosis Persons: Its Bearing on the Public Health, with Special Reference to the States of Texas and New Mexico." *Public Health Reports* 30 (17): 1225–55.

Tone, Andrea. 2001. *Devices and Desires: A History of Contraceptives in America.* New York: Hill and Wang.

Trujillo-Pagán, Nicole. 2013a. *Modern Colonization by Medical Intervention: U.S. Medicine in Puerto Rico.* Leiden: Brill.

———. 2013b. "Worms as a Hook for Colonising Puerto Rico." *Social History of Medicine* 26 (4): 611–32.

Turda, Marius. 2010. "Race, Science, and Eugenics in the Twentieth Century." In *The Oxford Handbook of the History of Eugenics,* edited by Alison Bashford and Philippa Levine, 62–79. Oxford: Oxford University Press.

Whalen, Carmen T. 2001. *From Puerto Rico to Philadelphia: Puerto Rican Workers and Postwar Economies.* Philadelphia: Temple University Press.

Wilkinson, Lise. 2000. "Burgeoning Visions of Global Public Health: The Rockefeller Foundation, The London School of Hygiene and Tropical Medicine, and the 'Hookworm Connection.'" *Studies in History and Philosophy of Biological and Biomedical Sciences* 31 (3): 397–407.

Worboys, Michael. 2000. "The Colonial World as Mission and Mandate: Leprosy and Empire, 1900–1940." *Osiris* 15 (2000): 207–18.

Zulawski, Ann. 2018. "Environment, Urbanization, and Public Health: The Bubonic Plague Epidemic of 1912 in San Juan, Puerto Rico." *Latin American Research Review* 53 (3): 500–16.

# 6

# Healthcare in the US Latinx Community

## Challenges, Disparities, and Opportunities

CHRISTOPHER D. MELLINGER

According to the 2010 US Census, the Latinx community is the largest minority population in the United States (Humes, Jones, and Ramirez 2011).[1] As a result, healthcare disparities in this community and the reasons for those disparities have often been researched by scholars, governments, and international organizations. Healthcare disparities (also called healthcare inequalities) are defined by the World Health Organization (WHO) as "avoidable inequalities in health between groups of people within countries and between countries" (WHO 2013). In the United States, disparities exist between the Latinx community and the non-Hispanic population. A 2004 report by the Centers for Disease Control and Prevention (CDC) indicated that Hispanics in the United States bore "a disproportionate burden of disease, injury, death, and disability when compared with non-Hispanic whites" (935). The report indicates higher incidence rates for heart disease, diabetes, HIV, and obesity while attributing these inequalities to socioeconomic factors, lifestyle behaviors, and access to preventive healthcare services. These discrepancies in healthcare outcomes across different racial and ethnic groups remain, despite efforts to eliminate or mitigate them by various agents, including the US Department of Health and Human Services (Chen et al. 2016; Vega, Rodríguez, and Gruskin 2009). This chapter examines challenges regularly encountered by the US Latinx community that have ultimately led to healthcare disparities and argues that language access and health literacy are key social determinants of health that must be acknowledged if discrepancies in health outcomes are to be overcome.

Redressing healthcare inequalities in the US Latinx population requires resolution to several challenges, including language services, health literacy, and access to health services. Each of these challenges will be discussed throughout this chapter along with some possible ways to address them. However, before delving into the specifics of each issue, it is important to acknowledge the diversity of the Latinx community in the United States. According to 2010 census data, there were over 50 million people in the United States who identified as Hispanic or Latino, representing a 43 percent increase from the 2000 census (Humes, Jones, and Ramirez 2011). These individuals are predominantly from Mexico, Puerto Rico, and Cuba, with smaller numbers from other countries in Central and South America. In addition, approximately three million people of Hispanic or Latino origin reported being more than one race. With so many countries of origin and a range of different racial identities, the Latinx community in the United States should not be considered or treated as a singular population, but rather one that represents many different cultures, customs, and traditions. This chapter addresses challenges at the broadest possible level faced by the diverse Latinx community, while acknowledging that some problems and solutions likely exist on a smaller scale.

The diversity seen in race and ethnic origin is also reflected in the languages spoken by the Hispanic population. For instance, 74 percent of Hispanics reported speaking a language other than English at home, with Spanish being most common despite a range of others being represented (Ryan 2013). Moreover, census data indicate that Spanish and English are used at various levels by these populations, with some people indicating high levels of proficiency in both languages, and others indicating strong proficiency in only one. The situation is further complicated by the presence of a sizable number of heritage language speakers of Spanish in the Latinx community in the United States. The term *heritage language* can take on many meanings given the complex relationship among race, ethnicity, identity, and language; however, a broad definition of the term includes a person who has a connection to a non-majority language (for a more extensive discussion, see Beaudrie and Fairclough, 2012). In many cases, this situation occurs when a person is raised speaking a language at home other than the one used in society. Language use in these communities also takes into account the context in which they are spoken, differences across different generations, and proficiency (Lynch 2012).

The demographic overview of the Latinx community in the United States is important to understand prior to discussing healthcare since these subpopulations have been shown to have different experiences accessing healthcare services. For instance, Weinick et al. (2004) analyzed data from the 1997 Medical Expenditure Panel Survey (MEPS) to understand whether specific groups use healthcare services differently in the United States. These surveys were conducted in either English or in Spanish, and comparisons were made both between demographic groups and between speakers of the two languages. The study concluded that Puerto Ricans are more likely to visit an emergency department when needed, whereas Mexican and Cuban populations are less likely to do so. While Weinick et al. (2004) are not able to determine the rationale for this difference, this observation may be linked to citizenship status or a lack of "real or perceived barriers to enrolling in public programs" (316). Discrepancies also existed between language preference; for example, English-only interviewees were more likely to have visits to outpatient clinics, emergency departments, and have access to prescription medications than Spanish-language interviewees. These examples demonstrate the interplay of language and ethnic origin and also emphasize that language must be considered when discussing the healthcare of the Latinx community in the United States.

The next sections review several of the challenges encountered by the Latinx community in relation to healthcare. First, language services that are offered to non-English-speaking patients will be presented as an initial step toward eliminating healthcare inequalities. While the ability to communicate in a preferred language is a critical step toward addressing healthcare inequalities, an important second challenge is health literacy. Information availability is not necessarily the same as an accurate understanding of the information. Therefore, healthcare disparities for the diverse Latinx community cannot be fully solved without addressing the issue of health literacy in addition to language access. The third challenge is that race, ethnicity, and language interact and pose substantial problems related to access to health services. The chapter concludes with a look toward the future and how these issues might be addressed.

## Language Access and Services

Patients who do not speak the same language as that spoken by a doctor or other healthcare provider are likely to need someone to help them navigate the healthcare system. One of the first solutions that comes to mind when someone thinks of how to help a non-English-speaking patient is a family member or friend who speaks the patient's language. However, untrained bilinguals are more likely to make mistakes that can make communication between the patient and the provider more difficult and can even result in suboptimal health outcomes for the patient (Flores et al. 2003; Flores 2005, 2006). These bilinguals are often referred to as ad hoc interpreters or language brokers, since they are performing the job of mediating between two languages without preparation or education to do so. Other ad hoc interpreters include:

> [A]n untrained person who is called upon to interpret, such as a family member interpreting for her parents, a bilingual staff member pulled away from other duties to interpret, or a self-declared bilingual in a hospital waiting-room who volunteers to interpret. Also called a *chance interpreter* or *lay interpreter.* (National Council on Interpreting in Health Care [NCIHC] 2008)

To avoid this situation, professional interpreters and translators are needed to provide language services to bridge the language and cultural gap in healthcare settings. At the most basic level, the distinction is made between *translation*—a task that is performed with written language and documents, and *interpreting*—a task involving spoken or signed language. The terms *translator* and *interpreter* refer to people who work primarily with either written or spoken/signed language, respectively, although the same person may perform both tasks, depending on skill level, education or certifications and context. While translation and interpreting are related in that they involve mediating between two languages, research on the topic shows that these skills differ and require distinct training and aptitude (Angelelli 2014, 2019). Professional interpreters are able to work in three different modes of interpreting—consecutive interpreting, simultaneous interpreting, and sight translation—and adhere to a code of ethics, understand specialized terminology, and remain an impartial party to facilitate communication (ISO 18841: 2018; Tipton and Furmanek 2016).

In the United States, approximately 25 million people (8.6 percent of the total population) speak English "less than very well" (Agency for Healthcare Research and Quality [AHRQ] 2012). That figure includes a portion of the Latinx community, because an estimated 12.5 million people who speak Spanish at home speak English "less than very well" (Castaño et al. 2007). Consequently, the need for translation and interpreting services in healthcare contexts is quite important. The Office of Minority Health in the US Department of Health and Human Services recognizes the nation's diverse population as well as the need to provide services appropriate for minority populations. As such, this office publishes the *National Standards for Culturally and Linguistically Appropriate Services (CLAS) in Health and Health Care* (*CLAS Standards*), which specifically calls for interpreting services to be provided to individuals who have limited English proficiency, along with printed materials in their languages.

Providing language services to non-English-speaking populations in the United States has been encouraged for a number of reasons, and healthcare interpreting scholars such as Roat and Crezee (2015) have identified four main lines of argument: 1) legal requirements, 2) quality of care and patient safety, 3) social justice, and 4) cost. The legal foundation for providing language assistance is found in Title VI of the Civil Rights Act of 1964, which states: "no person in the United States shall, on the ground of race, color, or national origin, be excluded from participation in, be denied benefits of, or be subjected to discrimination under any program or activity receiving federal funding assistance" (252).[2] As Roat and Crezee (2015) describe, the US Supreme Court has ruled on cases related to the provision of language services under Title VI and has affirmed these claims: "language is an inextricable aspect of country of national origin and therefore protected under Title VI" (239). There is an established consensus around the legal framework for providing language rights in healthcare (Chen, Youdelman, and Brooks 2007).

Quality of patient care is another important reason to provide language services. Even if a patient can communicate in both English and Spanish, language preference can diminish communication and understanding for limited-English proficient (LEP) individuals, and this fact contributes to healthcare disparities among the US Hispanic community. Patients who prefer speaking Spanish are less likely to receive routine medical care or have a primary healthcare provider (Pearson et al. 2008). Providing interpreting services can help overcome this potential barrier to preventive care (Jacobs et al. 2004). Therefore, language assistance not only satisfies legal requirements but can also improve patient outcomes.

In addition to the previously mentioned legal and clinical reasons, ethical and moral arguments are also made for providing language services in healthcare to members of the Latinx and other minority communities (see Jones 2010 for an extended discussion). Hilfinger Messias, McDowell, and Estrada (2009), for instance, describe how the US healthcare system "is not meeting the social justice mandate of equal and equitable access and treatment" (128). Their research, along with work by Angelelli (2004, 2019) and Hsieh (2016), illustrates how the interpreter's role is often viewed as being not only a conduit who interprets one language into another but also a cultural broker or advocate who resolves misunderstandings between speakers. Professional interpreters must be able to navigate complex situations to uphold their professional codes of ethics and avoid overstepping their professional boundaries so that patients are empowered to advocate on their own behalf. Nevertheless, these ethical questions further support the need for providing language assistance when needed.

Finally, there are financial reasons for providing language access services to LEP and non-English-speaking patients. In 2009, the Joint Center for Political and Economic Studies issued a report titled *The Economic Burden of Health Inequalities in the United States* which indicated that eliminating health disparities between 2003 and 2006 would have reduced direct medical expenses by $229.4 billion (LaVeist, Gaskin, and Richard 2009). In addition, 30.6 percent of direct medical expenses for African Americans, Asians, and Hispanics in the United States were the result of healthcare disparities. These figures illustrate how the costs for providing language assistance may ultimately result in savings if these disparities are addressed.

## Health Literacy

Language services are only the first step to resolving healthcare disparities in the US Latinx community; health literacy is another factor that causes disparities in health outcomes among minority communities. Here, the distinction needs to be made between literacy as it relates to specific language skills (i.e., reading, writing, speaking, and listening) and health literacy as the ability to understand concepts that regularly occur in healthcare. Ratzan and Parker (2000) define health literacy as "[t]he degree to which individuals have the capacity to obtain, process, and understand basic health information and services needed to make appropriate health decisions" (4). This definition shows how providing information in a particular language is not necessarily sufficient for people to be able to make informed decisions about their healthcare. Instead, individuals need to be able to comprehend the information that is provided and then act based on that information. Research has shown that monolinguals have difficulty with this task, even when working in their native language (Nutbeam 2000; Sørensen et al. 2012).

Much as variation exists within the Latinx community with regard to language use, there is also variation with regard to health literacy. In Kansas, a study on health literacy levels across a range of different communities found that members of the Hispanic community demonstrated a range of literacy (Chesser et al. 2016). Similar variation has been reported among the Latino community in California (Sentell and Braun 2012). This finding is not surprising, insofar as the US Latinx community is a diverse population that has a wide range of education levels. Nevertheless, overall health literacy levels are still relatively low compared to non-Hispanic communities, and the national average among Hispanics is lower than other groups in the United States (Showstack et al. 2019).

The link between health literacy and health outcomes among the Latinx community has been established by a number of empirical studies. Sentell and Braun (2012), for instance, find that LEP groups and those who had lower health literacy were at a higher risk for poorer health outcomes than groups with higher health literacy. Showstack et al. (2019) also find that LEP and low health literacy Latino patients may also be more prone to medical errors or to receive inadequate guidance. The findings of these studies suggest that the US Latinx community faces challenges when navigating the healthcare system not only in terms of their language use or preference but also in relation to health literacy rates.

To address these challenges, some healthcare providers are turning to technology as a potential solution. Chaet et al. (2016) offer a systematic review of consumer health information technology that was targeted toward the Spanish-speaking community. Many of these solutions aimed to present information about specific conditions but did not necessarily take into account diverse subpopulations of the Latinx community, such as the country of origin, different ethnic groups, or gender. The content included in these health information technologies is also not always tailored to the culture and subpopulations of the Latinx communities in the United States. As a result, efforts still need to be increased and additional solutions explored to better serve these communities.

## Access to Health Services

While language services and improved health literacy are two important steps toward decreasing healthcare disparities in the Latinx community, greater access to health services is necessary if these are to be fully addressed. As mentioned previously, the *CLAS Standards* call for language services to be provided to improve access to health services. These standards, however, extend beyond language services, with the principal aim of providing "effective, equitable, understandable, and respectful quality care and services that are responsive to diverse cultural health beliefs and practices, preferred languages, health literacy, and other communication needs" (*CLAS Standards*). Therefore, quality of care and services are directly linked to how responsive healthcare providers are to these many needs. For instance, the standards call for diverse hiring practices and continuing education for healthcare providers, staff, and leadership. In addition, healthcare entities ought to develop language access plans and allocate resources to make it possible to achieve culturally and linguistically appropriate services.

Despite the growing commitment to implementing these standards, studies show that policy and practice must be regularly reviewed to ensure disparities are being addressed. Non-English-speaking and LEP patients may face difficulty receiving the same quality of care, even when language services are provided (Pearson et al. 2008). For example, LEP patients in intensive care units have been shown to have longer stays, receive less comfort care, and receive fewer palliative care consultations (Barwise et al. 2018). Interpreters who work in these settings echo these concerns, suggesting that healthcare providers can change their approach to working with these patients to improve end-of-life quality (Norris et al. 2005).

Still larger systemic issues stymie efforts of the US Latinx community to access healthcare services. For instance, this population is less likely to have medical insurance (Flores and Lin 2013; Vega, Rodríguez, and Gruskin 2009). With ever-increasing costs for healthcare in the United States, a lack of health insurance can create a significant financial burden for patients, ultimately leading patients to avoid seeking medical attention unless absolutely necessary (Derose et al. 2009). When coupled with challenges that face the US Latinx community to obtain health insurance, medical treatment can be cost prohibitive.[3]

Bias in clinical settings is another issue that impacts access to health services and can manifest in the very documents that healthcare providers use to treat patients. For instance, a patient's medical record contains a range of information about their health, medications, and previous treatment, as well as more general information such as number of relatives and languages spoken. These records are vital to help physicians learn more about a person's previous care, particularly when they may not have been the healthcare provider who treated them previously. However, the way in which medical professionals describe their patients in the medical record potentially influences how others may view the patient. A recent experiment demonstrated that stigmatizing language in a medical record can cause medical professionals to have a more negative attitude toward the patient and can lead to less aggressive attempts to manage patient discomfort or pain (Goddu et al. 2018). Consequently, continued efforts are required to identify potential sources of implicit bias that may increase the likelihood of healthcare disparities among minority populations.

## Moving Forward: Challenges and Opportunities

The previous sections have discussed several of the challenges surrounding healthcare in the United States for the Latinx community; however, efforts are being made to improve the current situation. The *CLAS Standards* provide guidance on how to provide services that are appropriate for different cultures and in different languages. The CDC also describes how interpreters are a way for providers to help decrease barriers to healthcare. The provision of interpreters not only helps facilitate communication but is also a cost-effective means to decrease barriers to healthcare (Jacobs et al. 2004).

It is important to consider how these language services are provided to ensure they are effective. Three important steps for providing these services are 1) identifying who needs these services, 2) working with professional interpreters, and 3) choosing the communication modality (Karliner 2017). As noted earlier, the Latinx community is diverse, with different countries of origin, education levels, and language preferences. Language services should not be assumed to be necessary for every member of this population. An initial step to identifying who needs services might be taken by providers asking whether a patient prefers to use a language other than English or whether they would like the services of an interpreter (Karliner 2017). Working with professional interpreters is particularly important, given the training and experience needed to provide high-quality language services. Professional organizations in the United States, such as the National Council on Interpreting in Healthcare and the International Medical Interpreters Association, provide guidance on how to find professional interpreters and also support certification for a number of languages.

The communication modality—that is, whether the interpreter will be present physically or be accessible virtually by phone or video—also impacts communication between patient and provider. In some cases, remote interpreting is the only way to provide interpreting services or may be more cost effective; however, these remote services may make the job of the interpreter more difficult (Braun 2015; Karliner 2017). In addition, patients may be less likely to disclose information when working with a remote interpreter and may not be as satisfied with the services provided (Schwei, Rhodes, and Jacobs 2017). These choices need to be carefully considered when implementing the *CLAS Standards* to help ensure the best possible health outcomes and reduce the health disparities of minority communities in the United States.

Although there are challenges that are faced by the Latinx community with respect to healthcare in the United States, progress is being made as new legal requirements and policy guidelines are being written and implemented throughout the country. Interpreters and translators serve as a means by which non-English-speaking and LEP patients are able to access healthcare in a number of settings, while efforts are being made to improve accessibility of health information via translation and content originally written in Spanish. Larger systemic issues related to insurance and bias continue to be a challenge faced by the Latinx community, yet greater consciousness of these issues can help to address these situations. It remains crucial that support for language access and health literacy continue to grow in order to redress current healthcare disparities.

## Notes

1. In this chapter, the term *Latinx* will be used where possible to refer to the population in the United States that is Spanish-speaking or of Latin American descent, while being inclusive of a range of genders, ideologies, and perspectives (see Aldama and González 2018). The terms *Hispanic* and *Latino* are also used, in large part, interchangeably; however, these terms have different meanings. *Hispanic* is often a reference to being of Spanish-speaking descent while *Latino* refers to being a descendant of Latin American origin. When specific studies are cited, the language used in the original study has been maintained.

2. While Title VI of the Civil Rights Act of 1964 serves as the impetus for much of this discussion, subsequent cases such as *Madrigal v. Quilligan* have continued to define the obligations of hospitals and healthcare providers with respect to language services. See Dalton (chapter in this volume) for an extended discussion of this case.

3. Research conducted shows that specific barriers to accessing health insurance are numerous (e.g., full-time employment, immigration and citizenship status, legal and administrative requirements). While a full discussion lies outside the scope of the present chapter, see Alcalá et al. (2017) and Mathis et al. (2019) for more information.

## References

Agency for Healthcare Research and Quality (AHRQ). 2012. *Improving Patient Safety Systems for Patients with Limited English Proficiency: A Guide for Hospitals*. Rockville, MD: Agency for Healthcare Research and Quality.

Alcalá, Héctor E., Jie Chen, Brent A. Langellier, Dylan H. Roby, and Alexander N. Ortega. 2017. "Impact of the Affordable Care Act on Health Care Access and Utilization Among Latinos." *Journal of the American Board of Family Medicine* 30 (1): 52–62.

Aldama, Frederick Luis, and Christopher González. 2018. *Latinx Studies: The Key Concepts*. New York: Routledge.

Angelelli, Claudia V. 2004. *Medical Interpreting and Cross-cultural Communication*. New York: Cambridge University Press.

———. 2014. "Interpreting in the Healthcare Setting: Access in Cross-Linguistic Communication." In *The Routledge Handbook of Language and Health Communication*, edited by Heidi E. Hamilton and Wen-ying Sylvia Chou, 573–85. New York: Routledge.

———. 2019. *Healthcare Interpreting Explained*. New York: Routledge.

Barwise, Amelia, Carolina Jaramill, Paul Novotny, Mark L. Wieland, Charat Thongprayoon, Ognjen Gajic, and Michael E. Wilson. 2018. "Differences in Code Status and End-of-Life Decision Making in Patients with Limited English Proficiency in the Intensive Care Unit." *Mayo Clinic Proceedings* 93 (9): 1271–81.

Beaudrie, Sara M., and Marta Fairclough. 2012. "Introduction: Spanish as a Heritage Language in the United States." In *Spanish as a Heritage Language in the United States*, edited by Sara M. Beaudrie and Marta Fairclough, 1–17. Washington, DC: Georgetown University Press.

Braun, Sabine. 2015. "Remote Interpreting." In *Routledge Handbook of Interpreting*, edited by Holly Mikkelson and Renée Jourdenais, 352–67. New York: Routledge.

Castaño, M. Teresa, Joan L. Biever, Cynthia G. González, and Kathryn B. Anderson. 2007. "Challenges of Providing Mental Health Services in Spanish." *Professional Psychology: Research and Practice* 38 (6): 667–73.

Centers for Disease Control and Prevention (CDC). 2004. "Health Disparities Experienced by Hispanics–United States." *MMWR: Morbidity and Mortality Weekly Report* 53 (40): 935–37.

Chaet, Alexis V., Bijan Morshedi, Kristen J. Wells, Laura E Barnes, and Rupa Valdez. 2016. "Spanish-Language Consumer Health Information Technology Interventions: A Systematic Review." *Journal of Medical Internet Research* 18 (8): e214.

Chen, Alice Hm, Mara K. Youdelman, and Jamie Brooks. 2007. "The Legal Framework for Language Access in Healthcare Settings: Title VI and Beyond." *Journal of General Internal Medicine* 22 (Supp. 2): 362–67.

Chen, Jie, Arturo Vargas-Bustamante, Karoline Mortensen, and Alexander N. Ortega. 2016. "Racial and Ethnic Disparities in Health Care Access and Utilization under the Affordable Care Act." *Medical Care* 54 (2): 140–46.

Chesser, Amy K., Trisha V. Melhado, Robert B. Hines, and Nikki Keene Woods. 2016. "Identifying Health Literacy in Kansas Using the Behavioral Risk Factor Surveillance System (BRFSS)." *Journal of Family Medicine and Disease Prevention* 2 (2): art. 032.

*Civil Rights Act of 1964*, Public Law 88–352, 78 Stat. 241 July 2, 1964.

Derose, Kathryn Pitkin, Benjamin W. Bahney, Nicole Lurie, and José J. Escarce. 2009. "Immigrants and Health Care Access, Quality, and Cost." *Medical Care Research and Review* 66 (4): 355–408.

Flores, Glenn. 2005. "The Impact of Medical Interpreter Services on Quality of Health Care: A Systematic Review." *Medical Care Research and Review* 62 (3): 255–99.

———. 2006. "Language Barriers to Health Care in the United States." *New England Journal of Medicine* 355 (3): 229–30.

Flores, Glenn, and Hua Lin. 2013. "Trends in Racial/Ethnic Disparities in Medical and Oral Health, Access to Care, and Use of Services in US Children: Has Anything Changed Over the Years?" *International Journal for Equity in Health* 12: 10.

Flores, Glenn, M. Barton Laws, Sandra J. Mayo, Barry Zuckerman, Milagros Abreu,

Leonardo Medina, and Eric J. Hardt. 2003. "Errors in Medical Interpretation and Their Potential Clinical Consequences in Pediatric Encounters." *Pediatrics* 111: 6–14.

Goddu, Anna P., Katie J O'Conor, Sophie Lanzkron, Mustapha O. Saheed, Somnath Saha, Monica E. Peek, Carlton Haywood Jr., and Mary Catherine Beach. 2018. "Do Words Matter? Stigmatizing Language and the Transmission of Bias in the Medical Record." *Journal of General Internal Medicine* 33 (5): 685–91.

Hilfinger Messias, DeAnne K., Liz McDowell, and Robin Dawson Estrada. 2009. "Language Interpreting as Social Justice Work." *Advances in Nursing Medicine* 32 (2): 128–43.

Hsieh, Elaine. 2016. *Bilingual Health Communication: Working with Interpreters in Cross-Cultural Care*. New York: Routledge.

Humes, Karen R., Nicholas A. Jones, and Roberto R. Ramirez. 2011. *Overview of Race and Hispanic Origin: 2010*. Washington, DC: US Census Bureau.

ISO 18841. 2018. *Interpreting Services–General Requirements and Recommendations*. Geneva: International Organization for Standardization.

Jacobs, Elizabeth A., Donald S. Shepard, Jose A. Suaya, and Esta-Lee Stone. 2004. "Overcoming Language Barriers in Health Care: Costs and Benefits of Interpreter Services." *American Journal of Public Health* 94 (5): 866–69.

Jones, Cynthia M. 2010. "The Moral Problem of Health Disparities." *American Journal of Public Health* 100 (Supp. 1): S47–S51.

Karliner, Leah S. 2017. "Three Critical Steps to Enhance Delivery of Language Services in Health Care." In *Providing Health Care in the Context of Language Barriers: International Perspectives*, edited by Elizabeth A. Jacobs and Lisa C. Diamond, 20–34. Bristol, UK: Multilingual Matters.

LaVeist, Thomas A., Darrell J. Gaskin, and Patrick Richard. 2009. *The Economic Burden of Health Inequalities in the United States*. Washington, DC: Joint Center for Political and Economic Studies.

Lynch, Andrew. 2012. "Key Concepts for Theorizing Spanish as a Heritage Language." In *Spanish as a Heritage Language in the United States*, edited by Sara M. Beaudrie and Marta Fairclough, 79–97. Washington, DC: Georgetown University Press.

Mathis, Arlesia L., Matthew Dutton, Ivette A. López, Alan Becker, and C. Perry Brown. 2019. "After Implementation of the ACA—Coverage Gaps among Rural Latinos Still Remain." *Florida Public Health Review* 16: 64–70.

National Council on Interpreting in Health Care (NCIHC). 2008. *The Terminology of Health Care Interpreting*. NCIHC. www.ncihc.org/assets/documents/NCIHC%20Terms%20Final080408.pdf.

*National Standards for Culturally and Linguistically Appropriate Services (CLAS) in Health and Health Care*. (n.d.). U.S. Department of Health and Human Services Office of Minority Health. minorityhealth.hhs.gov/omh/browse.aspx?lvl=2&lvlid=53.

Norris, Wendi M., Marjorie D. Wenrich, Elizabeth L. Nielsen, Patsy D. Treece, J. Carey Jackson, and J. Randall Curtis. 2005. "Communication about End-of-Life Care Between Language-Discordant Patients and Clinicians: Insights from Medical Interpreters." *Journal of Palliative Medicine* 8 (5): 1016–24.

Nutbeam, Don. 2000. "Health Literacy as a Public Health Goal: A Challenge for Contemporary Health Education and Communication Strategies into the 21st Century." *Health Promotion International* 15 (3): 259–67.

Pearson, William S., Indu B. Ahluwalia, Earl S. Ford, and Ali H. Mokdad. 2008. "Language Preferences as a Predictor of Access to and use of Healthcare services among Hispanics in the United States." *Ethnicity & Disease* 18: 93–97.

Ratzan, Scott C., and Ruth M. Parker. 2000. "Introduction." In *National Library of Medicine Current Bibliographies in Medicine: Health Literacy*, edited by Catherine R. Selden, Marcia Zorn, Scott Ratzan, and Ruth M Parker. Bethesda, MD: National Institutes of Health.

Roat, Cynthia E., and Ineke H.M. Crezee. 2015. "Healthcare Interpreting." In *The Routledge Handbook of Interpreting*, edited by Holly Mikkelson and Renée Jourdenais, 236–53. New York: Routledge.

Ryan, Camille L. 2013. *Language Use in the United States: 2011: American Community Survey Reports* Vol. ACS-22. Washington, DC: US Census Bureau.

Schwei, Rebecca, Mary Rhodes, and Elizabeth A. Jacobs. 2017. "Understanding the Advantages and Disadvantages of the Diversity of Approaches to Overcoming Language Barriers in Medical Encounters." In *Providing Health Care in the Context of Language Barriers: International Perspectives*, edited by Elizabeth A. Jacobs and Lisa C. Diamond, 93–101. Bristol, UK: Multilingual Matters.

Sentell, Tetine, and Kathryn L. Braun. 2012. "Low Health Literacy, Limited English Proficiency, and Health Status in Asians, Latinos, and Other Racial/Ethnic Groups in California." *Journal of Health Communication* 17 (3): 82–99.

Showstack, Rachel E., Kelly Guzman, Amy K. Chesser, and Nikki Keene Woods. 2019. "Improving Latino Health Equity Through Spanish Language Interpreter Advocacy in Kansas." *Hispanic Health Care International* (171): 18–22.

Sørensen, Kristen, Stephan Van den Broucke, James Fullam, Gerardine Doyle, Jürgen Pelikan, Zofia Slonska, and Helmut Brand, for (HLS-EU) Consortium Health Literacy Project European. 2012. "Health Literacy and Public Health: A Systematic Review and Integration of Definitions and Models." *BMC Public Health* 12: art. 80.

Tipton, Rebecca, and Olgierda Furmanek. 2016. *Dialogue Interpreting*. New York: Routledge.

Vega, William A., Michael A. Rodríguez, and Elisabeth Gruskin. 2009. "Health Disparities in the Latino Population." *Epidemiologic Reviews* 31: 99–112.

Weinick, Robin M, Elizabeth A. Jacobs, Lisa Cacari Stone, Alexander N. Ortega, and Helen Burstin. 2004. "Hispanic Healthcare Disparities: Challenging the Myth of a Monolithic Hispanic Population." *Medical Care* 42 (4): 313–20.

World Health Organization (WHO). 2013. "Social Determinants of Health: Key Concepts." www.who.int/social_determinants/thecommission/finalreport/key_concepts/en/ Last accessed 16 May 2021.

# 7

# Eugenics and Doubly Marginalized Mexican and Chicana Women

Forced Sterilizations in Renee Tajima-Peña's
*No más bebés/No More Babies*

David S. Dalton

Renee Tajima-Peña's documentary *No más bebés/No More Babies* (2015) tells the story of numerous women of Mexican descent who were sterilized against their will while giving birth at the Los Angeles County-University of Southern California Medical Center during the 1960s and 1970s.[1] Hospital workers coerced women to sign permission forms for tubal ligation under duress—many patients were as many as eight centimeters dilated. Given that doctors performed this procedure in especially large numbers on women who did not speak English, many have suspected that the hospital operated on people without fully explaining what the procedure entailed. The documentary discusses the court case *Madrigal v. Quilligan*, which came about when several Mexican, Mexican-American, and Chicana women sued the hospital after learning that they had undergone nonconsensual tubal ligation. The hospital won this particular case, but the film suggests that this had less to do with justice and more with a host of issues that ultimately suppressed these women's voices. Despite the court decision, for example, *Madrigal v. Quilligan* spurred legislative changes that forced medical institutions to reevaluate their treatment of linguistic-minority patients (Manian 2018, 7). Tajima-Peña's documentary offers a counter history of sorts that recreates the political and legal dialogue surrounding the case. The director interviews numerous key figures, including Dr. Edward J. Quilligan—the man who oversaw hospital operations during the years in question—as well as a host of activists and women who underwent the sterilization procedures. What emerges is a tale of Mexican and Chicana women who learned that the local hospital was sterilizing them, but, given their double marginality as women and Latinas, they lacked support from both Chicano and Feminist activists because their interests did not comfortably align with those of either movement's agenda. In this documentary, Tajima-Peña denounces the conditions that allowed these sterilizations to occur in order to ensure that this never happens again.

The director takes advantage of the documentary mode to engage questions—and evidence—that may not be admissible in court. In this way, she seeks a form of societal justice that the legal system failed to deliver. Recent scholarship in many fields has discussed the role of media (film, literature, theatre) in achieving surrogate justice where the legal system itself cannot. William Acree (2006), for example, argues that media productions "can function as a purveyor of justice, as a space where trials take place, and as a means to come to terms" (42); this holds particularly true in those cases where the law has failed to punish unjust acts. Documentaries like *No More Babies* cannot create a legal substitute for previous rulings; rather, they allow for a degree of social closure—and even healing—as previously suppressed histories come to light. When we view the documentary through this lens, it becomes clear that, while Tajima-Peña cannot overturn Judge Jesse Curtis's decision not to hold the hospital liable, she can provide a clearer picture of the circumstances that made such a ruling possible. She also gives the victims of forced sterilization a platform from which to air their grievances. One of its most disconcerting characteristics is that, while the documentary focuses on a single event, it speaks to a broad historical referent in both California and the United States where eugenic practices operated within, and informed, state and federal laws (Manian 2018, 1–3; Rodríguez-Trías 1978, 10–12).

At its core, eugenics presupposes that certain people enjoy genetic traits and characteristics that make them superior to others (Paul 1995, 2). While scientists and humanists have now resoundingly discredited it, eugenics was seen as a scientifically rigorous, legitimate field of study until the mid-twentieth century. Colonizing powers from the West justified their position of relative privilege in global politics through Herbert Spencer's (1851) concept of social Darwinism and "survival of the fittest," which problematically conflated political dominance with biological superiority. Feelings of white supremacy, coupled with a "nativist impulse" (Gutiérrez and Fuentes 2009–2010, 90), sat at the heart of the coerced sterilization of Mexican and Chicana women in California. Rebecca M. Kluchin (2007) alludes to this fact when she argues that, in the Los Angeles sterilization cases, "race and ethnicity intersected with poverty to highlight social anxieties" (133).

The forced sterilizations reflected a drive to control California's growing Latino/a/x population.[2] Eugenics has long intersected with healthcare—or the lack thereof—in the United States (and beyond),[3] particularly as it relates to minority or marginal communities (Gutiérrez and Fuentes 2010). Tajima-Peña emphasizes that anti-Mexican and anti-immigrant attitudes within Southern California played a key role in shaping the attitudes necessary for a sterilization project to thrive. That said, what stands out in this particular case is that it occurred after the successes of the civil rights movement and a series of Supreme Court cases that had set a precedent against state-sponsored eugenics. As such, the County Clinic had to carry out its population-control program without explicitly invoking eugenics.

The legal machinations that made it possible to target Mexican and Chicana women for sterilization came from bipartisan consensus about the importance of expanding access to birth control. This reflected the shared goals of feminists and The Association for Voluntary Sterilization, a group that focused primarily on combating overpopulation through sterilization (Enoch 2005, 8). According to Alexandra Minna Stern (2005), eugenics during this time ceased to be merely the practice of curtailing "defective heredity" and became more focused on making population sizes manageable (1129–32). *Madrigal v. Quilligan* represented a tectonic shift in how Californians and Americans in general conceived of eugenics. Politicians and well-known philanthropists ranging from John D. Rockefeller III—father of the Democratic Senator John D. Rockefeller IV—to the Republican Richard Nixon had previously spoken about the benefits of family planning, contraception, and even sterilization.[4] While politicians invoked notions of empowerment, the documentary also explains that they gave grants to hospitals like the Los Angeles County Clinic so that they could lower the birthrate in their jurisdictions. *Madrigal v. Quilligan* thus underscored the tension inherent to a program focused on providing contraception to poor and minority women. When not handled carefully, these projects came to look a lot like social engineering. Medical providers absolutely can empower their patients if they provide adequate counseling for them to make decisions for themselves, but their actions become eugenic when they fail (deliberately or not) to explain the long-term ramifications of the procedure. *No More Babies* does not challenge the validity of concerns about overpopulation nor does it say that doctors should not assist poor women in seeking access to birth control. Rather, Tajima-Peña insists that individual women must be able to choose how many children they will have. In practice, the tubal ligations at the County Clinic were surgeries that (mostly white) doctors and nurses imposed on women of color.

The debates surrounding the legality of the sterilizations at the County Clinic revolved around whether or not they had occurred with women's consent. Because the hospitals had the necessary documents and signatures to show that their patients had, indeed, agreed to these procedures, it was difficult to find any smoking gun. Nevertheless, the records also showed that nurses and doctors had repeatedly requested permission to perform tubal ligations. This fact, coupled with the knowledge that medical personnel had made these requests while the women were under duress, made for a strong case that the policy had employed eugenic protocols. Indeed, an interview with Carlos Vélez-Ibáñez, an anthropologist and expert witness in the case, suggests that the hospital's defense ultimately centered not on whether or not the hospital had coerced women into accepting sterilizations but on an ethnographic argument that claimed that these medics could not know how harmful their actions would be on women from Mexican and Chicano/a/x communities. The professor emphatically states in the documentary that the hospital's lawyers twisted his words in order to exonerate the clinic. That being so, the film questions the morality of the court's decision by emphasizing its dependence on a misreading of legal testimonies. Tajima-Peña thus questions the ability of existing laws to fairly adjudicate cases of forced sterilization; indeed, the Latina plaintiffs found themselves at a legal disadvantage from the beginning. Beyond establishing the flawed reasoning that formalized the decision to side with the hospital, Tajima-Peña also lands a high-profile interview with Quilligan. Nearly forty years after the trial, the former director maintains that his facility always operated legally and ethically. Nevertheless, the documentary's retrial of the case plays by a different set of rules than does the courtroom; as such, it encourages its spectators to reevaluate Quilligan's claims.

The documentary has already prepared us for this interview by questioning the validity of the court's decision and by helping viewers to distinguish between what is legally permissible and what is morally correct. Tajima-Peña's editing challenges Quilligan's claims that his hospital acted ethically. The former hospital director asserts that a whistleblower, Dr. Bernard Rosenfeld, fed false allegations to lawyers, journalists, and policymakers. When pressed as to why anyone would have wanted to do this, Quilligan responds that he does not pretend to understand Rosenfeld's motivation. The director then cuts to Rosenfeld, who provides page after page of documented cases of suspicious sterilizations. Rosenfeld claims that the nurses and doctors would request permission every time they checked an incipient mother's cervix. Manian (2018) notes the insidious nature of these requests when she explains that healthcare providers often insinuated that they would not deliver the baby until the mother agreed to being sterilized (1). As Rosenfeld provides this information, he reiterates that he revealed the practices of his hospital because he believed that it had betrayed the trust of its patients. Tajima-Peña's juxtaposition of voices serves to discredit Quilligan and vindicate Rosenfeld. Furthermore, it underscores the documentary's thesis that the public at large cannot blindly trust health officials to advocate for the well-being of their patients. Rather, the people and the government must hold healthcare actors in check, especially if there are allegations of abuse. This belief leads to another critique that lies at the heart of *No More Babies*: beyond dealing with a clinic whose predatory sterilization policies constituted eugenics, Tajima-Peña also charges that neither the government nor activist groups were there to provide assistance and legal resources to women who were at risk of forced sterilization.

## Divisions within the Left: The Intersectional Interests of Mexican and Chicana Women

The movie emphasizes the fact that governments and the people themselves must work together to oversee healthcare providers and ensure that they provide needed care without depriving patients of their agency. One of the reasons that the sterilizations at the County Clinic continued for so long was that the victims were doubly marginalized along both gender and racial/ ethnic lines. They attempted to build alliances among Chicano and feminist activists, but their healthcare aims did not line up with those of their Chicano counterparts or their white feminist counterparts. That neither of the aforementioned groups incorporated the complaints of these victims into their platform emphasizes the fact that both were willing to sacrifice the needs of women of color for other, supposedly more pressing, issues within their respective movements. Indeed, the demands of the victims of the County Clinic often ran contrary to the goals of both the Chicano and especially the Feminist movements at large. Chicana women thus not only had to contend with eugenicist ideals that targeted them because of their race; they also had to navigate their subordinate position within both of the aforementioned movements due to their gender (the Chicano movement) and ethnicity (the Feminist movement).

The Chicano movement's lack of interest in the problem of forced sterilization presents perhaps the biggest puzzle. It certainly reflected the whims of a male-dominated movement whose priorities lay outside the realm of reproductive rights. Tajima-Peña includes several interviews with Gloria Molina, a woman who served as president of the Comisión Femenil Mexicana

Nacional—a Mexican-American women's organization that advocated for Chicana women when others would not—during the 1970s and 1980s. She explains: "when we raised these issues [of forced sterilization] to our brothers in the Chicano Movement, it was always considered a secondary issue." Chicano activists believed that the guarantee of female reproductive rights would not ensure gains in other spheres that they deemed more important. Tajima-Peña instructs us otherwise through her camerawork. Indeed, Molina's words take on a degree of irony as the director crosscuts between her interlocutor and borrowed footage of Chicano rallies in which male activists drew large crowds consisting of both Chicanos and Chicanas. In ignoring the needs of its women, then, the Chicano movement marginalized one of its most important demographics. The Chicana theorist Gloria Anzaldúa (1987) engages the fraught relationship between Chicanos and Chicanas directly in her writing when she says, "from the men of our race, we demand the admission/acknowledgment/disclosure/testimony that they wound us, violate us, are afraid of us and of our power. We need them to say they will begin to eliminate their hurtful put-down ways" (83–84). Her words resonate especially poignantly in the case of the forced sterilizations in Los Angeles County, where Chicano activists were missing in action.

Interestingly enough, healthcare sat at the heart of the Chicano movement of the 1970s and 1980s, but activists focused on working conditions for farmworkers rather than reproductive health for urban Chicanas. The fact that activists favored certain types of healthcare over others alludes to the peripheral role afforded to women—particularly those who lived in cities—within the movement at large. The focus on health in agricultural communities reflected the fact that the very nature of farm labor forced Chicano/a/x and Mexican workers of both genders to expose themselves to harmful chemicals. Nevertheless, the film also charges that, in ignoring the cases of forced sterilization, the movement ultimately turned its back on its women. Beyond testifying about the fissures between Chicano men and Chicana women, the film also makes room for reconciliation. On the one hand, it tells of women who suffered years of abuse and failed marriages after their sterilizations led their spouses and partners to view them as barren and thus worthless. On the other hand, it shows many women who finally tell their loved ones—many of whom are male—of the procedure that they suffered years earlier. The resulting conversations unanimously allow for a reconciliation across gender lines as men express support for the women in their lives. While perhaps a bit didactic, these conversations communicate the idea that Chicano men now understand that their Chicana counterparts were victims of predatory healthcare practices. That said, during the 1960s and 1970s, the divisions between men and women were such that Chicana women realized that they could not count on men to stand with them in solidarity. As such, many turned to leaders of the Feminist movement.

Once again, the sterilization victims found themselves with awkward bedfellows. At one point in the documentary, Molina explains that greater access to reproductive health was a principal aim of American feminists during those years. While white feminists certainly favored informed consent—or a "complete disclosure to a patient of the available choices and alternatives to sterilization" (McGarrah Jr. 1974, 6)—they tended to ignore how a woman's race or ethnicity could impede her ability to be properly informed (Enoch 2005, 9; *No More Babies*).[5] The incompatibility of white and Chicana experiences became obvious when the Chicanas suggested policy measures that would protect women against forced sterilization. These victims of forced sterilization claimed that medical personnel had pressured them into consenting to tubal ligation while under duress. In order to curtail such practices, they proposed a seventy-two-hour waiting period between giving consent and undergoing an operation. This met stiff opposition in feminist circles, which tended to view mandatory waiting periods as unnecessary roadblocks for women seeking reproductive healthcare. The competing interests between white feminists and women of color—feminist or not—made it difficult for them to find consensus despite the fact that they concurred that women should only be sterilized if they wanted to undergo the procedure.

While Chicana activists and victims of forced sterilizations found themselves in contention with white feminists, their disagreements tended to deal not with principle but policy. At issue was whether or not women would receive proper counseling from medical professionals. Feminist activists operated under the assumption that such professionals would act in good faith. Robert E. McGarrah Jr. (1974) emphasized that such was not the case when he observed that there had been reports of "medical staff efforts to 'sell' sterilizations to poor . . . patients" and patients of color (5). Clearly, activists across the country knew about the abuses that plagued women of color. As such, a cynic may argue that because these forced sterilizations happened mostly to poor women of color (Ladd-Taylor 2014, 193), they did not pose a threat to white feminists. Because these abuses went largely unnoticed in (white) feminist circles, legal attempts to curtail them met resistance; this, in turn, produced unintended consequences that facilitated the continued sterilization of Chicana women. The fissures between Chicanas and (white) feminists underscores the fact that any group's interests reflect a combination of factors that include both race and gender. What is good for women of one race or ethnicity may be harmful to women of another; this was especially evident regarding how women of different races viewed healthcare in the United States.

Tajima-Peña ultimately depicts the leaders of the Chicano and the Feminist movements as uninterested in the needs of Chicana women. Chicano activists focused on the rights of males to the exclusion of females, while feminist leaders focused so narrowly on reproductive rights that they looked the other way when faced with evidence that medics were selectively sterilizing women of color. As they avoided critical discussions about who could regulate birth control and sterilization, many groups inadvertently supported eugenic practices that ran directly counter to their purported agendas. This was not because they supported eugenics but because they refused to consider how their own inaction enabled such behaviors. Ultimately, women of Mexican descent had to work together in order to take their fight to the Los Angeles County-University of Southern California Medical Clinic. It is telling that the lawyer who represented the victims of forced sterilization was herself a young Chicana woman. As a member of the same demographic as her clients, she recognized both the gender-based and racial/ethnic discrimination that had enabled this practice in the first place.

In the end, Renee Tajima-Peña's *No Más Bebés/No More Babies* achieves surrogate justice through its provocative use of the documentary mode. The wide range of interviews juxtapose multiple voices and provide a platform for those women who suffered involuntary sterilizations at the hands of the doctors at the Los Angeles County-University of Southern California Medical Center. Beyond its powerful denouncement of the eugenicist logic that underpinned these acts of violence against Mexican and Chicana women, the film also condemns the relative silence of those who should have been the victims' strongest allies. Indeed, this multiplicity of criticism provides an interesting vantage point from which to theorize the efficacy of the so-called trial that the documentary carries out (Acree 2006). In the end, movies and other cultural products aim to achieve a political outcome when they put their society on trial. Tajima-Peña achieves this goal by filming certain reconciliations even as others remain elusive. For example, the film shows Chicana women and Chicano men coming together after the victims recount their experiences with the traumatizing sterilizations and how the effects of these have lingered throughout their lives. The shared embraces and kind words emphasize the shared solidarity that now exists between women and men of Mexican descent as they all come to grips with the trauma of the forced sterilizations. The film suggests that, to a lesser degree, a similar understanding has formed between white feminists and women of color. Nevertheless, Tajima-Peña provides no such opportunity for Edward J. Quilligan to absolve himself. Rather, the camera passes solemn judgment against him; even when he attempts to defend himself, Tajima Peña's editing undermines his claims. In its quest for surrogate justice, this filmic technique stretches far beyond a mere ad hominem attack. Rather, it serves to mobilize viewers and ensure that similar abuses do not happen in the future. In this way, the film's verdict, while not legally binding, attempts to leave a mark that will last well into the future. In order to ensure a more just society, all people must have access to healthcare without the fear that medical personnel will take advantage of them or discriminate against them.

## Notes

1. Throughout this chapter I refer to this medical center as the County Clinic.

2. In this chapter, I use the terms Latino/a/x and Chicano/a/x when referring to entire groups. That said, I use the term Chicano to refer specifically to men or to historically specific events like the Chicano Movement. I use the terms Latina and Chicana to refer to women.

3. See Nancy Leys Stepan (1991) for a discussion of eugenics in Latin America, for an example.

4. Indeed, Rockefeller and Nixon collaborated on the document "Population and the American Future: The Report of the Commission on Population Growth and the American Future" (1969), which viewed contraception and birth control as necessary steps to keeping the nation's population in check.

5. Benita Roth explores how women of different races created distinct forms of feminism in her book *Separate Roads to Feminism: Black, Chicana, and White Feminist Movements in America's Second Wave*.

## References

Acree, William. 2006. "The Trial of Theatre: *Fiat iustitia et pereat mundus*." *Latin American Theatre Review* 40 (1): 39–60.

Anzaldúa, Gloria. 1987. *Borderlands/La Frontera: The New Mestiza*. San Francisco: Spinsters/Aunt Lute.

The Center for Research on Population Security. 1969. *Population and the American Future: The Report of the Commission on Population Growth and the American Future*. Washington, DC.

Enoch, Jessica. 2005. "Survival Stories: Feminist Historiographic Approaches to Chicana Rhetorics of Sterilization Abuse." *Rhetoric Society Quarterly* 35 (3): 5–30.

Gutierrez, Elena R., and Liza Fuentes. 2009–2010. "Population Control by Sterilization: The Cases of Puerto Rican and Mexican-Origin Women in the United States." *Latino(a) Research Review* 7 (3): 85–100.

Kluchin, Rebecca M. 2007. "Locating the Voices of the Sterilized." *The Public Historian* 29 (3): 131–44.

Ladd-Taylor, Molly. 2014. "Contraception or Eugenics? Sterilization and 'Mental Retardation' in the 1970s and 1980s." *Canadian Bulletin of Medical History* 31 (1): 189–211.

Madrigal v. Quilligan. 1981. 639 F.2d 789, 1981 Cali. App. 9th Circuit.

Manian, Maya. 2018. "The Story of *Madrigal v. Quilligan*: Coerced Sterilization of Mexican-American Women." *University of San Francisco School of Law Research Paper No. 2018-04*: 1–15.

McGarrah, Robert E. 1974. "Voluntary Female Sterilization: Abuses, Risks, and Guidelines." *The Hastings Center Report* 4 (3): 5–7.

Paul, Diane B. 1995. *Controlling Human Heredity: 1865 to the Present*. New Jersey: Humanities Press.

Rodriguez-Trias, Helen. 1978. "Sterilization Abuse." *Women and Health* 3 (3): 10–15.

Roth, Benita. 2004. *Separate Roads to Feminism: Black, Chicana, and White Feminist Movements in America's Second Wave*. Cambridge: Cambridge University Press.

Spencer, Herbert. 1851. *Social Statistics*. London: George Woodfall and Son.

Stepan, Nancy Leys. 1991. *"The Hour of Eugenics": Race, Gender, and Nation in Latin America*. Ithaca: Cornell University Press.

Stern, Alexandra Minna. 2005. "Sterilized in the Name of Public Health: Race, Immigration, and Reproductive Control in Modern California." *Public Health Then and Now* 95 (7): 1128–38.

Tajima-Peña, Renee. 2015. *No más bebés/No More Babies*. Moon Canyon Films.

# PART III

## Healthcare in Central America and the Caribbean

# 8

## Cuba and the Cuban Healthcare System

KATHERINE HIRSCHFELD

In 1959, the government of Cuba was overthrown by a coalition of rebel groups that deposed an unpopular dictator and established a political alliance with the Soviet Union. Over the course of the next ten years, the entire Cuban economy—including the health sector—was transformed into a Soviet-style system organized by centralized planning. By the late 1960s, private medical practice in Cuba was outlawed, and healthcare was only available in government clinics and hospitals. Healthcare also became free at point of service, meaning that patients were never billed for accessing services. Many aspects of this Soviet-style system remain in place today, even as the Island has opened to foreign investment and international tourism.

Cuba was the only country in the Americas to undertake such a radical reconfiguration of its health system, and these policies fueled intense debates among scholars during the second half of the twentieth century. Sympathetic observers praised Cuba's state-run system as an effective remedy for the twin ills of poverty and inequality. Critics, including many Cuban exiles who left the Island, described various scenarios of economic ruin, political repression, and health decline resulting from the inefficiencies and irrationalities of centralized economic planning.[1] Over time, these disagreements expanded to frame larger conversations about healthcare and economic development in Latin America. Should Cuba's state-run health system be a model for the region? Or are Cuba's health improvements since 1959 a mirage maintained by political repression and falsification of health data?

This chapter presents a historical overview of health and healthcare in Cuba through the twentieth century with the goal of clarifying debates about the policies enacted after the 1959 Revolution. This longitudinal perspective is important because it establishes a more accurate starting point for making sense of health trends. Contemporary Cuban government publications, for instance, claim success by comparing the Island's "pre-revolutionary" health indicators with data from the "revolutionary" period.[2] This temporal framing, however, does not differentiate Cuba's three centuries under Spanish colonial rule from the Island's three decades as a US protectorate.

A more revealing and productive analysis of Cuban healthcare begins by exploring how Cuba's twentieth-century governments organized and maintained the public health programs put in place after the development of the germ theory of disease in the late 1800s. This improved timeline begins with an era of famine and mass mortality in the late colonial period, followed by rapid health improvements that coincided with the development of effective public health and sanitation policies.

### The Early Twentieth Century

Cuba's struggle for independence against Spain was more prolonged and destructive than in other Latin American countries. In the late 1800s, Spanish colonial officials confined entire villages of Cuban peasant farmers to concentration camps in order to cut off support for the Island's nationalist rebels. The resulting disruption in agriculture led to widespread food shortages, and lethal epidemics soon followed. Reports of mass mortality prompted US officials to send a public health officer named D. F. Brunner to monitor conditions and inspect steamships leaving Cuba so that dangerous pathogens would not spread to neighboring countries.

Once established in Havana, Dr. Brunner made regular visits to internment camps, morgues, and cemeteries so he could estimate the number of people dying every week from infectious diseases. His reports were horrific. In August 1897, he visited a concentration camp and counted 1,700 new arrivals. Three months later, he noted that 70 percent of those individuals had died, mostly of starvation.[3] He also observed epidemics of bubonic plague, malaria, dengue, typhoid, dysentery, yellow fever, and smallpox in rural and urban areas. At one point he estimated there were over three thousand malnourished people (including women and children) living on the streets of Havana.

The United States entered the war against Spain in the spring of 1898, and the conflict was resolved in just a few months. By August, Spain surrendered control of Cuba, Puerto Rico, and the Philippines to the United States, and these islands remained under US control. These events also coincided with the development of the germ theory of disease, and an aggressive set of public health and sanitation programs was put in place by US military forces stationed in Cuba and other territories under US neocolonial control between 1900 and 1910.

In 1899 the US Army created a Department of Health in Havana that included a quarantine service, an animal health service, and a street-cleaning and disinfection service. In February 1900, Dr. William Gorgas—a legendary sanitarian—was placed in control of the military's public health effort in Cuba, and he continued to intensify public health surveillance and sanitation work.[4] New orders were issued that established mandatory reporting for dangerous infectious diseases like leprosy, typhoid, smallpox, cholera, scarlet fever, and others. Once cases were identified, a military team was dispatched to implement quarantine and prevent further spread. The Army Corps of Engineers also worked to improve water systems, construct sewers, and pave dirt roads so that animal waste would no longer seep into household drinking water supplies. A military street-cleaning service was organized, and a house-to-house census was undertaken to inspect residences for mosquito breeding sites that could contribute to the spread of yellow fever, a lethal mosquito-borne disease that killed thousands of Spanish soldiers during the war.

These efforts led to rapid improvements in Cuba's health and mortality patterns. According to records published by a leading Cuban physician, the death rate in Havana declined from an all-time high of 91 per 1,000 residents in 1898 to only 16 per 1,000 in 1907.[5] This health transformation made Cuba increasingly attractive to international investors and foreign tourists in the 1910s and 1920s.

Cuba remained a US protectorate until 1933 due to the imposition of the Platt Amendment to the Cuban constitution. This legislation gave the United States the right to intervene in Cuba in the event of political instability or revolution, or if the Cuban government failed to maintain health and sanitation practices put in place by the US Army. The Platt Amendment was despised by Cuban nationalists, who saw it as a form of intrusive imperial domination that denied Cuban independence fighters control of their own country. But many Cuban health professionals remained in favor because Article Five of the Platt Amendment compelled the Cuban government to sustain the successful disease prevention programs put in place after the end of the war.

The United States did intervene in Cuban politics during the Platt era. There was a second US military occupation from 1906 to 1909, partly in response to an insurrection that threatened the stability of the government established under President Tomás Estrada Palma. US troops were deployed again in 1917 after a contentious national election led to an outbreak of violence in the eastern part of the country. Both of these insurrections interrupted public health programs and led to resurgent outbreaks of infectious diseases, including yellow fever. The United States also sent diplomatic representatives to reorganize some aspects of the Cuban government in response to allegations of graft and corruption.[6] All of these interventions increased anti-American sentiments on the Island and stoked nationalist opposition to US meddling in Cuban affairs.

## The Batista and Auténtico Eras

The Platt Amendment was finally abrogated in 1933 by President Franklin D. Roosevelt as part of his "good neighbor" policy toward Latin America. This pleased Cuban nationalists, but increased political instability on the Island. Multiple armed factions fought for control of the national government between 1933 and 1940. Cuba also developed into a lucrative offshore smuggling center for bootleg alcohol during the Prohibition years in the United States, and various international organized crime groups contributed to the violence and instability of Cuban politics. From 1932 to 1940 there were a number of bombings, insurrections, and general strikes that paralyzed transportation and commerce. More than ten different presidents cycled in and out of office in just eight years, with the shortest term of office being a single day.

All of this internal conflict and instability meant that Cuba's public health programs were repeatedly disrupted during the 1930s, and many preventable infectious diseases began to reappear. The health crisis was exacerbated by the economic crisis of the Great Depression, which led to widespread unemployment. There were newspaper reports of resurgent malaria and typhoid outbreaks during this time, but the exact scale of these epidemics is difficult to estimate since public health surveillance was also interrupted by political instability. Fortunately, an effective vaccine for yellow fever became available in the 1930s and prevented Cuba's most lethal endemic disease from re-emerging in epidemic form.

During the 1940s and 1950s political power in Cuba alternated between Fulgencio Batista (who controlled the military) and the Auténtico Party. While in power, Batista's supporters and the Auténticos used politics as a spoils system for patronage and personal enrichment. According to one journalist, an estimated US $400,000 per month was funneled to cronies in Batista's Ministry of Public Works, who did little or nothing to repair Havana's declining infrastructure (Phillips 1959a). There were also significant gaps in health and healthcare between rural and urban areas in Cuba in the

1940s and 1950s. Children in rural agricultural communities were described in one international report as afflicted by parasitic worms, lacking clean drinking water, and living in very poor-quality housing (International Bank for Reconstruction and Development Report on Cuba 1950).

All of this historical material suggests that health conditions in Cuba at the time of the 1959 Revolution were not as terrible as the current Cuban government has claimed. While there were significant rural–urban disparities in the 1950s, as well as socioeconomic and racial disparities in health and access to healthcare, Cubans did not suffer mass mortality from preventable infectious diseases after the colonial period.

### The Early Revolutionary Period

Fulgencio Batista suffered an electoral defeat in the late 1940s, then returned to power in a coup d'état in 1952. By the late 1950s, his increasingly authoritarian rule led to the formation of a powerful coalition of opposition groups. These anti-Batista activists included student leaders, labor organizers, politicians from the Auténtico Party, and pro-democracy activists from other countries in Latin America. The rebel band operating in the mountains of Eastern Cuba led by Fidel and Raúl Castro captured the most international attention, in part due to favorable media coverage in the *New York Times*. On January 1, 1959, the rebel coalition succeeded in driving Batista into permanent exile.

One of the first acts of the new Revolutionary government was to put the rebel army in charge of street cleaning and public works. A health census was conducted to identify households with mosquito breeding sites or other vector-borne disease risks, and repairs were made to municipal water and sewer systems. Ironically, these initiatives were similar to the ones organized by the US Army in the early 1900s, but the binary language and ideological oppositions of the Cold War has made these historical parallels difficult to recognize.

The new Revolutionary government also made significant investments in hospitals and health facilities. By 1963, after only four years in power, the Castro government had built over one hundred new rural health centers and approximately forty rural hospitals. Neighborhood watch organizations like the Committees for the Defense of the Revolution were also tasked with health outreach work, including registering births and deaths, epidemiological surveillance, and maternal health and education programs (Danielson 1979).

It is difficult to assess the impact of these revolutionary health policies because they coincided with increasing Soviet-style information control and criminalization of political dissent. Just a few months after Batista left Cuba, Fidel and Raúl Castro consolidated their power by arresting rivals and establishing personal control over the two most powerful organizations of the new government: the armed forces (FAR) and the Ministry of Agrarian Reform (INRA). Several months later, the Castro government issued a new decree authorizing INRA and the military to confiscate property from people engaging in "counterrevolutionary" activities (Phillips 1959b). This was several months after the *New York Times* observed: "Premier Castro bitterly criticizes anyone who opposes his policy and terms any opposition 'counter-revolutionary'" (Phillips 1959c, 6).

These authoritarian tactics forced political moderates into exile, and the Castro brothers forged a new alliance with pro-Soviet labor leaders who favored closer relations with the Soviet Union. A Soviet minister was invited to Havana and a central planning board was set up to "supervise and coordinate the economic affairs of the nation" (Phillips 1960, 1). These actions led the United States to intensify its efforts to overthrow the Castro government by supporting an invasion force that included military commanders from the Batista regime as well as former Castro allies who had originally worked to overthrow Batista. This ill-conceived force landed at the Bay of Pigs in April 1961 and was quickly defeated by the Cuban military. The threat of a second US intervention solidified Cuba's strategic alliance with the Soviet Union for the remainder of the Cold War. By 1965 the Communist Party was the only political party remaining in Cuba. In 1968 all remaining small businesses were nationalized in a final "revolutionary offensive." The healthcare system became fully controlled by the state at this time, with no remaining fee-for-service medical practitioners or independent associations of healthcare professionals.

## The Late Revolutionary Period

The time period from the late 1960s to the 1980s was characterized by ongoing expansion of hospitals and clinics and relative national prosperity as the Soviet Union provided Cuba with generous economic subsidies. Statistical health data published by Cuba's Ministry of Health (MINSAP) indicate continuous improvement in key indicators such as infant mortality and life expectancy. Leading causes of death listed in these MINSAP reports included heart disease, diabetes, and cancer, making Cuba's national health profile in the 1970s and early 1980s comparable to other industrialized countries at that time. There were no reports of malnutrition or epidemics of preventable infectious diseases.[7]

By the mid-1980s, most public health scholars and international health agencies described the Cuban healthcare system in very positive terms. Cuba was portrayed as a regional leader in public health, infectious disease control, and healthcare delivery. This reputation was further enhanced when Cuba developed a new Family Doctor program in the 1980s designed to improve primary care by integrating physicians into the communities they served. A network of neighborhood clinics with attached residences was constructed with the goal of improving patient compliance and strengthening epidemiological surveillance. Cuba also publicized a number of medical and scientific advances during these years, including development of a meningitis vaccine and several experimental treatments for degenerative diseases.

Other developments in the 1980s were more controversial and eroded international support for Cuba's health programs. Cuba was criticized, for instance, for imposing mandatory HIV testing on the entire population and denying citizens privacy regarding their HIV status (Gómez Dantés 2018). HIV positive Cubans were instead quarantined in special hospitals, even if they showed no signs of disease. Given the long latency period of the virus, this amounted to a lifelong prison sentence determined by a potentially unreliable health screening test. Gay rights activists also pointed out similarities between the Cuban government's anti-gay policies in the 1960s (which involved incarcerating gay men in forced labor camps) and the HIV quarantine policy in the 1980s.[8] There were also allegations of psychiatric abuses against political dissidents, similar to the practices observed in the Soviet Union (Brown and Lago 1992).

Cuba's controversial HIV policy softened in the 1990s, and HIV positive Cubans were eventually allowed to leave the AIDS *sanataria*. But a small number of human rights activists continued to point out ethical problems in the organization and delivery of healthcare. Family doctors, for instance, were expected to provide political reports to the Cuban government and to monitor their communities for signs of political dissent. Patients had no right to privacy in health clinics, and government officials often intruded on reproductive decision-making to keep the country's infant mortality rate artificially low (Berdine, Geloso, and Powell 2018). Cuba was also criticized for not following international protocols to guarantee patients' rights in medical research, and there were no protections against medical malpractice (Ullman and Spooner 2014). This was especially concerning since Cuba was expanding into new areas of biotechnology, pharmaceutical drug development, and vaccine trials without following international guidelines for obtaining informed consent from research subjects.

## The Post-Soviet Era

The Soviet Union collapsed in 1991, and the loss of Soviet subsidies plunged the Cuban economy into a deep economic and existential crisis. Fuel imports declined by 90 percent between 1989 and 1992. Many international observers doubted that the Castro regime could survive without Soviet support, and the United States quickly enacted punitive new trade sanctions designed to accelerate the collapse of the Castro regime. Cuba responded by declaring a "Special Period in Time of Peace," that essentially put the Cuban economy on a wartime footing, with increased rationing of consumer goods, accompanied by harsh crackdowns on public protests.

The economic crisis meant severe shortages of household essentials like soap, shampoo, laundry detergent, cooking oil, and cooking fuel for most of the 1990s. Municipal services like trash removal and street cleaning became irregular since there was not enough gasoline to power cars or trucks. Water and sewer systems broke down due to lack of spare parts. Irregular supplies of cooking fuel meant that Cubans could not boil contaminated drinking water to prevent gastrointestinal diseases. Agricultural production declined since tractors could not operate, and an epidemic of nutritional deficiency disease afflicted thousands of Cubans (New England Journal of Medicine 1995). Health clinics and pharmacies experienced widespread shortages of basic supplies like disinfectant, bandages, and aspirin. Patients' families were expected to provide sheets, towels, food, soap, and laundry service for the duration of hospital stays, an impossible economic burden given the scarcity of these items in the early 1990s. Many hospitals and clinics also relied on reusable glass syringes for injections, and sterilization equipment was often broken or unusable due to power outages.

The Cuban government responded to the economic crisis of the 1990s by enacting a series of economic reforms designed to increase hard currency reserves. A network of retail stores was opened that only accepted US dollars, and Cubans living in exile were encouraged to send remittances to support their families on the Island. These stores were operated by corporate entities controlled by the Cuban military and security services, who also operated luxury hotel chains and import-export companies in partnerships with international investors. Other Cuban military corporations opened fee-for-service health clinics and pharmacies that only accepted US dollars as payment. This created a stratified system of health services on the Island, with well-stocked clinics available for high-ranking government officials or anyone able to pay with hard currency. Cubans without these resources were left with few options for obtaining quality care or essential supplies.

All of these developments led to an array of major and minor disease outbreaks in the 1990s, including skin infections (from lack of soap), malnutrition, and gastrointestinal diseases caused by failing municipal water systems. Cuba also experienced new outbreaks of vector-borne diseases like dengue fever, which became increasingly prevalent throughout Latin America during the 1990s. Despite increasingly desperate conditions on the Island, the Cuban government continued to report improvements in population health indicators. Infant mortality declined and longevity appeared to increase, even in the worst years of the economic crisis. There was also increased authoritarian repression, including suppression of information. Despite partial privatization of some sectors of the economy, all mass media in Cuba remained controlled by the state, and these media outlets continued to reiterate the Cuban government's rigid ideology: Socialism in Cuba was declared an ongoing success, and any problems observed on the Island were attributed to US trade sanctions, counterrevolutionary saboteurs, or enemy imperialists. An epidemic of dengue fever in 1997, for instance, was described in Cuban media as an act of biological warfare by the United States, rather than a natural consequence of reduced vector control activities and failing municipal water systems.[9]

One of the unintended consequences of Cuba's increasing socioeconomic inequality in the 1990s was the development of a thriving informal economy in health supplies and health services. Many family doctors, for instance, disliked reporting on the political beliefs of their friends and neighbors and chose to engage in informal medical consultations and procedures in exchange for bartered goods. Because these transactions occurred in the informal economy, doctors and patients benefited economically and could avoid political surveillance. There was also an informal economy in pharmaceutical drugs, many of which were either sent from abroad or pilfered from Cuban hospitals and clinics to be re-sold on the black market. While these practices solved some of the problems faced by ordinary Cubans in need of medical care, they also created new health risks since there were no consumer protections for goods or services exchanged in the informal economy. The Cuban government does not publish data on the number of Cubans harmed by outdated or counterfeit medications, nor does it estimate the incidence of nosocomial infections arising from poorly sterilized hospital equipment or syringes.

Conditions in Cuba improved following the election of Hugo Chávez as President of Venezuela in 1999. Venezuela has some of the largest petroleum reserves in the world, and, as oil prices rose in the early 2000s, Chávez sent millions of barrels of subsidized oil to Cuba as a gesture of ideological solidarity. In return, Cuba sent thousands of healthcare workers to staff clinics in impoverished neighborhoods in Venezuela. Cuba also exported physicians to Brazil, Peru, Ecuador, and a number of African countries as part of a medical diplomacy program. In some ways these arrangements were altruistic, but there was also a commercial component. Cuba charged foreign governments substantial hard currency fees for this medical assistance, but doctors themselves were given only a small percentage as salaries, making healthcare workers a lucrative export commodity for the Cuban government. There were also criticisms that the export of physicians was creating new shortages in Cuba. One group of doctors recently accused the Cuban government of labor exploitation equivalent to human trafficking (Gámez Torres 2018).

Fidel Castro governed Cuba from 1959 until 2008, when he surrendered power to his brother Raúl. Under Raúl's leadership, Cuba retained a number of authoritarian features, but new policies allowed more small businesses to operate and made it easier for Cubans to leave the Island for international travel. Internet access, however, remains restricted for most Cuban citizens. A few courageous dissidents did begin challenging the state's information control through blogs and social media, even though these expressions often resulted in harassment from police and state security officials.

In 2012 one dissident journalist was jailed after accusing the Cuban government of suppressing information about deadly outbreaks of dengue and cholera in Eastern Cuba (Reporters Without Borders 2012). In 2017 Yoani Sánchez (one of the first independent Cuban bloggers to challenge the state's control of information) gave an interview at the University of Miami where she lauded the availability of primary care on the Island, but also observed that many hospitals and clinics were in a "calamitous" state of disrepair with no functional plumbing and shortages of essential supplies. She also observed that the low salaries doctors earn creates a culture of corruption that leads them to expect supplementary gifts or bribes from their patients, and that these conditions exacerbate the socioeconomic inequality on the Island (Gutierrez 2017).[10]

## The Post-Castro Era

Fidel Castro died in 2016, and his brother Raúl assumed the office of the Presidency until the spring of 2018. This time period was notable for the reopening of formal diplomatic relations between the United States and Cuba, and a state visit by President Obama. Unfortunately, these relations quickly became strained when reports emerged of US diplomatic personnel suffering unexplained "health attacks" in their residences while stationed in Cuba. Many US diplomatic personnel were recalled as a result, and recreational travel from the United States has declined. The punitive US trade embargo also remains in place.

In April 2018 Cuba experienced its first real change in leadership since 1959. A new President, Miguel Díaz-Canel, was chosen by the National Assembly in a historic transition. Raúl Castro also stepped down from his remaining leadership positions in the spring of 2021, marking a transition to a new post-Castro era on the Island. The Díaz-Canel regime's strong rhetorical emphasis on "continuity," however, suggests the new era will have much in common with the previous, and the Castro brothers' legacy will remain in place for the foreseeable future. Today this legacy includes dramatic expansion of hospitals and clinics over the course of six decades of dynastic authoritarian rule. Are the health benefits of this system worth the human costs? Until independent journalists are allowed free access to information in Cuba, this essential question will remain unanswered.

## Notes

1. For positive assessments of Cuban healthcare during the Soviet period, see Danielson (1977; 1979), Elling (1989), and Feinsilver (1993). Recent laudatory analyses can be found in works by Kirk (2015), Kristof (2019), and Whiteford and Branch (2009). For critical analyses, see Diaz-Briquets (1983, 1986) and Ullmann and Spooner (2014). For more nuanced ethnographic and other first-person accounts, see Brotherton (2012), Hirschfeld (2008), and Kath (2010).

2. The Cuban government produces an annual compilation of health data that is made available to foreign researchers through MINSAP, the Ministry of Health. These data are always presented in categories of "revolutionary" vs. "pre-revolutionary" time.

3. Dr. Brunner's correspondence and epidemiological reports from Cuba are located in RG 90, records of the US Public Health Service, located in the US National Archives facilities in College Park, Maryland.

4. A detailed assessment of the US Military's public health programs during the occupation of Cuba can be found in Brooke (1899).

5. These data are taken from multiple primary historical sources, including Barnet (1905, 1913), LeRoy y Cassá (1921, 1922), López del Valle (1924), Porter (1899), and Recio (1945).

6. Sources detailing problems of graft and corruption in Cuba during the early twentieth century include Chapman (1927), Commission on Cuban Affairs (1935). Jenks (1928) Mencia (1936), and Phillips (1935).

7. Many Western observers also believed that the Soviet healthcare system was highly effective in the 1970s and 1980s. After the collapse of the Soviet Union, however, these researchers learned that Soviet health statistics were regularly falsified, and Soviet authorities were skilled at concealing outbreaks.

8. For details of life in Cuba's Unidades Militares de Ayuda a la Producción [Military Units to Aid Production] (UMAP) camps, see the documentary film *Conducta impropia* (1983, dir. Néstor Almendros and Orlando Jiménez Leal).

9. One dissident Cuban physician publicized this outbreak to international media and received an eight-year prison sentence (see Mendoza 2001). Fidel Castro's speeches denouncing the dengue epidemic as an act of "biological aggression" were published in Cuba's communist party newspaper, *Granma*.

10. Yoani Sánchez's blog posts can be viewed at https://generacionyen.wordpress.com. She is also the founder of https://www.14ymedio.com/englishedition, an independent news agency in Havana.

## References

Almendros, Néstor and Orlando Jiménez Leal, directors. 1984. *Conducta Impropria/Improper Conduct*. Antenne 2.
Barnet, Enrique. 1905. *La sanidad de Cuba*. Havana: Imprenta Mercantil Teniente Rey.
———. 1913. *Consideraciones sobre el estado sanitario de Cuba*. Havana: Academia de Ciencias Médicas.
Berdine, Gilbert, Vincente Geloso, and Benjamin Powell. 2018. "Cuban Infant Mortality and Longevity: Health Care or Repression?" *Health Policy and Planning* 33 (6): 755–57.
Brooke, John. 1899. *Annual Report of Major General John R. Brooke, U.S. Army Commanding the Division of Cuba*. Havana.
Brotherton, Sean. 2012. *Revolutionary Medicine: Health and the Body in Post-Soviet Cuba*. Durham, NC: Duke University Press.
Brown, Charles and Armando Lago. 1992. *The Politics of Psychiatry in Revolutionary Cuba*. New Brunswick, NJ: Transaction Press.
Chapman, Charles. 1927. *A History of the Cuban Republic*. New York: Macmillan and Co.
Commission on Cuban Affairs. 1935. *Problems of the New Cuba*. New York: Foreign Policy Association.
The Cuba Neuropathy Field Investigation Team. 1995. "Epidemic Optic Neuropathy in Cuba: Clinical Characterization and Risk Factors." *New England Journal of Medicine* 333: 1176–1182. https://www.nejm.org/doi/full/10.1056/NEJM199511023331803.
Danielson, Ross. 1979. *Cuban Medicine*. New Brunswick, NJ: Transaction Books.

———. 1977. "Cuban Health Care in Process: Models and Morality in the Early Revolution." In *Topias and Utopias in Health*, edited by Stanley Ingram and Anthony Thomas, 307–33. The Hague: Mouton Publishers.
Díaz-Briquets, Sergio. 1986. "How to Figure Out Cuba: Development, Ideology, Mortality." *Caribbean Review* 15 (2): 8–11; 39–42.
———. 1983. *The Health Revolution in Cuba*. Austin: University of Texas Press.
Elling, Ray. 1989. "Is Socialism Bad for Your Health? Cuba and the Philippines: A Cross-National Study of Health Systems." *Medical Anthropology* 11: 127–50.
Feinsilver, Julie. 1993. *Healing the Masses: Cuban Health Politics at Home and Abroad*. Berkeley: University of California Press.
Gámez Torres, Nora. 2018. "Cuba Doctors who Worked in Brazil Sue International Organization Alleging Forced Labor." *Miami Herald*, November 30, 2018. https://www.miamiherald.com/news/nation-world/world/americas/cuba/article222441145.html.
Gómez Dantés, Octavio. 2018. "The Dark Side of Cuba's Health System: Free Speech, Rights of Patients and Labor Rights of Physicians." *Health Systems and Reform* 4 (3): 175–82.
Gutierrez, Barbara. 2017. "A Conversation with Yoani Sánchez." *University of Miami News*, http://cuba.miami.edu/people/a-conversation-with-yoani-sanchez/.
Hirschfeld, Katherine. 2008. *Health, Politics and Revolution in Cuba since 1898*. New Brunswick, NJ: Transaction Press.
International Bank for Reconstruction and Development. 1950. *Report on Cuba. Findings and recommendations of an economic and technical mission organized by the International Bank for Reconstruction and Development in collaboration with the Government of Cuba*. Washington, DC: Johns Hopkins Press
Jenks, Lelend. 1928. *Our Cuban Colony*. New York: Vanguard Press.
Kath, Elizabeth. 2010. *Social Relations and the Cuban Health Miracle*. New Brunswick, NJ: Transaction Press.
Kirk, John. 2015. *Healthcare Without Borders: Understanding Cuban Medical Internationalism*. Gainesville: University Press of Florida.
Kristof, Nicholas. 2019. "Why Infants May be More Likely to Die in America than Cuba." *New York Times*, January 1, 2019. https://www.nytimes.com/2019/01/18/opinion/sunday/cuba-healthcare-medicare.html.
LeRoy y Cassá, Jorge. 1921. "The History of Public Health in Cuba during the Past Fifty Years." *American Journal of Public Health* 11: 1048–52.
———. 1922. *Desenvolvimiento de la sanidad en Cuba durante los últimos 50 Años*. Havana: La Moderna Poesía.
López del Valle, José A. 1924. *Los adelantos sanitarios de la república de Cuba*. Havana: Imprenta y Papelaria 'La Propagandista.'
Mencia, Manuel. 1936. *La sanidad y la beneficia en Cuba: Reformas indispensables*. Havana: Molines y Compañía.
Mendoza, Dessy. 2001. *Dengue*. Washington, DC: Center for a Free Cuba.
Phillips, Ruby Hart. 1935. *Cuban Sideshow*. Havana: Cuban Press.
Phillips, R. Hart. 1959a. "Castro Regime Strikes at Graft through Drastic Cuban Reform." *New York Times*, January 28, 1959. https://timesmachine.nytimes.com/timesmachine/1959/01/28/issue.html.

———. 1959b. "Reporter Convicted and Ousted by Cuba." *New York Times*. December 23, 1959. https://timesmachine.nytimes.com/timesmachine/1959/12/23/81530267.pdf?pdf_redirect=true&ip=0. Accessed 7 October 2020.

———. 1959c. "Former Air Chief Hunted by Cubans." *New York Times*. July 2, 1959. https://timesmachine.nytimes.com/timesmachine/1959/07/02/89216934.pdf?pdf_redirect=true&ip=0.

———. 1960. "Castro's Regime Puts All Trade Under Controls." *New York Times* February 21, 1960. https://www.nytimes.com/1960/02/21/archives/castros-regime-puts-all-trade-under-controls-private-enterprise.html?searchResultPosition=1.

Porter, Robert. 1899. *Industrial Cuba*. New York: Putnams.

Recio, Alberto. 1945. "Enfermedades infecto-contagiosas que amenazan a Cuba." *Anales de la Academia de Ciências Médicas, Físicas y Naturales de la Habana.*

Reporters Without Borders. 2012. "Independent Journalists Hounded and Arrested, While Granma Reporter Gets 14 Years on Spying Charge." *Reporteros Sin Fronteras*. https://rsf.org/en/news/independent-journalists-hounded-and-arrested-while-granma-reporter-get-14-years-spying-charge.

Sánchez, Yoani. 2022. The Political Prison in Cuba, From Pepe to Luisma. *Generaciony*, January 28, 2022. https://generacionyen.wordpress.com.

Sánchez, Yoani. 2016. "Cuba Survives Fidel Castro." *14ymedio*. November 27, 2016. https://www.14ymedio.com/englishedition.

Ullman, Steven, and Mary Helen Spooner. 2014. *Cuban Health Care: Utopian Dreams, Fragile Future*. Lanham, MD: Lexington Books.

Whiteford, Linda, and Laurence Branch. 2009. *Primary Health Care in Cuba: The Other Revolution*. Lanham, MD: Rowan and Littlefield.

# 9

# Disaster Preparedness and Management in Cuba

## A Health-Based Approach

EMILY J. KIRK

Cuba's efforts regarding disaster preparation and management have received praise from, among others, the United Nations, World Health Organization, Red Cross, and Oxfam. Although the country has often been ignored in the international media and healthcare scholarship, Cuba has developed a comprehensive system to protect the country from natural disasters, including hurricanes, floods, fires, drought, earthquakes, and tornadoes. This is particularly significant given the increase in the ferocity and frequency of natural disasters globally. The cornerstone of the Island's approach is a clear emphasis on the protection of human lives, and the understanding that, by their very nature, hurricanes and other disasters represent threats to public health. In the view of the Cuban government and populace, failure to plan for disasters constitutes a public health failure.

Of particular note is that Cuba boasts very few lives lost during hurricane-related disasters—a sharp departure from its Caribbean neighbors. For example, when Hurricane Matthew made landfall in October 2016, over 1,000 deaths were reported in Haiti and, more than one month following the disaster, 1.4 million Haitians remained in need of emergency assistance. By contrast, despite severe floods in the provinces of Granma, Holguin, and Santiago de Cuba, and a reported cost of $2.5 billion (USD) in damages, officials evacuated 1.3 million people, and not a single death was reported. To add further context: 40 deaths were reported in the United States as a result of this storm (Kirk 2017, 93).

The cases of Hurricane Maria and Hurricane Irma offer further telling comparative examples. Hurricane Maria hit Puerto Rico in September 2017 as a category 5 storm (the highest category on the Saffir-Simpson scale) and was widely considered to be the worst natural disaster to ever hit the Island. The widespread devastation was reflected in the death toll associated with the disaster. US President Donald J. Trump and US State authorities reported 66 deaths as a result of the hurricane (Guha-Sapir and Checchi 2018), but researchers from George Washington University concluded that there had been approximately 2,975 deaths associated with the hurricane between September 2017 and February 2018. These deaths were both direct (such as drowning or being crushed by a falling building due to high winds during the hurricane) and indirect results (such as contaminated water and spread of disease after the hurricane) of Maria. Furthermore, the researchers concluded that elevated risk for citizens continued beyond the observation period of the study—in other words, ongoing associated deaths and health issues were expected (George Washington University 2018).

In the same month, a powerful category 5 hurricane also hit Cuba. Irma was record breaking as it was the first hurricane to maintain category 5 intensity for three consecutive days as it pummeled the Caribbean Island. Like Maria, Hurricane Irma was extremely destructive, yet minimal loss of life occurred in Cuba. For example, despite damages calculated at over US $13 billion, 158,554 houses damaged or destroyed, and nearly two million people evacuated (of a population of 11.2 million), only ten deaths were reported (*Cubadebate* 2017). Of particular note is that zero indirect deaths were reported in the months following the devastation. This is largely because of Cuba's particular disaster preparedness and management system, which includes comprehensive response and recovery plans, as well as the Island's notable and well-documented public healthcare system that focuses on preventive measures. For example, following each disaster, reports suggest that it typically takes no longer than five days to re-establish electricity, even in the most affected zones, and clean drinking water is always available. Indeed, in a 2002 Disaster Report, the International Federation of the Red Cross (IFRD) asked, "What is the secret of Cuba's success?" (Oxfam America 2004, 6). This chapter illuminates the specific approach employed in Cuba, how it evolved, and what makes it unique. Above all, Cuba's focus on health and well-being has played a key role in contributing to the Island's disaster preparedness. While healthcare and medical history research has largely overlooked the connection between natural disasters and healthcare, the Cuban model demonstrates the clear and impactful linkages. As scholarship pivots to focus on these connections, the Cuban case offers both a distinctive case study, and possible solutions.

## Evolution of a System

Like many aspects of revolutionary Cuba, the country's complex system of disaster preparedness and management cannot be understood as a monolithic structure, unchanged throughout the more than sixty years of revolution. Rather, it developed and evolved considerably over time, adjusting to challenges, adapting to needs, learning from failed or imperfect approaches, and utilizing available resources. The system's evolution since the early 1960s can be clearly mapped, as new and complementary strategies were continually developed and implemented.

Cuba's contemporary system is rooted in 1963, following Hurricane Flora which devastated the Island. Although only rated a category 2 on the Saffir-Simpson scale, the hurricane caused significant damage and over 1,200 deaths. Evacuations and rescue attempts were haphazardly organized, while crops and houses suffered substantial damage. The significant human and material losses suffered as a result of a lack of preparation and management sparked the Cuban leadership's desire to develop and establish a comprehensive preparedness plan (Mesa 2008, 5). Indeed, in addition to being remembered for its destruction, the hurricane must also be understood as the catalyst for a dramatically improved disaster preparedness system.

Following the chaos of Flora, officials thoroughly analyzed the problems they had encountered, and the leadership sought to improve the Island's reaction to natural disasters. By 1965, the Institute of Meteorology was founded and given the responsibility of detecting, monitoring, and communicating hazards such as hurricanes, high winds, and heavy rainfall (Castellanos Abella and Wisner 2019, 9). The Popular Defense (founded in 1962 with a view to maintain vigilance and protect the economic and political targets of the country) was reorganized into the National Civil Defense in 1966. While its predecessor was focused on military protection, the Civil Defense was organized to protect the populations from both military threats and further natural disasters. This included organizing warning systems, plans for evacuations and shelter facilities, as well as managing safe drinking water, transportation, and communication (Puig González, Betancourt Lavastido, and Álvarez Cadeño 2010, 33). From the late 1960s, the Civil Defense increasingly became the engine of Cuba's disaster preparedness and management approach.

Throughout the 1970s and 1980s the government continued to seek means of improving its disaster preparation approach. In particular, in 1976 the organizational structure of the Civil Defense was significantly improved. Although the leadership of the Civil Defense rested with the president, a strong and clear centralized organization format was instituted, with Civil Defense representatives at the national, provincial, and municipal levels of leadership. The aim was to improve the efficiency of organization and communication. Furthermore, at this time the Civil Defense was placed in charge of planning, organizing, and overseeing the protection, preparedness, response, and recovery of the Cuban population in times of disasters, particularly natural disasters (Defensa Civil 2017).

During this time, education also became a progressively more important component of the preparedness and management system. For example, in 1986, a weekend-long training activity called "Meteoro" was instituted (Llanes Guerra 2008, 42). Organized by Civil Defense, the idea was to include disaster preparedness and response training for all citizens across the country. Specific drills were included, as detailed plans for evacuation and safety were practiced for a wide variety of possible disasters—from floods, to fires and water contamination. Notably, participation was mandatory, and included both children and adults. Since its inception, Meteoro has continued every year, usually in the month of May, as communities prepare for hurricane season.

Cuba faced significant challenges at the beginning of the 1990s as a result of the collapse of the Soviet Union—its largest trading partner. An intense economic crisis followed in Cuba, which necessitated further changing the Civil Defense system as well as the organization of the Island's disaster preparedness. Specifically, in 1994 the Civil Defense and its role of protecting the population and economy was reaffirmed and expanded. During this time, the already clear emphasis on the importance of prevention was again intensified. For example, funding was allocated to the Civil Defense to support their plans and specifically their prevention measure. This is particularly significant given the country's economic crisis, and it highlights the national dedication to the protection of the population. In terms of natural disaster, the management system was reorganized to include different stages—normal, informative, alert, alarm, and recovery (Pardo Guerra et al. 2017). In essence, despite the crippled economy, the government continued to increase attention to disaster preparedness and management.

In 2004, Cuba was severely impacted by two major hurricanes—Ivan and Charley—within a relatively short period of time. Following the destruction caused by the two powerful hurricanes, it was determined that changes needed to be made to the Island's prevention and management system. Specifically, a process of analysis and improvement was undertaken. The following year, a new law was instituted, entitled Directive 1. The document outlined the changes that would be implemented, focusing primarily on prevention and risk reduction. For example, it included plans to incorporate disaster preparedness into all future socioeconomic planning, improve communication and knowledge dissemination, and required comprehensive risk assessments of organizations (Directiva No. 1 2005).

Directive 1 would become an impactful legal framework for the ongoing evolution of Cuba's disaster management system. In 2007, and with a view to continue the emphasis on prevention, the Directive was updated to include the establishment of Risk Reduction Management Centers (RRMC) for every provincial and municipal government with the aim of increasing research and decreasing the risks associated with specific regions (Pardo Guerra et al. 2017). The centers play an important role in data collection, knowledge dissemination, and communication. The Directive was again updated in 2010, continuing its focus on risk reduction and preventive measures.

Similar to the impact of hurricanes Ivan and Charley in 2004, the devastation caused by Hurricane Sandy in 2012 again prompted the government to reassess its disaster preparedness and management strategy and include subsequent improvements. Indeed, during Sandy, some 343,230 people were evacuated from the western province of Santiago de Cuba, $4.7 billion in damage was reported, 171,380 houses were damaged, and 11 deaths were reported (Carrasco Martín 2012). As President Raúl Castro noted, Santiago de Cuba, "look[ed] like a city that ha[d] been bombed" (qtd. in Galinsky 2012). As a result of the significant damage, the heads of various ministries including, among others, Energy and Mines, Water Resources, Construction, Industry, and Internal Market were stationed in the capital of Santiago de Cuba to oversee the recovery and reconstruction.

The severe impact, both physically and within the cultural memory of the population, prompted the government to continue plans for prevention through risk reduction as well as ongoing analysis and improvements of related strategies. For example, among contemporary advancements to the system are the Risk Assessment studies (known by the Spanish acronym, PVR), largely directed by the Ministry of Science, Technology, and Environment. The aim of these studies is to compile as much data as possible on the specific hazards in each municipality (169 in total) to determine necessary improvements to protect human lives and the economy. While the studies originally focused on hurricanes (and by extension floods and high winds), they were expanded to include other forms of hazards, such as fires, drought, epidemiological crises, and landslides (Pardo Guerra et al. 2017). Of particular note is the fact that the PVR studies are revised annually to ensure that population and economic data is up-to-date. These assessments are considered vital for Cuba's preventive strategy, as they provide comprehensive assessments on potential problems and disasters, as well as how to manage them to minimize disasters.

Prompted by Flora, Cuba's system has evolved significantly from the early 1960s. It has developed around the central contention of the importance of human lives and well-being to become one of the most well-organized approaches globally. Specifically, there are eight key components to Cuba's disaster and preparedness and management system that distinguish it from others.

## Eight Key Components of Cuba's Disaster Preparedness and Management System

**1.** *Prevention.*

The main pillar of the Island's approach is undoubtedly that of prevention. Similar to the viewpoint behind the country's healthcare system, the approach to disaster preparedness and management is rooted in prevention, as it is widely believed that this is less costly than a strictly recovery-based approach. As such, prevention is considered paramount in the comprehensive strategy to protect the population from natural disasters.

**2.** *A Comprehensive National Civil Defense System.*

The National Civil Defense system is very complex and, as noted earlier, has evolved since 1962. It has developed over the decades to become a strong and centralized form of prevention, preparedness, response, and recovery from disasters. It is organized from the highest level, the president, all the way down to individual community leaders, such as hospital directors or school principals. As Enrique Castellanos Abella and Benjamin Wisner (2019) explain:

> The country is vertically organized into national, provincial, municipal, and popular council levels [ . . . ] A municipality has a "municipal council of defense" led by its president with a vice president trained and responsible for day-to-day operations of civil defense. A province has a "provincial council of defense" which is also led by its president. In addition, there is a "national council of defense" led by the president of the Republic of Cuba. (9)

This centralized and sweeping model allows the country to implement preventive or protective changes more easily, while also facilitating data collection and research, as well as evacuations and recovery work. The impact of the National Civil Defense in Cuba's successful approach to disaster preparedness and management has saved countless Cuban lives.

3. *Education.*

Formal education (in schools, universities, etc.) and informal education (media representation, cultural memory, etc.) has been extremely important in preparing Cuba's population for disasters. In terms of formal education, children begin learning about natural disasters and how to protect themselves and their families in primary school up to the university level. In addition, specialized natural disaster-related training is included in many university curricula (Santos Pérez et al. 2018). For example, medical students are required to learn about the most common medical issues during and after a disaster, as well as elements such as water safety and disease prevention. There are often public service announcements and information on the state-controlled TV and radio, and disaster preparedness education has become commonplace in communities as members of the Civil Defense continue to educate on best practices. Moreover, the annual weekend-long educative exercise, Meteoro, requires all citizens to participate in drills to reinforce knowledge of where to go and what to do in the event of a given disaster. Safety information is a top priority during Meteoro, as the population is trained on a wide range of topics including safe evacuation procedures, food and water safety, and first aid.

4. *Support of Legal System.*

Cuba's approach is supported throughout the legal system. The Cuban legal system contains four types of laws: Law, Decree Law, Decree, and Resolution. Beginning in 1962, several laws were enacted to protect the lives of Cubans in times of disasters. As of 2008 there were three laws, seven decree laws, thirteen decrees, twenty-one resolutions, and one directive that focused on disaster risk reduction as well as the protection of lives and well-being (Llanes Guerra 2008). Among the most significant laws is Decree Law 170, which was ratified in 1997. It notes that the Civil Defense is responsible (using a system of prevention, preparedness, response, and recovery) for avoiding "human loss" and for "protect[ing] the population," as well as the economy and agriculture from natural disasters. In addition, the Cuban Constitution, which was instituted under the revolutionary government in 1976 (as well as amended throughout the years, most recently in 2019), expressly supports the protection of the population during times of disasters. For example, Article 96 of the initial 1976 version states that the government is responsible for the "protection of lives and property in case of natural disasters" (República de Cuba 1976). The broad legal structure has translated into an effective foundation for the protective role of the government and the necessary compliance of the population in times of disasters, including evacuation, mobilization, and participation.

5. *Proactive Response to Climate Change.*

Since 2011, significant changes have been undertaken to protect the Island and its population from the effects of climate change. Specifically, the government's *Tarea Vida* (Project Life) was ratified in 2017 (Figueredo Reinaldo and Doimeadios Guerra 2017). The Project is an extremely detailed plan to meet the increasing challenges faced as a result of climate change until the year 2100. The main issues faced by Cuba, like other Caribbean islands, include loss of coastline due to rising sea levels resulting in floods, saltwater intrusion, and soil erosion, as well as the increase in hurricanes, rainfall, and high winds. For example, it was reported that increasing sea levels could cause the loss of up to 5.45 percent of Cuba's coastal land by 2100 (Castellanos Abella and Wisner 2019; *Granma* 2017). In addition to increasing internal protective measures against climate change, Cuba has also been extremely active in participating in global accords that seek to mitigate climate change and reduce related risks from natural disasters. For example, Cuba actively participated in the United Nation's Office for Disaster Risk Reduction's (UNISDR) Sendai Framework for Disaster Risk Reduction, which focuses on the years 2015 to 2030. The central aim of the Sendai Framework is "The substantial reduction of disaster risk and losses in lives, livelihoods and health and in the economic, physical, social, cultural and environmental assets of persons, businesses, communities and countries" (UNISDR 2015).

6. *All Ministries Are Involved in Preparedness and Recovery.*

Originally based on legislation that was instituted in 1966 (Law No. 1194) which focuses on the Civil Defense, all ministries in the Cuban government are required to participate in disaster preparedness and recovery (Defensa Civil 2017, 15–17). Additional legislation and responsibilities continued to be included for the roles of all ministries. Each ministry is tasked with specific responsibilities before, during, and after a disaster. For example, the Ministry of Tourism is responsible for the protection of all foreign tourists, the Ministry of Transportation for mobilizing vehicles to assist with evacuations, and the Ministry of Public Health for protecting the health of the population, such as ensuring sufficient equipment is available, and testing water quality. The Council of Ministers, comprised of the ministers from each government ministry, works collaboratively to determine the most impactful means of disaster management. This is particularly significant when compared to other industrialized countries in the region. For example, in Canada, in times of natural disasters, the primary body responsible for information and recovery is Environment and Climate Change Canada, the central department that works on all environment-related issues. In addition to their coordinating efforts, the armed forces are at times brought in to assist. Similarly, in the United States, while there is some support offered by Federal Emergency Management Agency (FEMA) and the armed forces, government departments are not integral to the overall preparedness or recovery.

7. *Solidarity.*

A powerful component of the success of Cuba's model has been the implementation and fostering of solidarity. While a somewhat nebulous term, "solidarity" can be defined as a "relation forged through political struggle which seeks to challenge forms of oppression" (Featherstone 2012, 5) or "a question of basic morality" (Appiah 2006, 157). For Cuba, its distinct brand of solidarity has roots in its struggle against Spanish colonialism, and particularly the War of Independence (1895–1898), as well as US neocolonialism (1898–1959), as the country sought independence and its own national identity, or *Cubanidad*. In addition, the significant economic challenges faced by the population as a result of the US embargo (since 1962) and later the collapse of the Soviet Union (1991) cultivated a deeply rooted and culturally engrained understanding of the importance of solidarity. Solidarity in post-1959 Cuba is, in essence, the view that human lives matter and as such it is the role of all Cubans to protect one another. Solidarity has been tremendously important in the Island's approach to protecting the population in times of crises. This includes housing neighbors, cleaning debris, mobilizing, evacuating, and rescuing.

8. *Constantly Evolving.*

Since Hurricane Flora—the first major hurricane to hit post-1959 Cuba—the disaster preparedness and management system has continued to evolve. Today's internationally celebrated strategy is the product of decades of challenges and improvements. Analysis and risk reduction were central to ongoing advances. The sweeping approach used today continues to undergo evaluation as the Cuban government and population seek to perfect the system that protects lives and well-being.

## Conclusion

Since the 1960s, Cuba has undoubtedly developed an effective approach to dealing with natural disasters. Despite the success of Cuba's approach to disaster preparedness and management, challenges persist. Chief among these is the US embargo. Castellanos Abella and Wisner (2019) note that "the economic blockade has placed severe burdens on the Cuban economy and the ability of the state to accomplish recovery in a timely way despite considerable mobilization of human and other resources" (17). Another significant challenge is the cost associated with the damage, including structural damage. For example, between 2005 and 2016, hurricanes damaged 1,199,102 houses across the Island, and caused the total collapse of 147,710 houses. The total estimated cost of damage from hurricanes between 2005 and 2016 is $23.5 billion (Castellanos Abella and Wisner 2019). These figures are particularly significant when one considers that the Island's population is 11.2 million, and its Gross Domestic Product (GDP) is equivalent to that of Gabon. In addition to the damage, another major problem is that recovery can be very time consuming due to the annual hurricane cycle. In other words, it is challenging to completely rebuild an area that is hit repeatedly, while simultaneously negotiating the need to work in the most devastated areas, leaving other damaged (although to a lesser extent) areas waiting for materials and recovery procedures.

Nonetheless, overall, Cuba has created an impactful disaster preparedness and management system. A unique feature of this approach is the central theme of health and well-being—which ultimately translates to lives saved. Throughout the evolutionary process, the primary focus of the government, and by extension the Civil Defense, was the protection of the health of the population. The core value of their ever-evolving preventive approach, including the legal system, education, Civil Defense, view of climate change, inclusion of all ministries, and the role of solidarity, is the protection of health and well-being. In this case, using an approach rooted in health above all has been extremely impactful. Without doubt, while the system cannot be transplanted elsewhere, it offers lessons for other countries. The case of Cuban disaster preparedness and management suggests that health and well-being may indeed be strong arguments for, and drivers of, policy change elsewhere. Clearly, as natural disasters continue to increase in number and intensity, new and innovative means of protection are needed.

## References

Appiah, Kwame Anthony. 2006. *Cosmopolitanism: Ethics in a World of Strangers.* New York: W. W. Norton & Company.

Carrasco Martín, Juana. 2012. "Datos preliminaries del impacto del huracán Sandy a su paso por Cuba." *Mesa Redonda.* October 26, 2012. http://mesaredonda.cubadebate.cu/mesa-redonda/2012/10/26/datos-preliminares-del-impacto-del-huracan-sandy-a-su-paso-por-cuba/

Castellanos Abella, Enrique, and Benjamin Wisner. 2019. "Natural Hazards Governance in Cuba." *Oxford Research Encyclopedias.* http://oxfordre.com/naturalhazardscience/view/10.1093/acrefore/9780199389407.001.0001/acrefore-9780199389407-e-238

Cubadebate. 2017. "Información del Consejo de Defensa Nacional." *Cubadebate.* September 29, 2017. http://www.cubadebate.cu/noticias/2017/09/29/informacion-del-consejo-de-defensa-nacional/#.XLIKza2ZOt8

Defensa Civil. 2017. *La Defensa Civil Cubana.* Havana: Casa Editorial Verde Olivo.

Directiva No. 1. 2005. Directiva No. 1 del vicepresidente del consejo de defensa nacional República de Cuba Consejo de Defensa. June 1. [Law]. Nacionalhttp://www.sld.cu/galerias/pdf/sitios/desastres/directiva_vp_cdn_sobre_desastres.ultima_version.pdf

Featherstone, David. 2012. *Solidarity: Hidden Histories and Geographies of Internationalism.* London: Zed Books.

Figueredo Reinaldo, Oscar, and Dianet Doimeadios Guerra. 2017. "Tarea Vida: ¿Cómo enfrentará Cuba el cambio climático?" *Cubadebate.* 16 May. http://www.cubadebate.cu/especiales/2017/05/16/tarea-vida-como-enfrentara-cuba-el-cambio-climatico-video/#.XKdExq2ZOt8

Galinsky, Seth. 2012. "Hurricane Sandy: Cuba Gov't Leads Effort to Meet Needs and Rebuild." *The Militant* 76 (42). https://www.themilitant.com/2012/7642/764202.html

George Washington University. 2018. *Project Report: Ascertainment of the Estimated Excess Mortality from Hurricane Maria in Puerto Rico.* https://publichealth.gwu.edu/sites/default/files/downloads/projects/PRstudy/Acertainment%20of%20the%20Estimated%20Excess%20Mortality%20from%20Hurricane%20Maria%20in%20Puerto%20Rico.pdf

Granma. 2017. "Experts Warn of the Impact of Climate Change on Central Cuba." *Granma.* August 8, 2017. http://en.granma.cu/cuba/2017-08-08/experts-warn-of-the-impact-of-climate-change-on-central-cuba

Guha-Sapir, Debarati, and Francesco Checchi. 2018. "Science and Politics of Disaster Death Tolls." *British Medical Journal* 362: n. p.

Kirk, Emily J. 2017. "Dealing with the Perfect Storm: Cuban Disaster Management." *Studies in Political Economy* 98 (1): 93–103.

Llanes Guerra, José. 2008. "Cuba: Paradigma en la reducción de riesgo de desastres" [Report]. *PreventionWeb.* https://www.preventionweb.net/files/2558_CubaParadigmaenlareducciónderiesgodedesastres.pdf

Mesa, Guillermo. 2008. "The Cuban Health Sector & Disaster Mitigation." *MEDICC Review* 10 (3): 5–8.

Oxfam America. 2004. "Weathering the Storm: Lessons in Risk Reduction from Cuba."

An Oxfam America Report. www.proventionconsortium.org/themes/default/pdfs/CRA/Cuba.pdf.

Pardo Guerra, Ramón, Luis A. Macareño Velíz, Albo Parra Salinas, Gloria Gely Martínez, Wilfred Cobas Dávila, Raúl R. Costa Gravalosa, Humberto de la Rosa, Noel Pérez Lozano, and Marbelis Rodríguez Azahares. 2017. *Guía metodológica para la organización del proceso de reducción de desastres.* Defensa Civil Cuba and UNPD. https://www.preventionweb.net/files/59362_guiametodologicaparaorganizacionrrd.pdf

Puig González, Miguel Ángel, José Ernesto Betancourt Lavastido, and Rolando Álvarez Cadeño. 2010. *Fortalezas frente a huracanes (1959–2008).* Havana: Editorial Científico-Técnica.

República de Cuba. 1976. *Constitución Política de 1976.* http://pdba.georgetown.edu/Constitutions/Cuba/cuba1976.html

Santos Pérez, Santiago, Alfonso Núñez Leguen, Marbelis Rodríguez Azahare, Virginia Huergo Silveira, Milagros Santa Cruz Domínguez, Berta Lidia Castro, and Mayra Díaz Gaicía. 2018. *Buenas prácticas cubanas para la protección de niños y adolescentes en situaciones de desastres.* Havana: Sello Editor de la Educación Cubana.

United Nation's Office for Disaster Risk Reduction (UNISDR). 2015. *Sendai Framework for Disaster Risk Reduction. United Nations Office for Disaster Risk Reduction.* https://www.unisdr.org/we/coordinate/sendai-framework

# 10

## Stories of Giving Birth in Central America
### Class, Race, and Politics in Women's Health

SOPHIE ESCH AND ALICIA Z. MIKLOS

This chapter discusses what it means to give birth in Central America by focusing on the stories of three individuals: a white woman from Nicaragua, an Indigenous woman from Guatemala, and a mestiza from El Salvador. Marked by extreme social and economic stratification, the region offers poignant examples of how differences in class, race, and ethnicity result in disparate circumstances for women's reproductive health. We offer an overview of the institutional and community contexts of women's health and childbirth practices in modern Central America and look at different narratives and politics of childbirth. The case studies we examine begin with a reflection on obstetric violence and feminist resistance via Gioconda Belli's autobiography, *The Country under My Skin: A Memoir of Love and War* (2003) [*El país bajo mi piel* 2002]. The second case study highlights Indigenous childbirth practices and concerns as relayed by Rigoberta Menchú in her *testimonio*, *I, Rigoberta Menchú. An Indian Woman in Guatemala* (2009) [*Me llamo Rigoberta Menchú y así me nació la conciencia* (2007, originally published in 1983)] compiled and coauthored by Elizabeth Burgos. In the final instance, we examine the effects of draconian abortion laws on women's reproductive rights and well-being via the case of Teodora del Carmen Vásquez, who was sentenced to thirty years in prison in 2008 after the stillbirth of her daughter (Amnesty International 2018). All these examples relate to questions of family planning, defined as the plethora of educational and medical interventions that help people decide freely if, how, and when they want children. The question of the presence or absence of the state in women's lives and its positive or adverse impacts on the birth experience and aftermath, as well as feminist responses to the challenges that

Central American women face when giving birth, are of particular interest for our discussion.

## Giving Birth in Central America: Panoramic Overview

The institutional and community contexts of women's health and childbirth practices in modern Central America vary widely, as Central America encompasses many diverse cultures and sub-groups. Due to the region's institutional and religious history of colonization and long-standing economic disparity, stratification exists between different social classes, ethnicities, and races. Across these differences, however, Central American women share a history of reacting to the conditions of gender inequality that have limited their autonomy regarding their bodies and destinies. In Latin America, power emanating from the state, religious institutions, and the family have dictated women's behavior and health, with motherhood defining women's social worth and value (Romero Meza 2016, 56). Norms established by these male-centered institutions have held much power over how women experience reproductive health issues and problems. The story of birthing practices in Central America today is marked as a site of contention and power. Birth is an area in which women negotiate identities and grapple with patriarchal domination and its mandates over women. The feminist movements are tied to the revolutionary movements in the region and have opened discussions regarding shared responsibility over children and care work. Asserting women's rights to participate in the public sphere, feminist activists in Central America have identified forced pregnancy and motherhood as ways that men continue to exercise control over women and girls.

Statistics paint a general picture of where, how, and with whom Central American women go through the process of labor and birthing, as well as women and infants' chance of surviving this process. Commonly, experts use two main indicators to denote survival rates for birthing: maternal mortality rates (MRR) and infant mortality rates (IMR). These indicators are used by healthcare experts and international organizations to determine the quality of prenatal and perinatal care in a given country. IMR are measured by the number of deaths per 1,000 live births, while MMR are measured out of every 100,000 live births. Causes of maternal death in Latin America are attributed to hemorrhages, hypertensive disorders, and infections (Sistema de las Naciones Unidas en Honduras 2010, 124).

For Latin America overall, the United Nations reported 9 deaths per 1,000 for the neonatal mortality rate (pertaining to newborns) for 2018 and

14 per 1,000 for the infant mortality rate (pertaining to children under five years of age) for 2018 (UN Inter-agency Group for Child Mortality Estimation 2018, 17; 49). Those rates are higher in Central America, where the UN reports 19.9 deaths as the average between 2010 and 2015 (UN Data 2019). Belize reported 19.9, with Guatemala at 21.3, El Salvador at 16.8, Honduras at 17.2, Nicaragua at 18.3, Costa Rica at 8, and Panama reported 9.9 deaths per 1,000 live births. For comparison, countries like Haiti reported 46.8 and Ethiopia 49.6 deaths, while the United States reported 5.8 (Central Intelligence Agency [CIA] 2017).

Looking at the larger Latin American and Caribbean region in terms of MMR, the World Health Organization Data from 2015 shows Latin America with 60 and the Caribbean with 175 deaths per 100,000 live births. For 2015, Belize reported 28, Guatemala 88, El Salvador 54, Honduras 129, Nicaragua 150, Costa Rica 25, and Panama reported 94 (CIA 2017). For comparison, Haiti reported 359, Ethiopia 353, the United States 14, and Germany 6.

The probability of a mother or infant experiencing a healthy birth outcome depends on numerous factors, many of which involve the mother's socioeconomic conditions leading up to the pregnancy: education level, urban vs. rural environment, and marital status, among others. Upon becoming pregnant, access to prenatal and perinatal care and advice become vital contributors to healthy outcomes.[1] The biggest disparity in prenatal and perinatal care in Central America comes from a divided healthcare system: some have access to private hospitals, while others rely on public hospitals. The quality of public hospitals varies from country to country and between rural areas and urban centers. Costa Rica, for example, boasts an extremely well-funded network of public hospitals, and workers are required to register for public healthcare through the Caja or Bank of Costa Rican Social Security (Sáenz et al. 2011, 59–60). Access to a hospital or doctor during birth is certainly not the norm across Central America. A study on Honduras conducted by the United Nations shows that access to professional medical attention during birth was determined by social class: 30 percent of women in the first income quintile—that is the lowest income—had access to a doctor while giving birth. Meanwhile, 95 percent of women in the fifth income quintile—those with the highest income—had access to a doctor (Sistema de las Naciones Unidas en Honduras 2010, 124). In addition to inequalities in pre-, peri-, and postnatal care, the World Health Organization (WHO) also spoke out for the first time in 2014 about the prevalence of obstetric violence—"disrespectful and offensive treatment that women receive during childbirth at healthcare centers"—across the world (WHO 2014).[2]

The issue of medically dangerous or unwanted pregnancies opens up a discussion of state control of women's reproduction in the region. Within Latin America, Central America has the strictest abortion laws. In particular, in El Salvador and Nicaragua abortions are illegal even in cases of rape, danger to the mother's life, or deformation of the fetus. In El Salvador, it is common for medical institutions to suspect women of intentionally aborting when they have a medical emergency that endangers the fetus, and they often contact law enforcement in these cases. In Costa Rican law, abortions are illegal, except when the mother's life will be endangered by the pregnancy.

While it is possible to measure how many women gave birth with the assistance of a medical professional, it is much more difficult to assess the emotional and interpersonal factors shaping women's perceptions of birth. To capture the more subjective and personal dimensions of giving birth in Central America, we turn to literature, testimony, and mass media representations. Cultural texts such as these show how women of different class, ethnic, and racial identities navigate the personal and institutional worlds of maternity. A complex process physically, psychologically, and economically, pregnancy and childbirth integrate women into spaces of modern Western medicine—like clinics and hospitals—or into age-old cultural traditions in their home.

## Case Study 1: A White Upper-Class Feminist in Private and Public Hospitals in Nicaragua and Costa Rica—Obstetric Violence and Female Empowerment

What does giving birth have to do with revolution? Everything, according to Gioconda Belli, Nicaragua's most famous female poet and novelist and participant in the Sandinista Revolution (1970s–1980s). As a young woman, Belli, a member of a Nicaraguan upper-class family, joined the revolution in order to fight against the military dictatorship of the Somoza clan, smuggling arms and money and working on public relations materials. During that time, she also gave birth to several children. Her autobiography, *The Country under My Skin*, tells the story of her life as a woman, a revolutionary, a working professional, a mother, a feminist, a lover, and a friend. Her story interweaves questions of female liberation with those of national liberation, and, as such, it touches upon issues of womanhood, of class, and of revolutionary commitment in relation to her different experiences of giving birth in a private hospital in Nicaragua and a public one in Costa Rica. Belli is the mother of four children, and the dramatic experiences of the birth of her first and her third child figure with particular prominence in her autobiography. The prominence of these experiences invites us to consider the revolutionary struggle not only as the fight against dictatorship but also as a time when women clamored for equal access to individualized, dignified medical assistance during childbirth.

In 1967, at only nineteen years of age, Belli experiences her first childbirth as a moment of both humiliation and revelation. Delivering in a hospital is, for her, mostly violent and disempowering. She describes the intimacy-violating medical procedures in great detail: the shaving of her pubic hair, the application of an enema in combination with the hospital gown open to the back, the parade of doctors inspecting the dilation of her cervix, and the terminology employed in which her child is referred to as "the product" (Belli 2003, 21). She also finds utterly ridiculous the doctor who performs her abdominal expression, which is often referred to as the Kristeller maneuver—a controversial method in which a medical professional pushes down on the belly to accelerate the birth during the second stage of labor. The medical procedures contrast deeply with her own sensations and convictions; she marvels at the experience of childbirth despite the painful twelve-hour labor. As a cultural feminist, Gioconda Belli celebrates femininity and believes that there is a feminine essence. Giving birth connects her to this femininity, and she feels nature—"an age-old wisdom [that] controlled everything"—(Belli 2003, 21) taking over. She trusts her body and her instincts and lets herself be guided by nature. She describes birth as a primal experience in which, in the end, she receives her baby girl and smells her "like any animal smelling her newborn" (22). Images of nature and technology overlap in the narration, as if she were trying to reconcile the alienating, cold experience of the hospital with her own personal, intimate, primal, and uniquely feminine experience. This first childbirth, while traumatic, is ultimately positive since she manages to negotiate between the two worlds. Her optimism might be in part because of her young age and the novelty of the situation, but it could also depend upon the surroundings: she delivers her child in a private hospital accompanied by her family and personal doctor.

Her third experience at childbirth, now exiled in Costa Rica, and in a public hospital, is a completely different affair. She tells of a harrowing experience: overfilled hospital rooms, incompetent doctors, and an overall dismissive and patronizing attitude toward the pregnant women, their needs, and their intelligence. After five and a half months of pregnancy, she has contractions, goes to the hospital, and there, when a doctor puts his stethoscope "brusquely" on her belly, her amniotic sac breaks (Belli 2003, 188). Now at risk for a miscarriage, she has to stay at the hospital and subsequently contracts an infection. When the fetus is in distress, she has to undergo an emergency C-section. In what ensues, the hospital staff tells her twice that her baby has died. This happens first right after the C-section, until the medical personnel realize that he is still alive. Later, while Belli is in the ICU, a doctor informs her that her baby is dead. Moments later, a nurse stops by to tell the new mother about seeing her baby boy, alive. In the end, it is clarified that her baby is in fact alive. Her infection worsens, however, and, with the help of her own mother, who arrives from Nicaragua, she arranges a transfer to a private hospital where she is operated on again and hovers between life and death for a month. When she is finally able to visit her still-tiny preemie, she names him Camilo after a friend who has just died in the revolution.

The dreadful experience at the hospital is compounded by an ideological dilemma and an ensuing marital fight. Belli is used to the privileges of a private hospital setting, but going to a public hospital is more in tune with her and her partner's revolutionary commitment. When Belli's experience at the public hospital turns dire, her determination is challenged and her partner dismisses her anger at the poor treatment she has received as that of a spoiled upper-class woman. He disapproves of her decision to switch hospitals. She finds his "quasi-religious morality" and "attitude very typical of the left" (190). She does not share his belief "that the true revolutionary should endure the same injustices the masses had to cope with" (190). Instead, she wants everyone to enjoy better care; she wants to stop the mistreatment, not "democratize it" (190).[3]

Belli also highlights in both episodes how doctors tend to dismiss women's concerns, dignity, and fear. Belli herself tries to fight the cold, sterile, industrial, masculine hospital environment by focusing on her body, her power, her womanhood. The body in Belli's work is always a place of resistance (Inés Antón 2017, 162) and, as such, birth is represented as a moment of increased tenderness and danger, a moment of life and death, repeatedly disempowered through the hospital machinery, but which can be a moment of empowerment for a woman if she is in a safe environment, supported by doctors, nurses, and family members. Finally, the importance of these episodes is that they exist, and that they are being told. In a book about one of the most important Latin American revolutions of the twentieth century, these tales of childbirth figure prominently. Traditionally, stories of revolution focus on the battlefield and the mostly men who fight on them. Some may even present stories about love. Seldom do they ever highlight the challenges of childbirth. But even during war and revolution, children are born, and during that process, two lives hang in the balance: that of the mother and of the child. Belli shows that stories of childbirth are as much a part of the history of the Nicaraguan revolution as all the others; they are revolutionary stories of near death, of battles, of suffering, joy, and power.

## Case Study 2: An Indigenous Woman in Her Private Home in Guatemala—Community, Biopolitics, and Survival

The description of birth in the testimonio by Rigoberta Menchú, an Indigenous rights leader from Guatemala, is a very different one, but not any less political. As a testimonio and not an autobiography, it is far less concerned with the individual and, instead, it is all about community: Maya K'iche communal practices before and during childbirth and their relation to the survival of the community amid genocide. With *I, Rigoberta Menchú*, Menchú told her story and that of her people during the most violent years of the Guatemalan Civil War—the early 1980s—to call attention to the atrocities committed against the Indigenous population by the Guatemalan state and military. Menchú explains that at that moment in her life (at the age of 23 in 1982) she decides not to have a partner or children, because the fight for her people is far more pressing. Also, pregnancy and maternity are too dangerous since, at any time, she could be imprisoned, tortured, or killed (Burgos and Menchú 2009, 263–65).[4] Nonetheless, descriptions of Maya K'iche practices and rituals surrounding childbirth and maternity occupy an important place in Menchú's testimonio (7–19), and, in their context, contentious issues such as family planning and biopolitics in Guatemala emerge.

The community is paramount in the process, because, as Menchú (2009) explains, the child "belongs to the community not just to the parents" (8). Menchú clarifies that, traditionally, Maya women give birth at home, not at a hospital, where they are accompanied by members of the community (three married couples): the spouse, the godparents, and the husband and wife who serve as village leaders (the woman leader often occupying the role of midwife). Instead of having the mother give birth lying down, as is common in modern Western medicine, the woman delivers while standing, sometimes holding on to a rope that hangs from the ceiling to facilitate the birthing process. During and after pregnancy, emphasis is placed on putting the child in contact with nature. While pregnant, the expectant mother will go into the woods or the mountains to tell her future child about animals and plants, teaching it to respect nature and the community. The Maya describe themselves as people of corn, the most important agricultural crop in Mesoamerica. The child must learn that it comes from corn, that its mother ate this staple, and that it will be nourished similarly throughout its life. The mother also prepares the child for a life of suffering (Burgos and Menchú 2009, 8; 33). Only as part of the community will it be able to face this hardship. The child has to abide by community rules, integrate into the whole, be respectful, and take on the pain of existence, poverty, discrimination, and persecution (16–18).

Despite her recognition of the pain that Maya parents express about bringing another child into this world to suffer, Menchú is dismissive of family planning, which she sees as "a way of swindling the people, to get money out of them" (Burgos and Menchú 2009, 9). This is a brief comment in the testimonio, and Menchú does not elaborate further on this point (as put together by the anthropologist Elizabeth Burgos, who created the testimonio on the basis of interviews with Menchú). Yet behind this brief comment rises a mountain of contentious issues regarding reproductive rights, family planning, and biopolitics in Guatemala. For one, family planning attempts—which arrived in Guatemala via collaborations between local organizations and US aid as part of biopolitical aims of population control in the midst of the Cold War—were often met with resistance and suspicion in the country (Hartmann 2018, 126). Nationalist and left-wing groups saw it as undue US intervention, while Catholic groups perceived it as meddling in God's creation (Hartmann 2018, 129). In these debates, rumors and allegations of forced or involuntary sterilizations, especially of Indigenous women, were used to discredit family planning efforts (Hartmann 2018, 129–32). Given the absence of a substantial scholarly study on the issue of imposed sterilizations in Guatemala, the actuality and extent of these claims remains unclear (Clouser 2018, 778). For her part, Menchú never mentions the issue in her testimonio. Nonetheless, the general mistrust toward family planning should be seen not only in the context of traditional cultural systems (be it Catholic or Maya) but also in relation to the history of eugenics and health interventions without informed consent in Guatemala (for example, the US government-funded and supervised syphilis experiments in the 1940s in Guatemala),[5] and most importantly, the question of survival of Indigenous communities in the context of genocide during the Guatemalan civil war.

Menchú explains that the Maya see the birth of children as the survival of their community, of their knowledge, and of their way of life. As such, at a child's communal baptism, village leaders explicitly link the newborn to a shared destiny: "'Let no landowner extinguish all this, nor any rich man wipe out our customs'" (14). Menchú's skepticism toward birthing at hospitals and family planning thus points to multilayered issues at stake when it comes to providing culturally appropriate and acceptable healthcare services to diverse populations in Central America. It also underscores, once more, the highly political nature of conception, pregnancy, and childbirth that cannot be separated from the intersectional context in which they take place. Family planning services based on ample information and free will can provide important benefits for the community in relation to maternal and infant health outcomes, poverty, women's liberation, self-determination, sexual literacy, and well-being, but, in the wrong hands, these services can also be a tool of intrusive, destructive, and racist biopolitics.

### Case Study 3: A Mestiza Working-Class Woman, a Stillbirth, and a Prison in El Salvador

This section looks at the case of a mestiza woman in El Salvador, Teodora del Carmen Vásquez, who was sentenced to thirty years of prison after suffering an obstetric emergency in the bathroom at her workplace that resulted in the death of her baby. The Salvadoran Supreme Court commuted her sentence in 2018, after she had served ten years of her term. This case exemplifies state management and enforcement of strict policies of control over women's reproductive health in the Central American region. It illustrates how state agencies, with the support of medical professionals, enforce the legal prohibition on pregnancy termination by pursuing and investigating cases of miscarriage to determine whether a woman had some hand in inducing the episode. The courts, in turn, often interpret the law to treat women who have been hospitalized for miscarriages or suffered them at home just as harshly as women who had medically assisted or self-administered abortions.

In 1998, El Salvador amended its penal code to make abortion illegal in all circumstances, even when the mother's life is in danger, when she has been the victim of rape, or when the fetus is deformed (Kampwirth 2004, 103). Since then, at least forty-nine women have been convicted under these laws, serving decades-long sentences (Brigida 2018; Webber 2016). El Salvador's constitution, in fact, states that life begins at the moment of conception. In the region, Nicaragua shares a similarly strict law. Passed in 2006, the Nicaraguan law bans all abortions, reversing previous exceptions for those performed when the mother's life was in danger. Access to contraceptives and safe termination of pregnancy within these legal conditions constitute two of the most pressing issues regarding women's health in the Central American region.

Other Salvadoran women who have been affected by this law, tell the story of fainting or collapsing from an obstetric emergency and waking up handcuffed to a hospital bed (Webber 2016). These situations show how the nation's abortion law makes medical professionals complicit in law enforcement, creating a "culture of suspicion" (Webber 2016, n.p.) where healthcare workers fear losing their jobs for not reporting women who seek assistance for failed pregnancies (Webber 2016). The law can also lead institutions to treat women as potential criminals and expectant mothers to avoid seeking medical attention if they suffer pregnancy complications. According to Amnesty International (2018), in El Salvador: "women who suffer pregnancy-related complications resulting in miscarriages and stillbirths are routinely suspected of having an abortion. . . . Prosecutors often charge them with 'homicide' or even 'aggravated homicide,' which carries a penalty of up to 50 years in prison." That is precisely what happened to Teodora del Carmen Vásquez who received a 30-year sentence.

Public opinion and government pronouncements about Teodora Vásquez's case focused not on her wrongful conviction, nor on the potentially detrimental effects of the nation's abortion law in cases of obstetric distress, but rather on her successful rehabilitation into society. Even though the court commuted her sentence due to lack of evidence of willful termination, it refused to overturn the sentence itself. Official statements never conceded that Vásquez was wrongly convicted, as *El Faro* journalists point out (Ramos and Nóchez 2018). Headlines that appeared in mainstream newspapers in San Salvador cemented public opinion regarding the moral stance against pregnancy termination and fostered the presumption of Vásquez's guilt. *Diario el Mundo*, for example, used the headline: "This is How Teodora Vásquez was Liberated, Convicted of Killing her Baby" [*Así fue liberada Teodora Vásquez, condenada por matar a su bebé*] (Redacción 2018). *La Prensa Gráfica*, one of the capital's highest circulation newspapers, quoted the Vice Minister of Security in its headline: "Today We Turn Over a New Teodora to Society" [*Hoy entregamos a una nueva Teodora a la sociedad*] (Laguan and Abarca 2018).

Teodora Vásquez's case brings up several issues regarding women's access to reproductive care in El Salvador. By focusing on an extreme outcome of the abortion law—that a woman was persecuted and imprisoned for having a stillbirth—the press coverage indicates some recognition that the law could be problematic in instances of obstetric complications. The nation's interest in Teodora Vásquez's situation could, in fact, signal moderate societal acknowledgment of the strict nature of current abortion laws. While the controversy that this case generated could help—at least minimally—to push for the decriminalization of stillbirth, a number of deeper issues have been left untouched. Media and government discourses do not address, for example, the prohibition of abortions for women who have suffered sexual violence or whose very lives would be endangered by a pregnancy. Media representations of cases like this also tend to reinforce the societal appreciation of women as mothers above all else. Teodora Vásquez, for example, may be described in the press as one of the proverbial good ones—a good mother who certainly did not choose to abort her baby. Such coverage would thus seem to imply that motherhood is always desirable—if not obligatory—for all women, while elective abortions remain marginalized from the debate.

The press reportage that we analyzed also leaves out questions of privilege, access, and structural discrimination. This is a problematic exclusion, as it has been shown that a woman's socioeconomic class can determine if she will be prosecuted for stillbirth. Recently, for example, the Center for Reproductive Rights (2014) conducted a survey of 129 prosecution cases in El Salvador and found that the majority of the women were young, unmarried, and living in poverty or extreme economic dependence (41). The implications of this profile of prosecuted women are twofold. First, there is a correlation between poverty and pregnancy complications, because lack of resources makes it difficult for these expectant mothers to access healthcare if they experience symptoms of obstetric distress (Center for Reproductive Rights 2014, 41). Second, these women do not have the means to challenge their prosecution through proper legal counsel. This means that the Salvadoran state, in effect, criminalizes and imprisons women for lacking access to proper medical care. Middle- and upper-class women, on the other hand, can pay for a private clinic or go out of the country to have an abortion (Webber 2016). Additionally, as Teodora's own lawyer, Víctor Mata, explains, these more privileged women can more easily afford a lawyer to avoid jail sentences if they are suspected of aborting (Weiss and Patiño 2017).

Overall, Teodora Vásquez's conviction confirms the prevalence of reactionary views of women's reproductive health in a conservative, Catholic society. While mass media narratives acknowledge the criminalization of obstetric complications and emergencies, they tend to shy away from the controversial question of elective abortions. From a feminist perspective, the ultimate goal would be to grant women full reproductive rights, and this case shows that many struggles remain for women's and feminist groups in El Salvador. Between 2018 and the beginning of 2019, the Salvadoran Supreme Court began to change its stance. After commuting Teodora Vásquez's sentence, the tribunal began to reverse the sentences of other women imprisoned under similar circumstances. Despite these improvements, the situation in El Salvador brings into focus many unresolved issues: the existence of a law that criminalizes women seeking reproductive care, the rights and obligations of healthcare providers, and the continuation of cultural prejudices about childbearing. In the end, the many cases of imprisoned women in El Salvador show that the burden of these conflicts falls on poor, working-class women.

## Final Remarks

Overall, the three case studies in this chapter show that giving birth in Central America is a highly political issue. Through the struggles described in each situation, one can observe a society's divergent viewpoints on motherhood and womanhood and appreciate how the different categories that shape a woman's identity and experience in life—such as race and class—can impact her experience with childbirth. They also show that the region's revolutions of the 1970s and 1980s were often contentiously tied to questions of women's liberation. From these revolutionary experiences, autonomous women's movements formed across Central America in the 1990s, fighting for issues related to women's liberation. Gender-based violence and draconian abortion laws are among the biggest challenges faced by Central American women. Another consideration seen in the case studies presented is the common equation of womanhood with motherhood, although participation in revolutionary struggle has broken these molds to some degree. Other Central American voices have appeared that question the seemingly intrinsic link between womanhood and motherhood (Romero Meza 2016). Ultimately, reproductive rights and gender roles will continue to inspire intense debates within Central American societies.

## Notes

1. Prenatal or antenatal care is administered by an obstetrician or a midwife and includes advice on proper self-care and diet, weight checks to ensure appropriate weight gain, and monitoring from complications such as edema and preeclampsia. Prenatal care also includes access to proper vitamins, nutrition, and rest, conditions that can be difficult for poorer, working-class women to meet. The perinatal period is from 22 weeks of gestation to 7 days after birth and care received during this period is closely related to maternal health (WHO 2017).

2. On obstetric violence in Central America see Quintela Babio (2016). Gioconda Belli's autobiography (discussed later) also engages this topic.

3. Her experience in the public hospital does not mean that care in public hospitals is necessarily poor. In fact, Costa Rica is famous for having a relatively well-function-

ing public health system—but, since the care she receives there contrasts poorly to that which she receives in a private hospital, her experience shows the problem of underfunded and overcrowded healthcare systems.

4. Over a decade later she would get married and have a son.

5. For discussions of cases of forced sterilization in the United States, see the chapters by David S. Dalton and Benny J. Andres Jr. in this volume.

## References

Amnesty International. 2018. "El Salvador: Release of Woman Jailed for Stillbirth Must Signal End of Total Abortion Ban." February 15, 2018. https://www.amnesty.org/en/latest/news/2018/02/el-salvador-release-of-woman-jailed-for-stillbirth-must-signal-end-of-total-abortion-ban/.
Belli, Gioconda. 2002. *El país bajo mi piel. Memorias de amor y guerra.* New York: Vintage Español.
———. 2003. *The Country under My Skin. A Memoir of Love and War.* New York: Random House.
Brigida, Anna-Catherine. 2018. "Women Serving Decades-Long Prison Terms for Abortion in El Salvador Hope Change Is Coming." *Washington Post,* September 27, 2018. https://www.washingtonpost.com/world/the_americas/women-serving-decades-long-prison-terms-for-abortion-in-el-salvador-hope-change-is-coming/2018/09/26/0048119e-a62c-11e8-ad6f-080770dcddc2_story.html.
Burgos, Elizabeth, and Rigoberta Menchú. 2007. *Me llamo Rigoberta Menchú y así me nació la conciencia.* 20th ed. Mexico City: Siglo XXI Editores.
———. 2009. *I, Rigoberta Menchú. An Indian Woman in Guatemala.* Translated by Ann Wright. New York: Verso.
Center for Reproductive Rights. 2014. *Marginalized, Persecuted, and Imprisoned: The Effects of El Salvador's Total Criminalization of Abortion.* Center for Reproductive Rights; Agrupación Ciudadana por la Despenalización del Aborto Terapéutico, Ético y Eugenésico. https://www.reproductiverights.org/sites/crr.civicactions.net/files/documents/El-Salvador-CriminalizationOfAbortion-Report.pdf.
Central Intelligence Agency (CIA). n.d. "The World Factbook Country Comparison, Infant Mortality Rate." https://www.cia.gov/library/publications/the-world-factbook/rankorder/2091rank.html.
Clouser, Rebecca. 2018. "Reality and Rumour: The Grey Areas of International Development in Guatemala." *Third World Quarterly* 39 (4): 769–85. https://doi.org/10.1080/01436597.2017.1368380.
Hartmann, Annika. 2018. "Shaping Reproductive Freedom: Family Planning and Human Rights in Cold War Guatemala, 1960s–1970s." *Forum for Inter-American Research (Fiar)* 11 (3): 124–39.
Inés Antón, Tamara de. 2017. "Translating Central American Life Writing for the Anglophone Market: A Socio-Narrative Study of Women's Agency and Political Radicalism in the Original and Translated Works of Claribel Alegría, Gioconda Belli and Rigoberta Menchú." PhD diss., University of Manchester. https://www.research.manchester.ac.uk/portal/en/theses/translating-central-american-life-writing-for-

the-anglophone-market-a-socionarrative-study-of-womenas-agency-and-political-radicalism-in-the-original-and-translated-works-of-claribel-alegraa-gioconda-belli-and-rigoberta-mencha(9cab9568-fd8d-4107-9cf8-e09990d75c52).html.

Kampwirth, Karen. 2004. *Feminism and the Legacy of Revolution: Nicaragua, El Salvador, Chiapas.* Columbus: Ohio University Press.

Laguan, Jonathan, and Blanca Abarca. 2018. "'Hoy entregamos a una nueva Teodora a la sociedad': La reacción del viceministro de Seguridad tras la liberación de la salvadoreña acusada de matar a su bebé." *La Prensa Gráfica,* February 15, 2018. https://www.laprensagrafica.com/elsalvador/Hoy-entregamos-a-una-nueva-Teodora-a-la-sociedad-la-reaccion-del-viceministro-de-Seguridad-tras-la-liberacion-de-la-salvadorena-acusada-de-matar-a-su-bebe-20180215-0092.html.

Quintela Babio, Carmen. 2016. "Violencia obstétrica, el enemigo invisible dentro del sistema de salud." *Plaza Pública,* July 11, 2016. https://www.plazapublica.com.gt/content/el-enemigo-invisible-dentro-del-sistema-de-salud.

Ramos, Fred, and María Luz Nóchez. 2018. "Teodora recupera su libertad mas no su inocencia." *El Faro,* February 15, 2018. https://elfaro.net/es/201802/ef_foto/21486/Teodora-recupera-su-libertad-mas-no-su-inocencia.htm.

Redacción. 2018. "Así fue liberada Teodora Vásquez, condenada por matar a su bebé." *Diario El Mundo,* February 15, 2018. https://elmundo.sv/asi-fue-liberada-teodora-vasquez-condenada-por-matar-a-su-bebe/.

Romero Meza, Milagros. 2016. "Maternidades feministas: Experiencias y reflexiones en construcción." In *Las resistencias nuestras de cada día: Subversiones cotidianas a las violencias simbólicas,* edited by Ana Victoria Portocarrero and Edurne Larracoechea, 54–89. Antiguo Cuscatlán, El Salvador: UCA Publicaciones.

Sáenz, María del Rocío, Mónica Acosta, Jorine Muiser, and Juan Luis Bermúdez. 2011. "Sistema de Salud de Costa Rica." *Salud Pública de México* 53 (January): 156–67.

Sistema de las Naciones Unidas en Honduras. 2010. *Objetivos de desarrollo del milenio. Tercer informe de país: Honduras.* Sistema de las Naciones Unidas en Honduras. https://www.unicef.org/honduras/ODM5.pdf.

UN Data. 2019. "Infant Mortality Rate, for Both Sexes Combined." July 17, 2019. http://data.un.org/Data.aspx?d=PopDiv&f=variableID%3A77.

UN Inter-agency Group for Child Mortality Estimation, and United Nations Children's Fund (UNICEF). 2018. *Levels & Trends in Child Morality. Report 2018.* UNICEF, World Bank, World Health Organization (WHO), United Nations Population Division. https://data.unicef.org/wp-content/uploads/2018/09/UN-IGME-Child-Mortality-Report-2018.pdf.

Webber, Jude. 2016. "El Salvador's Anti-Abortion Laws: 'An Aggressive, Punitive Attack on Women.'" *Financial Times,* November 16, 2016. https://www.ft.com/content/68064cac-a484-11e6-8898-79a99e2a4de6.

Weiss, Jessica, and Andrea Patiño. 2017. "Fue condenada a 30 años por la muerte de su bebé en el parto: Ahora vuelve a juicio en El Salvador." *Univision,* December 5, 2017. https://www.univision.com/noticias/abortos/fue-condenada-a-30-anos-por-la-muerte-de-su-bebe-en-el-parto-ahora-vuelve-a-juicio-en-el-salvador.

World Health Organization (WHO). 2014. "Prevention and Elimination of Disrespect and Abuse during Childbirth." World Health Organization. September 3, 2014. http://

www.who.int/reproductivehealth/topics/maternal_perinatal/statement-childbirth/en/.

———. 2015. *Trends in Maternal Mortality: 1990 to 2015. Estimates by WHO, UNICEF, UNFPA, World Bank Group and the United Nations Population Division.* World Health Organization.

———. 2017. "More Women Worldwide Receive Early Antenatal Care, but Great Inequalities Remain." December 5 2017. http://www.who.int/reproductivehealth/early-anc-worldwide/en/.

# PART IV

## Healthcare in the Andean Region

# 11

## A Revolution in Healthcare?
The Politics of Public Health in Postrevolutionary Bolivia

Nicole L. Pacino

A social revolution in Bolivia in April 1952 brought the Movimiento Nacionalista Revolucionario [Revolutionary Nationalist Movement] or MNR to power and precipitated major changes to the country's political climate, social structure, and economy. The MNR vowed to make the country more modern, productive, and equitable. One of the promises that the MNR made to Bolivians was to improve people's quality of life. To this end, after 1952, the MNR dramatically expanded public health services, especially in rural areas. Newly built health centers and mobile units staffed by recently trained nurses and auxiliary medical personnel brought healthcare to areas of the country where such amenities had been virtually nonexistent. Yet, accessible healthcare in remote rural regions was not merely an altruistic offering by the MNR to its constituents; it was also paternalistic. This health infrastructure gave the government a presence in rural regions and an opportunity to secure political loyalty from voters enfranchised for the first time by a 1952 universal suffrage decree. This expansion of public health programs after 1952, therefore, helped the MNR consolidate political power and court rural voters.

This chapter addresses the following question: What is the relationship between politics and public health during moments of political and social upheaval? Specifically, I look at public health's pivotal role in Bolivia's postrevolutionary politics and explain how healthcare became a tool for state building and political consolidation. I will also briefly compare the Bolivian case to that of its neighbors, Perú and Ecuador, that experienced their own periods of state expansion during this time. This comparison highlights unique attributes of Bolivia's postrevolutionary moment while identifying patterns in the relationship between health and politics across the Andes in the mid-twentieth century. This case study demonstrates that healthcare is never truly altruistic or apolitical; instead, public health often serves political objectives.

## Public Health, Politics, and Revolution

There is a tendency to see politics and healthcare as unrelated—public health is objective, scientific, and evidence-based, while politics involves backdoor dealing, persuasion, and propaganda. However, the definition of public health itself highlights the relationship between politics and health: government entities are responsible for protecting the general population, preventing widespread threats to health, and promoting healthy living. Federal agencies such as the Centers for Disease Control and Prevention (CDC) and the Food and Drug Administration (FDA) in the United States rely on public authority to safeguard populations from health threats because people have to believe that these agencies are working to protect the public from everything from epidemics to foodborne illnesses. These agencies' reach and funding are tied to political processes, as politicians in the legislative and executive branches determine budgets and mandates (L. Brown 2010, 156–60).

Therefore, it behooves us, as Lawrence D. Brown (2010) suggests, to "study public health politically . . . [which means we need] to inquire how public institutions and actors (executives, legislatures, courts, bureaucracies, subnational governments) and stakeholders in the private and voluntary sectors (interest groups, the media) shape the formulation and implementation of policies and programs the public health field proposes and pursues" (157). For instance, government interventions into people's private affairs—such as what they eat, how and when they regulate fertility, and whether or not their children are vaccinated—extend the role of the national government beyond electoral politics and economic regulation. However, these same interventions tend to raise questions about government legitimacy and whether or not it has the right to encroach on personal liberty and dictate private decisions.

To study public health politically takes on added significance in the context of a social revolution or a moment of political upheaval or disruption. Social revolutions, like the one that happened in Bolivia in 1952, are relatively rare, but they are significant events that shed light on how political public health can be. Revolutions disrupt the ordinary functions of the state. They also lead to the implementation of new political systems, bring new groups of people to power, and enfranchise popular groups. Leaders who take power through social revolutions find themselves in a precarious position because the people that supported their movement will inevitably make demands upon the new political authority. Since common causes of social revolutions include poverty, inequality, political marginalization and repression, and economic hardship, it is likely that these groups will call for the new government to improve average citizens' general quality of life. Even if these demands do not directly include healthcare improvement and access, other social or economic changes might indirectly lead to better health outcomes (Eckstein 1982, 79–80). Would we expect, as some scholars have suggested, that countries that have had social revolutions would have better healthcare provision than those that had not? While there is some debate about the extent to which social revolutions have positively impacted healthcare, there does seem to be a correlation between social revolutions and improvements in health and welfare (Eckstein 1982; Horn 1983).

Certain trends are evident in Latin American countries where social revolutions occurred in the twentieth century.[1] First, healthcare indicators did generally improve; second, people increased pressure on the state to improve healthcare; and third, postrevolutionary governments pointed to these advancements as evidence of their commitment to bettering lives. For instance, the Mexican Revolution, which lasted from 1910 to 1920, changed people's expectations about what social services the government should provide. Both medical professionals and ordinary citizens demanded better access to healthcare for the country's most impoverished sectors (Soto Laveaga and Agostoni 2011; and Bliss and Hernandez Berrones in this anthology). Mexican doctors and government officials used public health to advance political objectives and even claimed responsibility for improvements in public health made prior to the Revolution (Birn 2006; Bliss 2010; Kapelusz-Poppi 2001). After Nicaragua's 1979 Sandinista Revolution, access to medical care improved despite the economic and political crises of the 1980s (Garfield and Williams 1989). Similarly, in spite of ongoing economic hardship, Cuba's health indicators are among the best in the world as a consequence of the health system implemented after Fidel Castro's victory in 1959 (De Vos 2005; Eckstein 1982). In Bolivia, thanks to government investment in social services, the popular perception among the Indigenous population was that the MNR improved quality of life even as economic inequality grew (Kelley and Klein 1981, 119).

Revolutions, therefore, allow us to examine the political uses of public health for two reasons. First, citizens of revolutionary societies often see these moments as opportunities to make demands on the state. Second, from the perspective of the state, healthcare provision is one means of showing its commitment to transforming society.

## The Bolivian Revolution

On April 9, 1952, revolution erupted in Bolivia's capital city of La Paz. The military government had prevented the MNR party from taking power after winning an election in 1951, leading to outcry and political mobilization. The MNR's revolution enjoyed widespread support from a variety of Bolivia's popular sectors, including students and miners. After three days of fighting and minimal bloodshed contained to Bolivia's principal cities, the MNR took control of the government on April 11, 1952 (Alexander 1958; Dunkerley 1984; Malloy 1970).

Between 1952 and 1964, the MNR government attempted to transform Bolivian society through three reforms: universal suffrage, nationalization of the tin mining industry, and agrarian reform. A universal suffrage decree, issued in July 1952, gave illiterate, female, and Indigenous Bolivians the right to vote for the first time and expanded the voting population from about 200,000 to over one million out of roughly three million inhabitants (Klein 1992, 232). 85 percent of registered voters participated in 1956 in the first post-Revolution presidential election, and support for the MNR in rural areas (approximately two-thirds of the population) was overwhelming (Alexander 1958, 57–79). In October 1952, the MNR government nationalized the tin mining industry and targeted foreign-owned corporations in order to reinvest mining profits in Bolivia's domestic economy (Malloy 1970, 72–78). Finally, in August 1953 came the Agrarian Reform Law. Before the Revolution, 5 percent of landholders owned 70 percent of agricultural land; the 1953 law redistributed this land to peasants so that they could become economically solvent and contribute to national development (Alexander 1958, 57–79). These reforms attempted to foster economic growth based on national production and move toward independence from foreign corporations. They also focused on economic diversification and investment in physical infrastructure, such as building roads.

Changing Bolivia's economic system was not the MNR's only priority. The party also wanted to improve daily living conditions and address centuries of social inequality that benefited a small wealthy class at the expense of working-class and Indigenous populations. Universal suffrage was one means of dismantling an exclusionary political system and opening new channels for civic participation. Social programs, such as a 1955 education reform (Contreras 2003) and the development of a national system of sanitary services, complemented these economic and political reforms. Expanding access to public health services was an early MNR priority tantamount to the economic and political reforms that defined the revolutionary era.

MNR leaders were both "genuinely committed to social reform" (Kelley and Klein 1981, 100) and a "reluctant band of revolutionaries" (Malloy 1970, 171); they wanted to radically transform Bolivian society but also wanted to control the process and were wary of giving popular groups too much power or influence. The trick for the MNR party was to balance the former, which led to increased investment in social services, with the latter, which caused it to co-opt some of Bolivia's more radical sectors, such as the miners. The MNR enacted its main political and economic reforms during a "period of initial radicalism" (Whitehead 2003, 29) between 1952 and 1956. The remaining years (1956–1964) have been called a "revolution in retreat" because the MNR tempered its policies and focused on consolidating power, fostering political loyalty, and convincing the US government to provide financial aid to the struggling country (Dunkerley 1984, 83–119). At this point, economic austerity measures and the MNR government's growing acquiescence to US political concerns made more radical allies, like the miners, vocal critics of the regime. A military coup in 1964 removed the MNR party from power and led to a period of military dictatorship and political repression.

Despite the MNR's growing political conservatism after 1956, the government continued to invest in expanding healthcare access in the countryside in the form of clinics, mobile units, and personnel. These initiatives supported, rather than diverged from, the party's attempts to consolidate political power and foster loyalty in the newly enfranchised Indigenous population.

## The Postrevolutionary Expansion of Healthcare

The basic framework for post-1952 public health programs built upon pre-revolutionary initiatives, but linked them to the politics of the postrevolutionary period (Larson 2003). Public health increased in national importance throughout the 1920s and 1930s and gradually became more centralized. In 1936, health was part of an institution that also focused on labor and social welfare. A separate Ministry of Health and Hygiene [Ministerio de Higiene y Salubridad] was created in 1938 (Zulawski 2007, 160). Prior to

1952, some basic health infrastructure existed, but it was generally only accessible in cities. The MNR sought to change this dynamic and dramatically expanded the healthcare system, especially in rural areas.

In 1900, only 142 registered doctors practiced medicine in Bolivia, and their services were limited to urban centers (Zulawski 2007, 27). Physicians tended to congregate in cities, where they had better pay, professional opportunities, and modern medical facilities. A 1953 report noted that "the entire medical profession was serving only one-third of the population" (Association of Schools of Public Health 1953, 1244). By 1955, the Public Health Ministry [Ministerio de Salud Pública] (MSP) reported that 795 registered doctors and 79 licensed midwives attended to Bolivia's approximately three million inhabitants, a fivefold increase since the beginning of the century (Ministerio de Salud Pública 1960–1961, 23).

The expansion of public health-related infrastructure in terms of institutions, personnel, and access to services helps document this process. In the early 1950s, the MNR focused on constructing buildings, such as hospitals, clinics, rural posts, and mobile units, and creating training programs for health workers. Both of these initiatives were possible due to the MNR's ongoing relationship with the Cooperative Inter-American Health Service [Servicio Cooperativo Interamericano de Salud Pública] (SCISP), which operated in Bolivia from 1942 to 1963 and was jointly funded by the United States and Bolivian governments, but operated under the Bolivian Health Ministry's auspices (Zulawski 2007, 105). SCISP emphasized apprenticeship training in rural areas for Bolivian doctors and nurses and helped build health centers outside of Bolivia's largest cities (Pacino 2016).

The first health center was built in La Paz in 1943. By 1952, when the MNR took power, there were nine health centers in six of Bolivia's nine provinces, and by 1959 there were eighteen fully operational ones across the country. Large health centers located in cities served sizable urban populations. Medium-sized health centers, stationed in provincial capitals, served populations of 8,000 to 40,000 inhabitants, each with a staff of 10 to 20 employees. Small health centers in remote locations served populations of 2,000 to 10,000 inhabitants with 5 to 10 employees each (A. Brown 1959, 11). Health centers provided preventive medical care, including maternal and infant health and immunizations, as well as treatment for diseases. These services expanded during the 1940s and 1950s; while the program served just 1,000 people in 1943, in 1955 it treated 57,275 individual patients. By 1956, SCISP estimated that its programs reached one-fifth of Bolivia's total population (National Archives and Record Administration 1956). To supplement the health center program, mobile brigades staffed by a doctor, a sanitary inspector, and a vaccinator traveling in a vehicle equipped with a projector and educational films extended preventive care beyond health center sites. They visited dispensaries run by auxiliary nurses to give immunizations and provide emergency medical attention, screened health-related films, and distributed health literature to encourage families to recognize symptoms and seek medical treatment (A. Brown 1959, 14).

SCISP also helped the MNR train auxiliary medical personnel to further expand health services to remote areas. To augment the lack of doctors, training programs for midwives, nurses, sanitary inspectors, social workers [*visitadoras sociales*], and even school teachers increased the number of licensed individuals associated with national public health. In 1954, the MNR mandated an obligatory year of rural service for doctors and nurses to ensure that underserved populations had access to medical care (Flores Céspedes and Centro de Investigaciones Sociales 1976, 78). This growing corps of trained medical personnel operated in an increasing number of hospitals, health centers, rural sanitary posts, and mobile units.

In the late 1950s, new institutional and administrative programs combined different public health programs and streamlined their execution. For instance, the National Health Service [Servicio Nacional de Salud] was formed in 1958 to coordinate all public health activities overseen by state institutions (Mendizábal Lozano 2002, 215). The Sanitary Code [Código Sanitario], also enacted in 1958, codified the functions of various state public health entities and defined health as both a "primordial state responsibility" and a "fundamental right of the people" (Ministerio de Salud Pública 1958, 3). The 1961 Constitution incorporated this language and, for the first time, guaranteed health as a basic right, differentiating it from the 1938 Constitution, which defined health as the state's responsibility, but not a fundamental right of citizenship (Mendizábal Lozano 2002, 208).

Morbidity and mortality rates show that access to rural healthcare did improve during the MNR's tenure: in 1960, MNR leaders pointed to a network of rural health centers, disease eradication projects, and medical training programs as evidence of its commitment to improving Bolivians' lives (Movimiento Nacionalista Revolucionario 1960, 98–105). In 1960, there were about 3,700 Bolivians per doctor (down from about 20,000 per doctor in 1900), and the population per hospital bed was 580. Infant mortality rates also declined from 123 deaths per 1,000 live births between 1945 and 1949 to 76.5 deaths per 1,000 live births in 1965, meaning more children survived beyond the first year of life in the 1960s than in previous decades (Eckstein 1982, 82–83). Reported incidences of disease also decreased during this period. Between 1952 and 1960, the number of reported cases of malaria, smallpox, tuberculosis, polio, syphilis, and diphtheria declined significantly, and smallpox was considered completely eradicated as of 1960 (Pan-American Health Organization 1962; Pan-American Sanitary Bureau 1954, 19).

## Public Health and the Consolidation of Political Power

Health centers, training programs, and disease control efforts gave the MNR a feasible way to advance its public health agenda and spread state presence into rural areas. After 1952, MNR leaders wanted to fulfill promises of national progress and transformation, expand the reach of the national government, and generate political loyalty. The government sought to extend its presence into rural Bolivia in many ways, including state-sponsored peasant unions and road-building projects (Alexander 1958, 172–175; Malloy 1970, 203–215; Rivera Cusicanqui 1987). An expanding medical infrastructure in the form of clinics, mobile units, and licensed personnel also created state presence and fostered political loyalty through paternalistic means. In places with vast territory and dispersed populations like Bolivia and Mexico, public health incursions were often the first state-sponsored activity in the countryside, and national governments gained legitimacy by providing services to rural communities (Birn 1998, 44).

Despite the political utility of these programs, the MNR government did not impose them upon rural communities. Both the MNR and Bolivia's rural population politicized public health in the 1950s for their own purposes. While the MNR used public health initiatives to expand state influence and cultivate political loyalty from rural populations, rural communities demanded access to available state services, often for the first time, under the MNR government. Thousands of letters sent to the MNR authority by rural communities throughout the 1950s document the same general requests for government services: access to a medical professional (doctor, nurse, or vaccinator) and/or medicines and construction of a medical facility, either by the state or through funds for the community to build their own (Pacino 2019). Written correspondence from Health Minister Julio Manuel Aramayo demonstrates that the government responded to these demands, or at least acknowledged them. Even when Aramayo only promised to take them under consideration for the following budget, or allotted less money than requested, he acknowledged that national leadership could not ignore these demands. If the MNR desired to consolidate its power in rural areas, it needed to attend to rural inhabitants' requests. The overall result was better access to healthcare for rural citizens and a visible state presence in these regions in the form of public health infrastructure and licensed medical professionals.

## Public Health and Politics in the Andes

Like Bolivia, Perú and Ecuador experienced similar moments of political instability and social reform in the 1950s and 1960s, although the conditions were different from those in Bolivia. Bolivia's situation can be characterized as a "revolution from below;" Perú's "revolution from above" occurred when General Juan Velasco Alvarado seized power in a coup d'état in 1968. In contrast to other military coups that occurred in Latin America during the mid- to late twentieth century,[2] Velasco Alvarado headed a left-leaning military government and used state power to enact land reform and nationalize foreign-owned industries, most notably in the oil sector (Eckstein 1982, 44). Unlike Bolivia, where miners and peasants pushed the MNR's reforms to become more radical than they originally intended, in Perú the masses were mostly passive participants in the process of social change (Aguirre and Drinot 2017, 6). Velasco Alvarado was eventually ousted by another military coup in 1975.

Like in Bolivia from the 1950s to the 1970s, Perú's healthcare sector went through a period of professionalization, expansion, and reorganization. During the 1950s and 1960s, training programs for doctors, administrators, nurses, and other auxiliary health personnel proliferated, often with the assistance of the Peruvian SCISP (Bustíos Romaní and Arroyo Aguilar 2018). The military government also enacted a series of laws between 1969 and 1975 to better organize and consolidate health services, including a Sanitary Code in 1969 that was similar to Bolivia's 1958 law (Bustíos Romaní 1985, 1–2). Velasco Alvarado placed great emphasis on maternal and infant care initiatives because he saw population as a source of wealth and economic development. For this reason, he reversed family planning initiatives popularized during the 1960s in favor of a pronatalist agenda. By 1974, all labor, delivery, and postpartum care in Ministry of Health facilities were free (Necochea López 2014, 114 and 121). Like in Bolivia, these initiatives were paternalistic rather than altruistic; they served the military government's political and economic objectives.

In comparison with Bolivia, Perú's health indicators show slightly better ratios of population per doctor (2,400 in 1960 and 1,820 in 1976) and population per hospital bed (580 in 1960 versus 450 in 1970). Infant mortality also declined during Velasco Alvarado's time in office, from 74 to 65 deaths per 1,000 live births between 1965 and 1970, although this trend was already evident before 1968 (Eckstein 1982, 82–83). According to these measures, healthcare access was slightly better in Perú than in Bolivia during this time period.

We know less about how political upheaval affected healthcare organization and access in Ecuador during the mid-twentieth century. Ecuador's leftist military coup came earlier than Perú's. Known as the July Revolution, a group of reform-minded junior army officers led a bloodless coup and established a military junta as the ruling political authority in 1925. The 1920s through the 1940s were also a period of state building and public health expansion, specifically in the realms of disease control and maternal and infant health (Clark 2012, 2015). Little has been written about how public health fared in the period after 1950, although Ecuador did have its own reformist governments. President José María Velasco Ibarra, a populist who held office five times between the 1930s and the 1970s (only completing one full term), emphasized infrastructure development, including building hospitals (Lauderbaugh 2012, 110–20). Although Velasco Ibarra initiated the discussion about agrarian reform during one of his presidencies, a military junta that deposed Velasco Ibarra and his successor finally enacted agrarian reform in 1964. In this way, social reform in Ecuador, like in Perú, came in the form of top-down decrees from a ruling military junta.

**Contemporary Context**

A series of unexpected events rocked Bolivia during October and November 2019. Evo Morales, Bolivia's first Indigenous president, ran for re-election on the ticket of his party, the Movement Towards Socialism [Movimiento al Socialismo] (MAS) despite controversy over his eligibility to do so. The election, which was held on October 20, appeared to give Morales the necessary margin of victory to avoid a run-off with his closest rival. However, a twenty-four hour pause in the result reporting generated reports of fraud and vote tampering that prompted weeks of protest across the country from diverse sectors, including Morales opponents and former supporters. Calls for his resignation originated from popular sectors, most notably the trade unionists. Morales also lost the support of the police and military. After agreeing to hold new elections, Morales and his vice president, along with several other MAS officials, resigned on November 10. The serial resignations left a power vacuum, as the positions in the traditional order of succession were vacated. After several days, Jeanine Áñez, opposition party member and highest-ranking Senate official after the resignations, assumed the presidency on November 12 without congressional approval, but with the blessing of the national court. Violence and repression ensued in the following days. Despite the interim government's only mandate to hold new elections, the new government vowed to roll back many of the major reforms of the Evo years.

During his tenure in office, which lasted from 2006 to 2019, Morales oversaw a series of policies and reforms designed to better acknowledge and incorporate the country's diverse Indigenous peoples into political life. A new national health policy, the Family Community Intercultural Health Policy [Salud Familiar Comunitaria Intercultural], implemented in 2008, aimed to address major inequities in healthcare access in a majority Indigenous nation (Bernstein 2017). This innovative policy looked to pair Indigenous medical practices with biomedical approaches to make healthcare more approachable, accessible, and culturally sensitive, and has been described as an attempt to "decolonize" healthcare. However, it was hard to implement and led to mixed results (Johnson 2010). There has been some improvement in eradicating inequities, although as a pathway to universal health coverage and primary care access, it is an imperfect and unfinished process (Heaton et al. 2014). Despite the limited successes of the intercultural health program, the initiative made progress in addressing historical inequities in terms of access to quality medical care and making public health more culturally sensitive. Those gains were potentially under threat from the interim government (Hartmann 2019).

New elections were scheduled for May 2020, but the interim government postponed them due to lockdown orders issued in response to the COVID-19 pandemic. The elections were rescheduled for September 6, but were postponed again until October 18. Critics claimed that Áñez, who ran in the general election, kept postponing the election in a bid to remain in power. Her government also came under scrutiny for its handling of the pandemic—as of May 2021, Bolivia, which has a population of roughly 11 million, has registered more than 300,000 cases and 13,000 deaths, according to the World Health Organization's COVID-19 dashboard (World Health Organization 2020).

The general election was finally held on October 18, 2020, and the MAS candidate, Luis Arce, won the election outright. Official observers documented no evidence of fraud. The extent of Arce's win shocked most political observers, but it is a good example of the politics of public health. It is quite possible that the interim government's handling of the pandemic undercut its already tenuous legitimacy and bolstered support for a flailing MAS party. It is far too early to predict what will happen to the healthcare programs initiated by the Morales government, but it is reasonable to conclude that a new MAS administration will continue or even expand the programs of the previous one.

## Conclusions

A few general trends in public health provision are evident in the Andes in the mid-twentieth century. First, reformist governments looked to expand access to healthcare to marginalized regions and populations. Second, these moments of public health expansion focused on maternal and infant health initiatives and disease treatment and prevention. Finally, Andean governments built infrastructure to provide services to needy populations, including hospitals and other edifices in remote regions.

Reform-minded governments oversaw these healthcare improvements, but only in Bolivia did they come about as a result of a social revolution with popular participation. Since the MNR came to power with the support of a broad cross section of Bolivian civil society, the party had to cater to the demands of popular sectors. Public health expansion was not merely imposed upon rural populations; evidence shows that rural communities embraced, and even demanded, these government-sponsored initiatives. It is clear that public health programs fulfilled some of the MNR's other objectives, like giving the national government more of a presence in rural regions and encouraging Bolivians in these areas to vote for the party that acted in their best interests. However, healthcare access improved and indicators rose as a result of a combination of state programs and popular demand. In comparison, in Perú and Ecuador improved healthcare access was a top-down initiative imposed by left-leaning military governments. There is currently little evidence that these military rulers, who came to power through political coups, responded to popular demand in the realm of healthcare.

The public health reforms undertaken in these three cases were neither completely altruistic nor apolitical. Regardless of the type of government in power, expanding public health programs helped bolster state legitimacy, gain popular support, and showcase government intent to provide for its citizens' well-being. This reality is especially evident in the context of Bolivia's social revolution, as the MNR had to navigate between its own political ambitions and the demands placed upon it by popular groups empowered by the 1952 revolution. When we "study public health politically" (L. Brown 2010, 157) we can better see the connections between politics, health programs, and health outcomes, showing that they are inextricably linked.

## Notes

1. Theda Skocpol's (1979) definition is that "social revolutions are rapid, basic transformations of a society's state and class structures; and they are accompanied and in part carried through by class-based revolts from below" (4). This definition is based in Marxist theory, as was the dominant scholarly trend at the time, and subsequent theorists of revolution have revised it to include not just the "Great Revolutions" Skocpol identified (France, Russia, China), but also a variety of armed insurrections, guerrilla organizations, and social movements. The key factor for something to be labeled a social revolution is the participation of popular sectors of society. In Latin America, beyond the examples identified in this paragraph, which were all armed insurrections that took state power, we could point to Guatemala 1944–1954 and Chile 1970–1973 as examples of social revolutions that took place within existing democratic institutions.

2. See, for example, Guatemala 1954, Bolivia 1964 and 1971, Brazil 1964, Chile 1973, Argentina 1976, and El Salvador 1979.

## References

Aguirre, Carlos, and Paulo Drinot. 2017. "Introduction." In *The Peculiar Revolution: Rethinking the Peruvian Experiment under Military Rule*, edited by Carlos Aguirre and Paulo Drinot, 1–23. Austin: University of Texas Press.

Alexander, Robert J. 1958. *The Bolivian National Revolution.* New Brunswick, NJ: Rutgers University Press.

Association of Schools of Public Health. 1953 "Programs and Problems in Professional Education and Inservice Training of Health Personnel." *Public Health Reports* 68 (12): 1243–49.

Bernstein, Alissa. 2017. "Personal and Political Histories in the Designing of Health Reform Policy in Bolivia." *Social Science & Medicine* 177: 231–38.

Birn, Anne-Emanuelle. 1998. "A Revolution in Rural Health?: The Struggle over Local Health Units in Mexico, 1928–1940." *Journal of the History of Medicine* 53: 43–76.

———. 2006. *Marriage of Convenience: Rockefeller International Health and Revolutionary Mexico.* Rochester, NY: University of Rochester Press.

Bliss, Katherine Elaine. 2010. *Compromised Positions: Prostitution, Public Health, and Gender Politics in Revolutionary Mexico City.* University Park: Pennsylvania State University Press.

Brown, Antonio. 1959. *Resumen de las actividades del SCISP en Bolivia, 1942–1959.* La Paz: Ministerio de Salud Pública.

Brown, Lawrence D. 2010. "The Political Face of Public Health." *Public Health Reports* 32 (1): 155–73.

Bustíos Romaní, Carlos. 1985. *Atención médica y su contexto, Perú, 1963–1983.* Lima: Ministerio de Salud.

Bustíos Romaní, Carlos, and Ruth Arroyo Aguilar. 2018. "Profesionalización de la salud pública y la capacitación de sanitaristas en el Perú: 1935–1968." *Anales de la Facultad de Medicina* 79 (3): 252–61.

Clark, A. Kim. 2012. *Gender, State, and Medicine in Highland Ecuador: Modernizing Women, Modernizing the State, 1895–1950*. Pittsburgh: University of Pittsburgh Press.
———. 2015. "New Arenas of State Action in Highland Ecuador: Public Health and State Formation, c. 1925–1950." In *State Theory and Andean Politics: New Approaches to the Study of Rule*, edited by Christopher Krupa and David Nugent, 126–41. University Park: University of Pennsylvania Press.
Contreras, Manuel E. 2003. "A Comparative Perspective on Education Reforms in Bolivia, 1950–2000." In *Proclaiming Revolution: Bolivia in Comparative Perspective*, edited by Merilee Grindle and Pilar Domingo, 259–86. Cambridge: Harvard University Press.
De Vos, Pol. 2005. "'No one left abandoned': Cuba's National Health System since the 1959 Revolution." *International Journal of Health Services* 35 (1): 189–207.
Dunkerley, James. 1984. *Rebellion in the Veins: Political Struggle in Bolivia, 1952–82*. London: Verso Editions.
Eckstein, Susan. 1982. "The Impact of Revolution on Social Welfare in Latin America." *Theory and Society* 11 (1): 43–94.
Flores Céspedes, Gonzalo, and Centro de Investigaciones Sociales. 1976. *Las condiciones de salud de la población boliviana*. La Paz: Ediciones CIS.
Garfield, Richard, and Glen Williams. 1989. *Health and Revolution: The Nicaraguan Experience*. Oxford: Oxfam.
Hartmann, Chris. 2019. "Bolivia's Plurinational Healthcare Revolution will not be Defeated." *NACLA*. December 19, 2019.
Heaton, Tim B., Benjamin Crookston, Renata Forste, and David Knowlton. 2014. "Inequalities in Child Health in Bolivia: Has Morales Made a Difference?" *Health Sociology Review* 23 (3): 208–18.
Horn, James J. 1983. "The Mexican Revolution and Health Care, or the Health of the Mexican Revolution." *Latin American Perspectives* 10 (4): 24–39.
Johnson, Brian B. 2010. "Decolonization and its Paradoxes: The (Re)envisioning of Health Policy in Bolivia." *Latin American Perspectives* 37 (3): 139–59.
Kapelusz-Poppi, Ana María. 2001. "Rural Health and State Construction in Post-Revolutionary Mexico: The Nicolaita Project for Rural Medical Services." *The Americas* 58 (2): 261–83.
Kelley, Jonathan, and Herbert Klein. 1981. *Revolution and the Rebirth of Inequality: A Theory Applied to the National Revolution in Bolivia*. Berkeley: University of California Press.
Klein, Herbert S. 1992. *Bolivia: The Evolution of a Multi-Ethnic Society*. Oxford: Oxford University Press.
Larson, Brooke. 2003. "Capturing Indian Bodies, Hearths, and Minds: The Gendered Politics of Rural School Reform in Bolivia, 1910–52." In *Proclaiming Revolution: Bolivia in Comparative Perspective*, edited by Merilee Grindle and Pilar Domingo, 183–209. Cambridge: Harvard University Press.
Lauderbaugh, George. 2012. *The History of Ecuador*. Santa Barbara, CA: Greenwood.
Malloy, James M. 1970. *Bolivia: The Uncompleted Revolution*. Pittsburgh: University of Pittsburgh Press.

Mendizábal Lozano, Gregorio. 2002. *Historia de la salud pública en Bolivia: De las juntas de sanidad a los directorios locales de salud.* La Paz: OPS/OMS.
Ministerio de Salud Pública. 1958. *Código Sanitario de la República de Bolivia.* La Paz: Editorial Don Bosco.
Ministerio de Salud Pública. *Informe de Labores, 1960–1961.* Archivo Nacional de Bolivia (Sucre), Presidencia de la República, 1659.
Movimiento Nacionalista Revolucionario. 1960. *Programa de Gobierno Movimiento Nacionalista Revolucionario: Tercer Gobierno de la Revolución Nacional (1960–1964), aprobado por la VIII Convención del MNR* La Paz: Movimiento Nacionalista Revolucionario.
National Archives and Record Administration. 1956. "Notes for a Brief Interpretation of the Servicio Cooperativo Interamericano de Salud Pública in Bolivia," August 17, 1956. Records of the US Foreign Assistance Agencies, 1948–1961, ICA-USOM, 1955–1960, P 219, box 9, Record Group 469, National Archives and Record Administration, Washington DC.
Necochea López, Raúl. 2014. *A History of Family Planning in Twentieth-Century Peru.* Chapel Hill: University of North Carolina Press.
Pacino, Nicole. 2016. "Stimulating a Cooperative Spirit?: Public Health and US-Bolivia Relations in the 1950s." *Diplomatic History* 41 (2): 305–35.
———. 2019. "Bringing the Revolution to the Countryside: Rural Public Health Programmes as State-Building in Post-1952 Bolivia." *Bulletin of Latin American Research* 38 (1): 50–65.
Pan-American Health Organization. 1962. "Summary of Four-Year Reports on Health Conditions in the Americas, 1957–1960." Washington, DC: Pan-American Health Organization, July 1962.
Pan-American Sanitary Bureau, XIV Pan American Sanitary Conference, VI Meeting Regional Committee, Santiago, Chile, 1954. "Summary of Reports of the Member States, 1950–1953," Sept. 10, 1954. Rockefeller Archive Center, Rockefeller Foundation collection, record group 2.1954, series 200, box 21, folder 148.
Rivera Cusicanqui, Silvia. 1987. *Oppressed but not Defeated: Peasant Struggles among the Aymara and Qhechwa in Bolivia, 1900–1980.* Geneva: United Nations Research Institution for Social Development.
Skocpol, Theda. 1979. *States and Social Revolutions: A Comparative Analysis of France, Russia, and China.* Cambridge: Cambridge University Press.
Soto Laveaga, Gabriela, and Claudia Agostoni. 2011. "Science and Public Health in the Century of Revolution." In *A Companion Guide to Mexican History and Culture,* edited by William Beezley, 561–74. Oxford: Blackwell Publishing.
Whitehead, Laurence. 2003. "The Bolivian National Revolution: A Twenty-First Century Perspective." In *Proclaiming Revolution: Bolivia in Comparative Perspective,* edited by Marilee Grindle and Pilar Domingo, 25–53. Cambridge: Harvard University Press.
World Health Organization. 2020. WHO Coronavirus Disease (COVID-19) Dashboard. Accessed September 28, 2020. https://covid19.who.int/?gclid=EAIaIQobChMIya-s5tXu6wIViODICh0zkQVgEAAYASAAEgItMfD_BwE
Zulawski, Ann. 2007. *Unequal Cures: Public Health and Political Change in Bolivia, 1900–1950.* Durham: Duke University Press.

# 12

## Maternal and Child Health in the Andean Region

Renata Forste

Drawing upon demographic data, this chapter highlights improvements in maternal and child health in the Andean region, as well as continuing challenges. This region includes the countries of Bolivia, Colombia, Ecuador, Peru, and Venezuela. Although there have been improvements in maternal and child health in South America over the past fifty years, the highest mortality rates are still found in the Andean region, particularly in Bolivia (Kent 2010a; UNICEF 2019); overall, Latin America continues to be one of the most unequal regions of the world in terms of income inequality (Lustig 2015). Additionally, the Andean region includes many of the poorest countries in South America, and within countries, there are profound economic disparities (Messina and Silva 2017).

The greatest challenges to maternal and child health in the Andean region are linked to high levels of poverty, particularly in rural, Indigenous communities (GTR 2017; Shin, Aliaga-Linares, and Britton 2017). Many rural, Indigenous families lack access to quality health services, and have limited educational and economic opportunities (GTR 2017). Many of the conditions in impoverished communities, such as poor nutrition and low maternal education, negatively influence maternal and child health outcomes (Heaton and Forste 2003; Shin, Aliaga-Linares, and Britton 2017; UNICEF 2019). Other conditions influencing health include access to quality reproductive care, skilled birth attendants, and prenatal care (Adsera and Menendez 2011; Frost, Forste, and Haas 2005; Heaton and Forste 2003). Women in this region often have low status, lack physical security, and have limited autonomy due to poor educational and economic opportunities (Frost, Forste, and Haas 2005; WomanStats Project 2019). The status of women has a profound influence on the well-being of not only mothers but also children.

This chapter outlines demographic trends in maternal and child mortality, fertility and reproductive health, as well as education and women's status in the Andean region. The first section focuses on measures of mortality, including infant mortality rates, life expectancy at birth, and maternal deaths. Important factors related to health and well-being, such as improvements in nutrition and vaccination are discussed, as well as the link between reproduction and mortality in the region. The second section highlights trends in fertility such as the total fertility rate, contraceptive use, and access to skilled birth attendants—factors important in reducing infant and maternal deaths. Last, the larger socioeconomic context of the Andean region is examined, including school enrollments, economic development, and measures of women's status as they relate to the health and well-being of women and children.

## Child and Maternal Mortality

Child and maternal mortality vary among the countries of the Andean region as shown in table 12.1. Rates in the Andean region are generally higher than those of the rest of South America. Based on indicators reported in 2019, the highest child and maternal mortality rates are in Bolivia (see table 12.1). Infant mortality rates measure the number of infant deaths before the age of one per 1,000 live births, and the child mortality rate is the number of deaths under age five per 1,000 live births. Child deaths are lowest in Colombia and highest in Bolivia (see table 12.1). Recently (in 2019), infant mortality rates increased in Venezuela because of the political turmoil and economic sanctions the country is experiencing. By comparison, the infant mortality rate in South America as a whole is similar to rates in Colombia, Ecuador, and Peru (Population reference Bureau [PRB] 2019). High rates of child mortality in Bolivia underscore the link between poverty, particularly in Indigenous communities, and poor child and maternal health. In contrast, recent declines in health in Venezuela emphasize the importance of political stability for child and maternal well-being. Although rates remain relatively high in parts of the Andean region, there have been improvements over time.

In 1970, the infant mortality rate ranged from 54 deaths per 1,000 births in Venezuela to 156 deaths in Bolivia (PRB 2014). As shown in table 12.1, rates dropped to 27.9 deaths per 1,000 births in Venezuela and 33.2 deaths in Bolivia by 2019. Infant mortality had been even lower in Venezuela (14.1 deaths per 1,000 births in 2011) until the most recent rise of economic and political conflict. Under Hugo Chávez (1999–2013), infant mortality rates

Table 12.1. Maternal and child health measures, Andean region (2015–2019)

| Country | Bolivia | Colombia | Ecuador | Peru | Venezuela |
|---|---|---|---|---|---|
| **CHILD HEALTH** | | | | | |
| Neonatal mortality per 1,000 births (2018) | 19.0 | 8.5 | 11.2 | 7.5 | 10.3 |
| Infant mortality rate per 1,000 births (2019) | 33.2 | 12.7 | 15.4 | 17.2 | 27.9 |
| Under five mortality rate per 1,000 births (2018) | 42.0 | 14.8 | 18.1 | 21.9 | 34.7 |
| **MATERNAL HEALTH** | | | | | |
| Maternal mortality per 100,000 births (2015) | 206 | 64 | 64 | 68 | 95 |
| Female life expectancy at birth (2019) | 73.1 | 79.7 | 80.5 | 76.7 | 74.7 |

*Source*: 2019 Census Bureau International Database; 2018 World Health Statistics, WHO

declined until 2012 when they began to rise steadily to current levels, nearing 28 deaths per 1,000 births in 2019 (see table 12.1). Efforts in the Andean region to increase access to medical care for women and children, as well as to improve standards of living, have been essential in reducing infant mortality in the region. In particular, increased access to potable water and sanitation removal have improved child survival. Increased maternal education has also reduced infant deaths—as more educated mothers seek healthcare and provide nutritionally for their infants—relative to less educated mothers (Frost, Forste, and Haas 2005; Heaton and Forste 2003).

Neonatal deaths account for about half of infant deaths in the region, as most infant mortalities (about 75 percent) occur in the first week of life (UNICEF 2019). Neonatal mortality rates measure the number of infant deaths in the first twenty-eight days of life per 1,000 births. Access to prenatal care, maternal education, and a skilled birth attendant are critical to further reduce infant deaths in the Andean region. Respiratory infections and diarrhea are the primary preventable causes of child illness and mortality (Huicho et al. 2016; Kent 2010a). These illnesses are also closely tied to poverty and poor child nutrition (Shin, Aliaga-Linares, and Britton 2017; UNICEF 2019). Even in urban areas, children living in poverty experience poor nutrition as they consume cheap, low-quality foods (Lipus et al. 2018).

Maternal education and breastfeeding practices, in addition to immunizations and child nutrition, are important protections against child mortality (Heaton and Forste, 2003; Frost, Forste, and Haas 2005). With the importation of vaccinations and other health practices in the region, infant and child mortality rates have declined dramatically since the 1970s, but inequality within countries continues to contribute to poor health outcomes (GTR 2017). Children with the highest likelihood of morbidity and mortality are those living in poverty, living in rural, Indigenous communities, and born to mothers with little education. In the Andean region, children of mothers with low education are 3.5 times more likely to die than are children of more educated mothers (UNICEF 2019).

The United Nations Countdown to 2015 and 2030 reports for Bolivia and Peru underscore the improved rates of child immunization in the region with 86 to 95 percent of children receiving at least partial immunizations by 2014 (Countdown to 2015; Countdown to 2030). Vaccinations are lower among children living in poverty but have continued to increase over time, especially immunizations against tuberculosis and measles (Kent 2010a). Rates of stunting (a measure of chronic malnutrition) have also declined from 37 percent of children under five moderately or severely stunted in Peru (1992) and 44 percent in Bolivia (1989) to lows in 2012 near 18 percent. But again, child undernutrition is much higher in rural or remote areas in Peru and Bolivia, where Indigenous communities are concentrated, relative to children in urban areas (PAHO/WHO 2015).

Peru and Bolivia also report high levels of exclusive breastfeeding, with 64 percent or more of infants under six months exclusively breastfed (Huicho et al. 2016). Breastfeeding is important for infant survival because it is more nutritious, sanitized, and cheaper than commercial formula infant feeding products (American Academy of Pediatrics 2012). Breastfeeding also helps lengthen intervals between births in communities where women do not use modern contraception. Longer birth intervals enhance the health of mothers and their children (Forste 1995; Forste 1998). Even with these health improvements, Bolivia continues to have the highest infant mortality rates in Latin America, with close to double the number of infant deaths in Colombia, Ecuador, or Peru (Kent 2010a; PRB 2019), due, in part, to very large, rural, poor, Indigenous populations in Bolivia (Heaton and Forste 2003).

Closely linked to infant mortality is maternal mortality. Maternal mortality is defined by the World Health Organization (WHO) as the death of a woman while pregnant or within forty-two days of the termination of pregnancy (WHO 2015). The maternal mortality rate indicates the number of maternal deaths in a year per 100,000 live births. Overall, maternal mortality rates in Latin America dropped from 124 deaths per 100,000 live births in 1990 to 60 in 2015 (GTR 2017; WHO 2015). The rates in the Andean region in 1990 ranged from 94 maternal deaths per 100,000 births in

Venezuela to 425 maternal deaths in Bolivia. The second highest rate in 1990 after Bolivia was Peru, with 251 maternal deaths per 100,000 births (WHO 2015). Maternal deaths have declined dramatically in Bolivia over the past 35 years, to 206 deaths per 100,000 births, whereas they remained steady in Venezuela over the same time period. As highlighted in table 12.1, Peru's maternal mortality rate also declined significantly to 68 deaths, and Colombia's and Ecuador's were even lower at 64 maternal deaths per 100,000 births in 2015 (PRB 2016; WHO 2015).

Although rates have declined over time, Bolivia continues to have the highest levels of maternal mortality in South America (PRB 2016). A national study in Bolivia in 2011 found that 68 percent of maternal deaths were among Indigenous women (GTR 2017). Indigenous mothers were three to four times more likely to die from complications during pregnancy, childbirth, or postpartum, compared to non-Indigenous women (GTR 2017; UNICEF 2019). Often Indigenous women find that healthcare providers are not sensitive to their culture and unable to communicate in their language (GTR 2017). Language barriers, as well as cultural practices that give the control of healthcare decision-making to men in the household, limit Indigenous women's access to quality care (PAHO/WHO 2015).

Primary causes of maternal mortality in Latin America (2013) are hemorrhaging or excessive bleeding (23 percent) and hypertension or high blood pressure (22 percent) (WHO 2015). Additional causes include embolism (3 percent), sepsis (8 percent), and abortions (10 percent), with other causes categorized together as "other direct" (15 percent) or "indirect causes" (19 percent). Most maternal deaths in the Andean region are preventable with improved access to quality healthcare (GTR 2017). Access to prenatal care, good maternal nutrition, and a skilled birth attendant are essential for improved maternal health. In addition, the proportion of Cesarean-section births has been increasing in countries such as Bolivia and Peru. This practice can save lives, but it can also put women and infants at greater risk of mortality if performed unnecessarily (GTR 2017).

The United Nations Human Rights Council in 2009 issued a resolution highlighting that "preventable maternal death constitutes a grave human rights violation and is a social, rather than an individual, problem" (GTR 2017, 9; United Nations 2012). Maternal mortality has a profound impact on the well-being of families: Following the death of a mother, her newborn is less likely to survive, older children are less likely to stay in school, and the family is likely to experience greater economic difficulties (GTR 2017). Thus, maternal mortality not only cuts short the life of a woman but also puts her children and family at greater risk of poverty and poor health outcomes.

Measures of life expectancy at birth follow a similar pattern as infant mortality rates in the Andean region. Life expectancy at birth is heavily weighted by infant mortality, and it is a summary measure of age-specific mortality rates for a given year. The measure indicates the average life expectancy of an infant born during a given year if exposed to current age-specific mortality rates across his or her lifespan. Life expectancy in 1970 ranged from 46 years in Bolivia, to 65 years in Venezuela (PRB 2014). In 2019, life expectancy had increased to 73.1 for women in Bolivia (see table 12.1). The rates in Peru, Ecuador, and Colombia were relatively similar in 2019—76.7 to 80.5 years for women. These rates mirror those of overall rates in South America—79 years for women (PRB 2019). The rates in Venezuela have recently declined and are similar to Bolivia, with 74.7 for women (see table 12.1). Recent declines in health in Venezuela are in response to current political and economic turmoil in the country and reflect increases in infant mortality following the end of the Chávez government.

## Fertility and Reproductive Health

The total fertility rate (TFR) is a summary measure of current age-specific fertility rates for a given year and indicates the number of children a woman would have across her childbearing career if exposed to those age-specific rates. The TFR in Bolivia in 1970 was 6.6 births per woman, and in Venezuela, it was 5.4 births (PRB 2014). Over the past five decades, fertility rates in Bolivia have dropped more than half to 2.5 births per woman, and 2.3 births in Venezuela, as highlighted in table 12.2. The lowest fertility rates are currently in Colombia at 1.96 births per woman (see table 12.2). This rate is below replacement level (2.1 births per woman), or the fertility level at which the population replaces itself (Lundquist, Anderson, and Yaukey 2015). Survey data highlight that most women in Bolivia desire 2.0 children, but without increased use of modern contraception, this ideal will not be reached (Kent 2010a). Access to contraception in Bolivia continues to vary greatly by income—those in the bottom income distribution have an unmet need 3.6 times greater than the unmet need of women in the highest income group (GTR 2017; Kent 2010a).

In 2010, contraceptive use was lowest in Bolivia, with only 35 percent of women reporting the use of modern methods, compared to 68 percent in Colombia (PRB 2010). By 2019, modern contraceptive use among women in a union increased to 45 percent in Bolivia and 76 percent in Colombia (see table 12.2). Rates for the other Andean countries ranged from 55 percent in Peru to 72 percent in Ecuador (PRB 2019). Modern contraceptive

Table 12.2. Fertility and reproductive health measures, Andean region (2015–2018)

| Country | Bolivia | Colombia | Ecuador | Peru | Venezuela |
|---|---|---|---|---|---|
| TOTAL FERTILITY RATE | 2.53 | 1.96 | 2.12 | 2.07 | 2.28 |
| percent married women using modern contraception | 45% | 76% | 72% | 55% | — |
| percent married women using all methods | 67% | 81% | 80% | 75% | 75% |
| ADOLESCENT FERTILITY RATE | | | | | |
| Births per 1,000 women aged 15 to 19 | 69 | 75 | 75 | 68 | 86 |

Source: 2019 Census Bureau International Database; 2018 World Health Statistics, WHO report; 2017 and 2019 World Population Data Sheets, Population Reference Bureau

use among women aged 15 to 49 includes methods such as the pill, IUD, condoms, and sterilization. The percent using modern contraception is reported for women in a union, either formally married or cohabitating (PRB 2019).

Many women, however, continue to rely on traditional contraceptive methods that have a high failure rate, such as herbal medicines, periodic abstinence and withdrawal (Kent 2010a; Kent 2010b). Modern contraceptive use is highest among educated women and those with higher socioeconomic status, whereas Indigenous, economically impoverished, and less educated women generally lack access to family planning services (GTR 2017; Kent 2010a). Data from 2013 highlight the relationship between wealth and contraceptive use. In Bolivia, among women in the richest quintile (top fifth of the income distribution), 47 percent reported modern contraceptive use. In contrast, only 23 percent used modern methods among women in the poorest quintile (lowest fifth of the income distribution). The gap between rich and poor was smaller in Colombia, with 75 percent of women in the top-wealth quintile using modern contraception, compared to 69 percent in the bottom quintile (PRB 2013).

Although overall fertility has declined in countries in the Andean region, the adolescent fertility rate has been steadily increasing over the past twenty-five years in both rural and urban areas, particularly in Colombia. Adolescent mothers generally come from lower socioeconomic backgrounds and experience greater likelihoods of domestic violence and child mortality (Urdinola and Ospino 2015). Peru and Bolivia have also experienced decreases in national fertility, while adolescent fertility has increased

Table 12.3. Percentage of women married or cohabiting by age (15 to 29 years), Bolivia (1989–2012)

| Bolivia | 1989 | 2001 | 2012 |
|---|---|---|---|
| **FORMAL MARRIAGE** | | | |
| 15 to 19 | 6.4 | 3.6 | 1.9 |
| 20 to 24 | 34.9 | 21.6 | 12.9 |
| 25 to 29 | 59.3 | 43.8 | 19.0 |
| Average Age at First Marriage | 22.2 | 23.3 | 24.1 |
| **CONSENSUAL UNION** | | | |
| 15 to 19 | 6.1 | 9.2 | 9.7 |
| 20 to 24 | 18.8 | 24.4 | 27.4 |
| 25 to 29 | 15.7 | 23.7 | 30.7 |

*Source*: 2017 World Marriage Data, United Nations

among Indigenous and rural populations (Flórez Nieto and Núñez 2002; PAHO/WHO 2015). Table 12.2 shows that adolescent fertility (births per 1,000 young women aged 15 to 19) is highest in Venezuela at 86 births, and lowest in Peru (68 births) and Bolivia (69 births), with rates in Colombia and Ecuador in between (WHO 2018).

Changes in patterns of family formation influence adolescent childbearing. Over the past several decades, age at marriage in Latin America has increased, yet women continue to form unions at about the same age. More women enter informal or cohabiting unions at earlier ages, rather than formal marriage (Covre-Sussai et al. 2015; García and de Oliveira 2011; Kent 2010b). To illustrate this trend, data on formal marriage and consensual unions among women in Bolivia between 1989 and 2012 are presented in table 12.3. In 1989, about 6 percent of girls ages 15 to 19 were formally married, and about 6 percent were in consensual unions. By 2012, the percentage of young girls in formal marriage had dropped to 1.9 percent, whereas the percentage of girls cohabiting increased to 9.7 percent. As shown in table 12.3, the percent of women entering formal marriage at earlier ages declined between 1989 and 2012, and age at first marriage increased. In contrast, the percent cohabiting increased in each age category over the same period. This same pattern is found in other Andean countries.

Women in Latin America with less than secondary schooling generally substitute cohabitation for marriage as a way to cope with poverty given that cohabitation requires no formal ceremony and no legal obligations. In contrast, more highly educated women remain single longer and form cohabiting unions prior to formal marriage (Covre-Sussai et al. 2015). Indigenous and rural women are more likely to form traditional cohabitating partnerships characterized by high levels of fertility, low female independence, high economic dependence, and early age of union formation. In contrast, more educated and urban women form cohabiting partnerships as a trial marriage, characterized by greater economic independence, older age of union formation, and lower fertility (Covre-Sussai et al. 2015; García and de Oliveira 2011).

Overall, this pattern of early sexual activity and later marriage has increased the number of unplanned pregnancies and births for single women, leading to high rates of single motherhood in Latin America (Kent 2010b). The percentage of all births to unmarried women is 55 percent in Bolivia (2008), 76 percent in Peru (2012), and 84 percent in Colombia (2009–10). According to Lippman and Wilcox (2013), the Andean region has some of the highest cohabitation rates and highest nonmarital fertility rates in the world, which has implications for the number of children living in female-headed households and in poverty.

Reproductive services, such as contraception, prenatal care, and a skilled birth attendant, are critical to the survival of infants and mothers, yet rural and poor communities in the Andean region have limited access to healthcare. The percentage of births attended by skilled personnel in 2005 ranged from 59 percent in Peru, to 95 percent in Venezuela (PRB 2005). Rates for Bolivia were at 65 percent, for Ecuador 69 percent, and for Colombia 86 percent. By 2018, rates had increased among Andean countries from 85 percent to 95 percent (WHO 2018). The Morales government in Bolivia made healthcare a priority and increased access to maternal care, including the number of births attended by a skilled professional (Heaton, Forste, and Knowlton 2008). Overall, Indigenous women, those in poverty, or women with little education, are less likely to access a skilled birth attendant than non-Indigenous or more educated mothers (GTR 2017).

The reproductive care of women in Bolivia is highlighted in the Countdown to 2030 report tracking the United Nations Sustainable Development Goals. According to the report, only 45 percent of the demand for family planning services is being met, whereas 75 percent of women are receiving prenatal care (four or more prenatal visits) (Countdown to 2030). As noted previously, the percentage of mothers in Bolivia receiving prenatal care has increased over the past few decades as the government increased efforts to provide access to healthcare in Indigenous communities (Heaton, Forste, and Knowlton 2008). The United Nations report notes that nearly 85 percent of births in Bolivia are attended by skilled personnel, with 77 percent receiving postnatal care (Countdown to 2030).

The 2015 Countdown report for Peru shows that 89 percent of the demand for family planning is satisfied, 95 percent of pregnant women receive prenatal care, and 90 percent of births are attended by skilled personnel. Postnatal care is received by 93 percent of mothers (Countdown to 2015). Although in Peru access to prenatal care for pregnant mothers is high, there continues to be a large gap between access in urban and coastal regions and rural and remote areas (PAHO/WHO 2015). Access to reproductive care also varies by education and residence. Women without formal schooling have more than twice the unmet need for contraception than do women with at least a high school degree (GTR 2017).

Although national fertility rates have declined and access to reproductive healthcare increased overall in the Andean region, less-educated, Indigenous, and rural women continue to lack access to quality healthcare, creating major discrepancies in maternal and child health. To address these healthcare gaps, Bolivia and Ecuador have trained and utilized traditional midwives as part of their health provider teams and have supported coordination between traditional midwives and health facilities. In addition, Bolivia and Peru have attempted to adopt birthing practices integrated with the local Indigenous culture—including vertical or squatting delivery positions (GTR 2017). Such efforts are important to improve the health of women and their infants in rural and Indigenous communities and increase the likelihood that Indigenous women will utilize available health services.

## Educational and Economic Opportunity

Educational and economic indicators underscore the inequality and economic variation between and within countries in the Andean region. Table 12.4 shows the variation in gross national income in 2018—ranging from $7,670 in Bolivia to $17,900 in Venezuela. Gross national income per capita is calculated as income in purchasing power parity (GNI PPP) divided by the mid-year population and reported in current international dollars. Compared with the GNI PPP of the Andean region noted above, that for South America is $16,059 (PRB 2019). This is much lower than high income countries such as the United States where GNI PPP is $63,390, but much higher than low income countries where average GNI PPP is only $2,225 (PRB 2019).

This variation in national income is also reflected in health expenditures per capita across the region. Bolivia spends only 197 US dollars per capita on healthcare, compared to $973 spent in Venezuela (see table 12.4). Interestingly, Ecuador has a lower gross national income than the other Andean

Table 12.4. Educational and economic measures, Andean region

| Country | Bolivia | Colombia | Ecuador | Peru | Venezuela |
|---|---|---|---|---|---|
| Current health expenditures per capita (2015 US$) | 197 | 374 | 530 | 323 | 973 |
| Gross national income per capita PPP (2018) | $7,670 | $14,490 | $11,410 | $13,810 | $17,900 |
| Percent of population living in urban areas | 69% | 77% | 64% | 78% | 88% |
| Secondary school enrollment ratio (female) (2009/2016) | 86 | 102 | 109 | 96 | 93 |
| Secondary school enrollment ratio (male) (2009/2016) | 87 | 95 | 105 | 96 | 86 |
| Tertiary education enrollment ratio (female) (2009/2016) | — | 60 | 45 | 43 | — |
| Tertiary education enrollment ratio (male) (2009/2016) | — | 52 | 35 | 39 | — |
| Women as percent of nonfarm wage earners | 37% | 46% | 38% | 37% | 44% |
| Gender ratio labor force rate (2013) | .79 | .70 | .66 | .81 | .65 |

*Source*: 2018 World Health Statistics; 2015, 2017 and 2019 World Population Data Sheets, Population Reference Bureau

countries excluding Bolivia, but spends more on healthcare than Colombia or Peru. There have been improvements in economic development in the region; for example, the percentage of the population living below the poverty line in Peru declined from 48 percent in 2000 to 24 percent in 2013 (Huicho et al. 2016). However, continued improvements in economic standards in the Andean region are needed to further the health and well-being of women and children.

As a common measure of education, the enrollment ratio indicates the number of students enrolled in school compared to the population in the applicable age group as a percentage. It can exceed one hundred if the number of students enrolled exceeds the population of the relevant age group (PRB 2017, 20). The secondary school enrollment ratio for boys is 105 percent in Ecuador, compared to 87 percent in Bolivia (see table 12.4); for girls the ratio is 109 percent in Ecuador and 86 percent in Bolivia. Rates in Colombia, Peru, and Venezuela are in between those of Ecuador and Bolivia, except that rates for boys in Venezuela are more similar to boys in Bolivia (PRB 2017). In Peru, the percentage of women with fewer than four years of formal schooling declined from 22 percent in 2001 to 7 percent in 2013

(Huicho et al. 2016). Thus, at least 85 percent of boys and girls in the Andean region are enrolled in secondary schools, in contrast to South America as a whole, where rates are 96 percent for males, and 101 percent for females (PRB 2017, 13). Although school enrollment has increased in the Andean region over time, rates in rural areas, especially among Indigenous females, are low compared to their urban and male peers (PAHO/WHO 2015).

Enrollment numbers for tertiary education (postsecondary) are much lower than are numbers for secondary school enrollment, as shown in table 12.4. Available data show enrollment ratios in tertiary education at 35 percent for males in Ecuador, 39 percent in Peru, and 52 percent in Colombia; for females the ratios are 43 percent in Peru, 45 percent in Ecuador, and 60 percent in Colombia (PRB 2017, 13). Data on tertiary enrollments are not available for Bolivia and Venezuela. Overall in South America, postsecondary enrollment ratios are 47 percent for men and 63 percent for women. Gender differences mirror those in the United States, where more women are enrolled in postsecondary education than men (Pew Research Center 2013). Thus, tertiary enrollment rates in the Andean region generally lag behind those in South America as a whole, especially for women.

Countries in the Andean region generally have lower levels of education relative to the rest of South America, but even within each country, there is variation by race and ethnicity. Using data from the 2010 AmericasBarometer, Telles and Steele (2012) found that individuals with darker skin color had lower levels of educational attainment relative to those with light skin color. This finding was especially evident in Bolivia. Bolivians with light skin color averaged 12.5 years of education, compared to 9 years among those with dark skin. This relationship between skin color and education was independent of social class, age, gender, residency, and country (Telles and Steele 2012). This study further underscores how Indigenous populations in the Andean region experience not only greater poverty but also educational inequality.

Another factor influencing maternal and child well-being in the Andean region is the physical security of women. Data from the WomanStats project (2019) indicate that women in many Andean countries lack physical security (for example, Peru and Columbia), and others in the region (for example, Venezuela, Ecuador, and Bolivia) have very low levels of physical security. Physical security includes laws against domestic violence, rape, and marital rape, as well as the enforcement of such laws. In addition, the measure includes social norms or taboos against reporting such crimes. Low rates of physical security in Andean countries further threaten maternal and child well-being in the region. Women that lack physical security have less decision-making power related to both their own healthcare and the health of their children, resulting in poor health outcomes (Frost, Forste, and Haas 2005; Heaton and Forste 2008).

More recently in the Andean region, however, reductions in socioeconomic and urban–rural inequalities have led to declines in the proportion of the population living below the poverty level and to increased maternal education—all factors that improve the health and well-being of mothers and their children (Huicho et al. 2016). Previous research underscores how the local socioeconomic environment, more than access to healthcare services, is a primary determinant of health outcomes in the region (Shin, Aliaga-Linares, and Britton 2017). This suggests that increasing access to quality healthcare may not be sufficient to improve maternal and child health, unless accompanied by improved living standards. Although Latin America continues to be one of the most unequal regions in the world in terms of disparities in income, economic development between 2000 and 2010 helped reduce the gap between rich and poor, particularly in Bolivia and Ecuador (Lustig 2015). Efforts to reduce further wage inequality and increase financial stability in the Andean region will be critical to further improve maternal and child health in the region (Messina and Silva 2017).

## Conclusion

Historically in South America, the Andean region has lagged behind in terms of maternal and child well-being. Since the 1990s, economic development and greater access to healthcare have lowered fertility rates and reduced mortality rates in the region—improving the health and well-being of women and children. Yet, within the Andean region, Bolivia continues to lag behind the other countries in terms of healthcare access and economic development. In large part this is because of inequalities between rural and urban centers, as well as between Indigenous and non-Indigenous communities. In Bolivia, as well as in the other Andean countries, the impoverished, rural, Indigenous communities are where women and children lack access to educational and economic opportunity and continue to suffer the most.

Despite improvements in maternal and child health in the Andean region over the past several decades, more work is needed to reach Indigenous and rural communities. Language and cultural barriers to healthcare among Indigenous women, particularly in rural areas, go beyond just economics and healthcare availability. Increased education of Indigenous, rural women is one way to empower women and give them greater access to decision-making that will improve their own health and that of their children (Frost, Forste, and Haas 2005; Heaton and Forste 2008). Health improvements need to be universal and equitable in order to further reduce maternal and child mortality to levels found in neighboring countries such as Chile, Brazil, and Argentina (Huicho et al. 2016). Moving forward, this will require greater access to reproductive and maternal healthcare, an increase in the status of women, reductions in poverty, and improvements in economic well-being in the region (Huicho et al. 2016; Shin, Aliaga-Linares, and Britton 2017).

## References

Adsera, Alicia, and Alicia Menendez. 2011. "Fertility Changes in Latin America in Periods of Economic Uncertainty." *Population Studies* 65 (1; March): 37–56.

American Academy of Pediatrics. 2012. "Breastfeeding and the Use of Human Milk." *Pediatrics* 129 (3; March): e827-e841.

Countdown to 2015. *The 2015 Report: Peru*. http://countdown2030.org/documents/2015Report/Peru_2015.pdf.

Countdown to 2030. *Country Profiles: Bolivia*. http://profiles.countdown2030.org/#/cp/BOL.

Covre-Sussai, Maira, Bart Meuleman, Sarah Botterman, and Koen Matthijs. 2015. "Traditional and Modern Cohabitation in Latin America: A Comparative Typology." *Demographic Research* 32 (32; May): 873–914.

Flórez Nieto, Carmen Elisa, and Jairo Núñez. 2002. "Teenage Childbearing in Latin American Countries." Washington DC: Inter-American Development Bank, Documento CEDE 2002-01. https://doi.org/10.2139/ssrn.312155.

Forste, Renata. 1995. "Effects of Lactation and Contraceptive Use on Birth-Spacing in Bolivia." *Social Biology* 42 (1–2): 108–23.

———. 1998. "Infant Feeding Practices and Child Health in Bolivia." *Journal of Biosocial Science* 30 (1; January): 107–25. https://doi.org/10.1017/S0021932098001072.

Frost, Michelle Bellessa, Renata Forste, and David Haas. 2005. "Maternal Education and Child Nutritional Status in Bolivia: Finding the Links." *Social Science & Medicine* 60 (2; January): 395–407.

García, Brígida, and Orlandina de Oliveira. 2011. "Family Changes and Public Policies in Latin America." *Annual Review of Sociology* 37 (1; August): 593–611.

Regional Task Force for the Reduction of Maternal Mortality (GTR). 2017. "Overview of the Situation of Maternal Morbidity and Mortality: Latin America and the Caribbean." *Latin American and Caribbean Task Force for the Reduction of Maternal Mortality*, December 2017. https://lac.unfpa.org/sites/default/files/pub-pdf/MSH-GTR-Report-Eng.pdf.

Heaton, Tim, and Renata Forste. 2003. "Rural-Urban Differences in Child Growth and Survival in Bolivia." *Rural Sociology* 68 (3; October): 410–33.

———. 2008. "Domestic Violence, Couple Interaction and Children's Health in Latin

America." *Journal of Family Violence* 23 (3; October): 183–93. https://doi.org/10.1007/s10896-007-9142-7.

Heaton, Tim, Renata Forste, and David Knowlton. 2008. "Tendencias en desigualdades estructurales de la salud infantil en Bolivia." In *Salud Comunitaria en Bolivia—Desafios hacia la Equidad* edited by Kathya Córdova Pozo 42–59. Cochabamba: Bolivia South Group, Instituto de Investigación

Huicho, Luis, Eddy Segura, Carlos Huayanay-Espinoza, Jessica Niño de Guzman, Maria Clara Restrepo-Méndez, Yvonne Tam, Aluisio Barros, Cesar Victora, and the Peru Countdown Country Case Study Working Group. 2016. "Child Health and Nutrition in Peru within an Antipoverty Political Agenda: A Countdown to 2015 Country Case Study." *Lancet Global Health* 4: 414–26.

Kent, Mary Maderios. 2010a. "In Bolivia, Slow Fertility Decline and Some Improvements in Health Indicators." Population Reference Bureau. https://www.prb.org/bolivia/.

———. 2010b. "Many Peruvians Rely on Traditional Family Planning Methods." Population Reference Bureau. https://www.prb.org/perufamilyplanning-2/.

Lippman, Laura, and W. Bradford Wilcox. 2013. "World Family Map 2013: Mapping Family Change and Child Well-Being Outcomes." *Child Trends*. https://www.childtrends.org/publications/world-family-map-2013-mapping-family-change-and-child-well-being-outcomes.

Lipus, Adam, Juan Leon, Susana Calle, and Karen Andes. 2018. "It Is Not Natural Anymore: Nutrition, Urbanization, and Indigenous Identity on Bolivia's Andean Plateau." *Qualitative Health Research* 28 (11; March): 1802–12.

Ludquist, Jennifer, Douglas Anderson, and David Yaukey. 2015. *Demography: The Study of Human Population*. Long Grove: Waveland Press, Inc,.

Lustig, Nora. 2015. "Most Unequal on Earth." *Finance & Development* 52 (3; September): 14–16.

Messina, Julian, and Joana Silva. 2017. *Wage Inequality in Latin America: Understanding the Past to Prepare For the Future*. Washington, DC: World Bank Group.

PAHO/WHO, Partnership for Maternal, Newborn and Child Health, World Bank and Alliance for Health Policy and Systems Research. 2015. "Success Factors for Women's and Children's Health: Peru." Geneva: World Health Organization.

Pew Research Center. 2013. "On Pay Gap, Millennial Women Near Parity—For Now." *Pew Research Center*. December 11, 2013. https://www.pewsocialtrends.org/2013/12/11/on-pay-gap-millennial-women-near-parity-for-now/.

Population Reference Bureau (PRB). 2005. *2005 Women of Our World*. Washington, DC: Population Reference Bureau. https://www.prb.org/wp-content/uploads/2005/03/WomenOfOurWorld2005.pdf.

———. 2010. *2010 World Population Data Sheet*. Washington, DC: Population Reference Bureau. https://www.prb.org/wp-content/uploads/2010/11/10wpds_eng.pdf.

———. 2013. *Family Planning Worldwide 2013 Data Sheet*. Washington, DC: Population Reference Bureau. https://www.prb.org/wp-content/uploads/2013/11/family-planning-2013-datasheet_eng.pdf.

———. 2014. *2014 World Population Data Sheet*. Washington, DC: Population Reference Bureau. https://www.prb.org/wp-content/uploads/2015/11/2014-world-population-data-sheet_eng.pdf.

———. 2015. *2015 World Population Data Sheet*. Washington, DC: Population Reference Bureau. https: scorecard.prb.org/2015-world-population-data-sheet/

———. 2016. *2016 World Population Data Sheet*. Washington, DC: Population Reference Bureau. https://www.prb.org/wp-content/uploads/2016/08/prb-wpds2016-web-2016-1.pdf.

———. 2017. *2017 World Population Data Sheet*. Washington, DC: Population Reference Bureau. https://www.prb.org/wp-content/uploads/2017/08/WPDS-2017.pdf.

———. 2019. *2019 World Population Data Sheet*. Washington, DC: Population Reference Bureau. https://www.prb.org/datasheets/.

Shin, Heeju, Lissette Aliaga-Linares, and Marcus Britton. 2017. "Misconceived Equity? Health Care Resources, Contextual Poverty, and Child Health Disparities in Peru." *Social Science Research* 66 (August): 234–47.

Telles, Edward, and Liza Steele. 2012. "Pigmentocracy in the Americas: How is Educational Attainment Related to Skin Color?" *AmericasBarometer Insights* 73: 1–8. https://www.vanderbilt.edu/lapop/insights/IO873en_v2.pdf.

UNICEF. 2019. *Maternal and Child Health*. https://www.unicef.org/bolivia/07_UNICEF_Bolivia_CK_-_concept_note_-_Maternal_and_Child_Health_low.pdf.

United Nations, Department of Economic and Social Affairs, Population Division. 2017. *World Marriage Data 2017* (POP/DB/Marr/Rev2017).

United Nations, Human Rights Council. 2012. "Technical Guidance on the Application of a Human Rights-Based Approach to the Implementation of Policies and Programmes to Reduce Preventable Maternal Morbidity and Mortality of Children Under 5 Years of Age." *The Office of the United Nations High Commissioner for Human Rights*. https://documents-dds-ny.un.org/doc/UNDOC/GEN/G14/071/24/PDF/G1407124.pdf?OpenElement.

United State Census Bureau. 2019. *International Data Base*. https: census.gov/programs-surveys/international-programs.html

Urdinola, Piedad, and Carlos Ospino. 2015. "Long-Term Consequences of Adolescent Fertility: The Colombian Case." *Demographic Research* 32 (55; June): 1487–1518.

WomanStats Project. 2019. "Physical Security of Women." *WomanStats Maps*. http://www.womanstats.org/maps.html.

World Health Organization (WHO). 2018. *World Health Statistics 2018: Monitoring Health for the SDGs, Sustainable Development Goals*. Geneva: World Health Organization.

World Health Organization (WHO). 2015. *Trends in Maternal Mortality, 1990 to 2015: Estimates by WHO, UNICEF, UNFPA, World Bank Group and the United Nations Population Division*. November 11, 2015. https://reliefweb.int/report/world/trends-maternal-mortality-1990–2015-estimates-who-unicef-unfpa-world-bank-group-and.

# 13

## Transsness and Disability in Discourses of Access to Healthcare in the Colombian Press (2000–2019)

JAVIER E. GARCÍA LEÓN AND DAVID L. GARCÍA LEÓN

In 2016, Colombian filmmaker Jorge Caballero produced the 70-minute documentary *Paciente* [Patient], which explores the life of Nubia, a middle-aged woman who looks after her cancer-stricken daughter. Nubia fights daily against bureaucratic obstacles to ensure that her child receives everything necessary to survive. Although one could read the film as a celebration of human resilience in the face of misfortune, it also critiques the neoliberal-era Colombian healthcare system. Similarly, transgender people in the country face stigma-related barriers and multi-level violence within the Colombian healthcare system.[1] Like Nubia in *Paciente*, trans women and men experience obstacles that put their lives at risk when accessing medicine and treatments. Trans people are not alone facing healthcare-related obstacles. Disabled individuals also encounter burdens when accessing health services in Colombia. Although the number of disabled people who are registered in the healthcare system steadily increased from 409,000 in 2009 to 600,000 in 2014, specialized care (for example, diagnostic tests and medicines for chronic and high-cost diseases) is not guaranteed for them (Correa-Montoya and Castro Martínez 2016, 79).

Inspired by these situations, our chapter explores the relationship between transness, disability, and healthcare in Colombian media. In particular, we examine the linguistic and discursive construction of access to the healthcare system by these two groups as both face similar barriers when accessing healthcare services in the country. We explore how *El Tiempo* (*ET*), Colombia's most widely read newspaper, portrays access to healthcare for trans individuals and disabled people. Our case study shows that

*ET* creates a spectacle out of social actors' subjectivity by reducing their lives to a dramatic and sensational story that conceals the role of the state in debilitating the healthcare system and, therefore, the lives of trans and disabled individuals in the country. In other words, we argue that *ET* masks the sociopolitical and materialist aspects of being disabled and trans. Thus, this chapter seeks to a) contribute to the intersection between transness and (dis)ability in Latin America, and b) question how the predominant discursive constructions of access to healthcare for trans and disabled people in the region adds to these groups' discrimination and oppression.

To achieve this goal, we briefly characterize the current healthcare system of Colombia and the main barriers that trans and disabled people face when accessing healthcare services. Second, we explore the representation of access to healthcare by trans and disabled people in the Colombian press exemplified by the coverage in *El Tiempo*. This case study offers an empirical glimpse that in no way represents the whole depiction of access to healthcare by minority groups, nor do we imply that our analysis can be generalized beyond the remit of the specific corpus analyzed here. On the contrary, through this exploratory qualitative study we aim to shed light on how the Colombian digital press has portrayed access to healthcare by disabled and trans people, as this issue has been underexplored from an intersectional approach. Finally, in our closing remarks, we reflect on the COVID-19 pandemic and its effects on trans and disabled individuals.

## The Neoliberal Colombian Healthcare System

According to the latest census published in 2018, Colombia is a middle-income country with a population of just over 48 million. Women make up 52.2 percent, while men represent 48.8 percent.[2] Colombia's population is predominantly urban, and the country has experienced a considerable and continuous decline in the number of people living in rural areas, as well as in those suffering extreme poverty (2.89 million) (Departamento Administrativo Nacional de Estadística [DANE] 2018). However, unemployment has increased slightly (from 12 percent in 2018 to 13 percent in 2019), and there has been a dramatic increase in self-employment (from 33.8 in 1990 to 53.6 percent in 2015) (Prada and Chaves 2019, 314). Colombia's total health expenditure as a percentage of the gross domestic product (GDP) increased from 5.8 percent in 1990 to 6.8 percent in 2013. Additionally, Colombia has endured an armed conflict for more than fifty years. In 2016, the government and the largest guerrilla group, Fuerzas Armadas Revolucionarias de Colombia (FARC), signed a peace accord. Nevertheless, violence and conflict still persist due to multiple factors that have jeopardized the implementation of the Peace Agreement.

At the beginning of the 1990s and following the Washington Consensus (1989), most Latin American countries underwent numerous social reforms meant to modernize their economies and their state apparatus (Panizza 2009, 11). These reforms followed the demands of international organizations such as the World Bank, which urged countries to align to the neoliberal policies of the Global North (for example, fiscal stability, reductions of state intervention, and more participation in the global market). In Colombia, President César Gaviria's (1990–1994) policy of "Economic openness and modernization of the State" [Apertura económica y modernización del Estado] led the country to a transformation that not only impacted the economic sector but also provided guidelines for modifying the healthcare system.[3] Before the implementation of this policy, the Colombian healthcare system faced several challenges: a) fragmentation, with over a thousand institutions involved; b) low levels of coverage since around 25 percent of the population did not have access to health services; and c) a worrisome financial deficit (Buitrago 2015, 56–57).

In 1991, and as a result of the National Constituent Assembly [Asamblea Nacional Constituyente], Colombia adopted a new Constitution in which social security was recognized as an inalienable right and healthcare was declared a public service borne by the state. At the same time, Gaviria's "Economic openness" [Apertura económica] urged the country to reduce economic protectionism and to open its markets to the globalized world. In 1993, the Colombian Congress approved Gaviria's bill to reform the healthcare system. Researchers such as Yudi Buitrago (2015) have argued that *Ley 100*, as the bill was later known, received support from different social actors, including the most recognized University Faculties of Medicine [Facultades Universitarias de Medicina] and the Colombian Association of Scientific Societies [Asociación Colombiana de Sociedades Científicas], among others. All of them agreed that the reform was important because it would contribute to build a more fair and equal society and to universalize healthcare access (65). *Ley 100* also meant an overhaul of social values toward health and community. Individual choice was a key element of the reform as it meant detaching the new system from negative social perceptions toward state services, usually conceived as monopolistic, corrupt, and inefficient. This rhetoric supported the idea that several institutional actors (for example, private and public hospitals and health service providers) should be involved during the implementation phase as they would contribute to a more competitive market from which citizens could benefit.

*Ley 100* reshaped the conditions under which citizens could access healthcare services. It created mandatory universal health insurance called the General System of Social Security in Health (known by its Spanish acronym, SGSSS). According to María-Luisa Escobar et al. (2009), SGSSS functions under a combination of payroll contributions and general taxations. That is to say, it is a two-tier scheme where the employee/employer enrolls in what is called the contributory regime, while low-income citizens benefit from the fully subsidized regime (4).[4] Additionally, as Escobar et al. (2009) explain, "beneficiaries enroll with public or private insurers (health funds), have legal rights to an explicit package of health benefits, and receive care from a mix of public and private providers" (4). From 2000 to 2015, this dual system produced a significant increase in coverage from 58.8 percent of the Colombian population to 94.5 percent. In 2015, 48.2 percent of the general population was affiliated with the contributory system and 42.4 percent to the subsidized program. While this plan has been positively evaluated for its results in coverage, access to quality health services remains poor (Agudelo Calderón et al. 2011; Gallego, Ramírez, and Sepulveda 2005; Giedion and Villar 2009; Molina, Vargas, and Muñoz 2010; Rodríguez Moreno and Vivas Martínez 2017; Vargas, Vázquez, and Mogollón 2010). The new system is complex and many for-profit organizations (for example, private healthcare providers) have created multiple administrative barriers to limit the real use of the services guaranteed by the SGSSS. To access healthcare, many Colombians, especially those of low income, have had to use judiciary interventions against insurance companies. As Prada and Chaves (2019) explain: "Although the government pretentiously claims that health insurance is purportedly part of the welfare state, it is clear that the system deepens inequality and the segmentation of the population according to income and social position, as one consequence of neoliberal policy implementation" (322).

The World Health Organization (WHO) (2011) has identified specific barriers that disabled people encounter when trying to access healthcare services in the country. These include physical and attitudinal challenges, obstacles to accessing public transportation, information and communication, and to accessing informational technology, as well as difficulties to gain education and work and employment. In the Colombian case, 6.4 percent of the population has a disability, which is more than 3 million citizens (Correa-Montoya and Castro Martínez 2016, 32). However, the proportion may be higher if we follow the overall rate of WHO, which estimates that 15 percent of the general population is a more accurate calculation. Therefore, the number of disabled Colombians could be approximately 7.2 million people (Correa-Montoya and Castro Martínez 2016, 32). Of disabled people, 70 percent are affiliated with the subsidized program, while the remaining 30 percent are enrolled in the contributory system.[5] These statistics contrast strongly with the general non-disabled population. In 2015, 48.2 percent of these individuals were affiliated with the contributory system and 42.4 percent to the subsidized one (Correa-Montoya and Castro Martínez 2016, 76). In other words, the fact that a significant number of disabled people use the subsidized scheme reflects that "they and their families are part of the poorest and most vulnerable group in Colombia and that in most cases such families are not part of the formal labor market" (Correa-Montoya and Castro Martínez 2016, 76).

All Colombians face barriers when accessing healthcare. Those challenges can be particularly acute for disabled individuals despite existing legislation that criminalizes discrimination and harassment against them.[6] It is for this reason that Gómez Perea et al. (2018) have noted that, despite a legal guarantee to health services, disabled people have no real access to rehabilitation procedures, they face delays in therapies, and they interact with healthcare providers who often lack knowledge of, and information about, disability issues. Moreover, this population is especially vulnerable due to other factors that intersect with healthcare. Disabled people face stronger discrimination in the labor market, generally have a lower level of education, and live mainly in marginalized areas (Pinilla-Roncancio 2015, 119). All of these factors increase their debilitation, in Jasbir K. Puar's (2017) terms, and they limit the quality and quantity of the healthcare services they receive.

Similarly, transgender people cope with several healthcare barriers. These include, for example, nonbinary restrooms in hospitals, management of electronic healthcare records designed in binary discourse (male/female), and financial barriers as trans populations suffer a disproportionate level of unemployment leading them to be reluctant to seek medical care. At another level, educational barriers include a lack of knowledge and training on trans issues on the part of health professionals that negatively impact the service provided to trans individuals (Roberts and Fantz 2014, 983). Specifically, in the Colombian case, Ritterbusch, Correa Salazar, and Correa (2018, 1836) identified several inadequacies within the system. Trans women experience a lack of coverage for surgeries, gender biases in procedural actions leading to medical errors, verbal abuse, profiling, and discriminatory language from health professionals. Authors also highlight that "there is no healthcare protocol tailored to the needs of the trans population in general, and to those individuals who suffer from intersectional multi-level violence, including historical victimization within the armed conflict" (Ritterbusch, Correa Salazar, and Correa 2018,1843). Indeed, even the peace agreement ignored the needs of LGBTQI+ individuals, and the voices of disabled people while incorporating a gender-based approach that focused on cis women and ethnic minorities (Biel Portero and Bolaños Enríquez 2018; Rivas Velarde, Garzon, and Shakespeare 2019).

Due to the systemic social oppression that transgender people face, trans patients also have specific healthcare needs. They possess a higher risk of contracting HIV than the general population, a higher tendency for drug and alcohol consumption, and stronger suicide attempt rates. Silva-Santisteban et al. (2016) have noted that the Colombian government has implemented limited HIV prevention strategies for men who have sex with men and transgender women, namely HIV information material and condom promotion and distribution (4). Additionally, access to HIV/STD testing centers for key populations (trans women and sex workers) is almost nonexistent outside of major cities like Bogotá and Medellín. Healthcare and counseling services also tend to focus mainly on aspects related to sexual behavior and sex reassignment (Lasso Báez 2014, 114). As a consequence, health professionals ignore other mental and physical issues that require attention when working with trans individuals.

As we can see, trans and disabled people share a series of commonalities when trying to access the Colombian healthcare system. Neither group has benefited from the implementation of *Ley 100*. Additionally, trans and disabled people also encounter additional social barriers that jeopardize their right to employment, education, and housing. Access to healthcare in the country has become a key element of the systemic oppression that both groups face in times where minorities are being (discursively) commodified in the press. It seems that the Colombian healthcare system is based on a neoliberal perspective that ignores the specific needs of these two populations. That is to say, it is built around a focus on the investment/coverage level to the point of ignoring structural and community-level issues. As Núria Homedes and Antonio Ugalde (2005) have noted, after closely following the World Bank reform plans, a large percentage of the Colombian population remains uncovered, access to healthcare remains subject to an ability to pay expensive copays, and healthcare equality has suffered (91).

## The Discursive Construction of Access to Healthcare by Disabled and Trans People in *El Tiempo*

As several explorations have shown (Grue 2015; Van Dijk 2009), the way that media discourses represent minorities—such as transgender and disabled people—strongly affects how the citizenry understands these communities. The decisions made by media producers concerning how trans and disabled people should be depicted are key as they feed and contribute to consolidating paradigms of representation. Furthermore, Zottola (2018) has shown that analyzing news media language is useful in identifying how media discourses influence and shape people's understanding of society at large (240). In this section, we explore the representation of access to healthcare by trans and disabled people in the Colombian newspaper *El Tiempo* (*ET*) during the last two decades to determine the relationship among media, representation, healthcare, transness, and (dis)ability; we find that news reports tend to promote dominant discourses that privilege ableism and cisheteronormativity. This case study aims to start a dialogue among transness, disability, and healthcare in Latin America by exploring the Colombian case from an intersectional and multidisciplinary approach.

Previous scholarly work from the North American, European, and Latin American academies has shown that newspapers and audiovisual journalism tend to portray disabled individuals within two tropes: the "tragic victim" or the "resilient hero" (Garland-Thompson 1997; Grue 2015). By doing so, the media secures attention from the general public and exploits the image of disabled individuals. In terms of mental healthcare in the Colombian press, for instance, Gutiérrez-Coba et al. (2017) have found that there is a lack of knowledge about mental health that denies most citizens the opportunity to learn about this form of disability beyond mere statistics or facts.[7] Conversely, most (trans) scholars (García León 2019, 2021; Gossett, Stanley, and Burton 2017; Halberstam 2005; Irving 2013; Serano 2013; Zottola 2018;) have argued that the current trans media representation is a trapdoor. Trans people shown in several newspapers, films, and TV shows continue to be spectacularized, portrayed as victims of gender-based violence or as entrepreneurs who commodify their bodies. Trans and disabled scholars/activists have also argued that representations are mainly produced by able cisgender journalists, centering gender binary and ability as the principal narratives and excluding trans and disabled experiences and expertise (Grue 2011; Ryan 2009).

To the best of our knowledge, most studies on healthcare and representation in the press have focused on health and illness in the media at large (Lupton 1999), healthcare and palliative care (Carrasco et al. 2019), or healthcare reforms in specific nations such as Canada and Australia (Benelli 2003; Collins et al. 2006; Lewis et al. 2018). Additionally, most of the work with a gender perspective has explored how media sensationalizes HIV/AIDS by associating this condition with homosexuality, illicit drug use, and promiscuity (Lupton 1999, 260–61). While a variety of research has focused on trans and disabled representation in newspapers, very few scholars from the North American and European academies (and essentially none from within Latin America) have questioned how cisgender, able-bodied journalists depict access to healthcare by disabled and trans people.

The data for this exploratory qualitative study is part of a larger study concerning the representation of trans and disabled people in Colombian media. For this project, news articles published between January 2000 and December 2019 were chosen based on three criteria: first, the articles were published by *El Tiempo* (*ET*); second, the articles specifically addressed trans and disabled people accessing healthcare services (this means that articles referring to LGBTQI+ individuals at large were excluded); and finally, the articles refered to local news related to local (Colombian) trans and disabled people. All items were downloaded from *ET*'s online platform and were retrieved using search terms such as: *discapacitado(a), transgénero, transsexual, trans, travesti, enfermo,* etc. All articles incorporated into this study—25 in total—were manually checked to ensure the relation to the topic of access to healthcare. The data analyzed for the present exploration constitute a representative sample of the newspaper. Based on Critical Discourse Analysis, Queer Linguistics, Trans and (Critical) Disability Studies as well as Cultural Studies of Representation, the questions that guided the analysis were: First, how is access to healthcare by trans and disabled people represented in news articles? Second, to what extent do these news articles sustain or transform the current representation of trans and disabled individuals in the Colombian press?

The representation of trans and disabled people accessing healthcare can be characterized as a spectacular and voyeuristic depiction of these people's bodies or health conditions. This type of representation exoticizes the social actor's subjectivity by reducing their life to a dramatic and sensational story. For trans women, the stories created by *ET* focus on a stereotypical representation of their femininity, as well as on the depiction of purportedly unsanitary practices. That is to say, the language used by *ET* makes trans women seem unsanitary due to their practice of certain body modifications. *ET*'s discussions of disabled people seeking healthcare tends to reduce their experiences to their impairment within a narrative of misery. Both groups share some commonalities when being represented. First, their need for healthcare is individualized/personalized through stories of struggle that allow the newspaper to conceal the state's responsibility in providing healthcare within a human-rights framework. Second, the reports use passive constructions and similar linguistic strategies to hide perpetrators of discrimination and violence toward these groups. Finally, the news articles do not address trans-crip-times to access healthcare, that is to say, the "additional" time often needed by disabled individuals "to perform certain tasks and the energy, emotional strain and temporal burden experienced in ableist societies" (Kafer 2013, 25–46).

When representing how trans women access healthcare, *ET* focuses on the tactics trans women employ to modify their bodies under dire circumstances. The newspaper is particularly interested in the depiction of practices such as the injection of fluids or oils in illegal clinics as access to hospitals and health services are limited or denied. Although this form of representation may be understood as a way of denouncing the struggles that trans women face, it lies in a voyeuristic and sensationalized discourse that, on the one hand, depicts trans women as unsanitary bodies and, on the other, negates the responsibility of the state in offering adequate health services to this community. The following two fragments are an excellent example of these two discursive strategies:

(1) Murió travesti tras inyectarse aceite de cocina en los glúteos y silicona para el pelo en el pecho
La Fiscalía de Santa Marta busca a otro travesti que se dedica a realizar esos implantes, que en los últimos tres meses han cobrado la vida a dos personas en esta ciudad.

[A transvestite died after injecting cooking oil into the buttocks and silicone for chest hair.
The Santa Marta Prosecutor's Office is looking for another transvestite who engages in performing these implants, which in the last three months have killed two people in this city.] (*El Tiempo* [*ET*] 2007)

(2) Las clínicas de garaje donde transgeneristas cambian su cuerpo.
Se inyectan fluidos y aceites para lograr la fisonomía de una mujer. Sus vidas penden de un hilo.

[Garage clinics where transsexuals change their bodies.

They inject themselves with fluids and oils to achieve the physiognomy of a woman. Their lives are hanging by a thread.] (Malaver 2014)

In (2), the journalist begins describing Yomaira as a trans woman who underwent several "illegal" medical procedures that caused her significant health conditions. Words such as "underworld," "frantic impulses," "caverns of doom," "deformation," ("bajo mundo," "impulsos frenéticos," "antros de perdición," "deformación,") are used not only to picture the places Yomaira visited to change her body but also the locations she attended daily. This semantic field creates a sense of disgust in the reader by associating Yomaira with illegality and sickness. In other words, Carol Malaver (2014) depicts Yomaira as an unsanitary citizen whose desire for body modification evinces a type of pathological self-destructiveness. Briggs and Mantini-Briggs (2003) state that "Public health officials, physicians, politicians, and the press depict some individuals and communities as possessing modern medical understandings of the body, health, and illness, practicing hygiene, and depending on doctors and nurses when they are sick. These people become sanitary citizens" (10). Consequently, individuals like Yomaira, who are depicted as incapable of using modern medical services, become unsanitary subjects.

Instead, Yomaira's incapability needs to be understood within a broader social framework of healthcare services and access that *ET* omits. Trans women are denied participation in the sanitary system as it is regulated by cisheteronormative guidelines. While cisgender women have access to the healthcare system to modify and take care of their bodies as well as employ aesthetic practices such as diets and cosmetics consumption, trans women are discursively and socially punished for trying to achieve current hegemonic beauty standards. This idea can be corroborated by the way that *ET* represents medical procedures. Journalists tend to construct them as whims and fancies instead of the medical needs of transgender women. Expressions such as the ones in the excerpts included below (see 3, 4, and 5) seem to assert that trans women undergo risky procedures due to vanity. What is more, the discourse in these sentences negates a deeper explanation of body modification (for example, beauty standards or the need to have a body that agrees with the inner gender identification).

(3) Su vanidad le pedía más [cambios corporales].

[His vanity demanded more [bodily changes]] (Malaver 2014).

(4) Un momento de vanidad se convirtió en el preludio de su tragedia.

[A moment of vanity became the prelude to her tragedy] (Malaver 2014).

(5) Esa vida de impulsos frenéticos lo llevó a Bogotá cuando solo tenía 20 años. No tenía dinero, pero sí, la convicción de ser mujer. "Llegué a consumir hormonas. Los travestis de la peluquería me contaron que eso se podía hacer. Se consiguen en cualquier droguería."

[That life of frantic impulses led him to Bogotá when he was only 20 years old. He had no money, but yes, the conviction of being a woman. "I got to consume hormones. The transvestites from the hair salon told me that that could be done. They are available at any drugstore."] (Malaver 2014).

By choosing who to cover and who can speak, journalists enable certain voices to frame the news without appearing to do so. In (5), when Malaver (2014) allows Yomaira to speak, her statement is framed within the narrative of whim and fancy. Indeed, the article uses the masculine object pronoun (lo) to discursively disassociate Yomaira's female gender identity. Such practices occur frequently throughout the text and recur regularly in other articles published by *ET*. Additionally, source attribution relies heavily on medical professionals and experts on LGBTQI+ issues whose statements reinforce the idea of trans women as unsanitary citizens. As we can observe in the next excerpt (6), even though the expert offers a human-rights perspective on access to health procedures, the journalist opts for quoting the expert's description of the effects some substances have on the bodies of trans women, thus reinforcing a voyeuristic gaze. Serano (2007) notes that journalists particularly emphasize trans women's artifices and corporealities evoking the "idea that trans women are living out some sort of sexual fetish" (44). This phenomenon is consistent with previous studies of source attribution in the Colombian press. Sánchez Buitrago and Lichilín Piedrahita (2005), have found that sourcing in news outlets is insufficient. Indeed, news stories frequently exclude people from marginalized communities as sources despite the fact that they are experts of their own experiences.

(6) "Mejor morir como mujer que vivir con el cuerpo de un hombre"
Es parte de la realidad que ha palpado a diario Pedro Julio Pardo Castañeda estos 10 años en la dirección ejecutiva de Santamaría Fundación, desde donde se promueve la autodeterminación de

mujeres trans para el ejercicio de su ciudadanía plena, el respeto y garantía de sus derechos humanos y acceso a los servicios del Estado, en especial de salud, "Son sustancias abrasivas, extrañas al cuerpo, en poco tiempo los efectos se reflejan en la piel, se forman brotes grandes, el aceite a veces llega al torrente sanguíneo, se produce embolia cerebral o pulmonar y sobreviene un evento cardiorespiratorio," dice Pardo.

["Better to die as a woman than to live with the body of a man'
It is part of the reality that Pedro Julio Pardo Castañeda has felt every day these 10 years in the executive management of the Santamaría Fundación, from where the self-determination of trans women is promoted for the exercise of their full citizenship, respect and guarantee of their human rights and access to state services, especially health. "They are abrasive substances, foreign to the body, in a short time the effects are reflected on the skin, large outbreaks form, the oil sometimes reaches the bloodstream, it produces cerebral or pulmonary embolisms and a cardiorespiratory event ensues," says Pardo.] (*ET* 2015b).

Physical modifications carried out by trans women are not inherently excessive; rather, they follow social ideas about the (feminine) body. Nevertheless, these journalists fail to depict other elements related to access to healthcare. *ET* thus focuses on the technologies/tactics trans women use rather than portraying the dominant logic of sexual identity, corporeality, and citizenship. Similarly, discourses toward accessing healthcare by disabled people tend to rely on images that exploit disabled bodies by reducing them to their impairment within a narrative of misery and struggle. This ultimately reinforces voyeuristic perspectives for understanding sexual and disabled minorities.

One of the main characteristics of the corpus studied is that disabled people clamor for privatized healthcare providers to guarantee access to treatment. Headlines usually focus on medical conditions to attract a reader's attention and invoke feelings of pity. This emphasis is particularly problematic as it does not tackle the role of the state. Rather, these articles depend on an individualization of healthcare that conceals the structural, social, and systemic barriers that are the result of a cis-ableist mentality. This mentality has been reinforced as neoliberal policies have taken root in Colombia over the last several decades. As other scholars have noted, individualized representations of disability hide an extended web of meanings based on neoliberal economics, (trans)national transformations as well as politics of inequality that impact disabled people (Antebi and Jörgensen 2016, 3). Our exploration of trans and disability representation adheres to the idea that disability representation in Latin America is based on a tension "between disability defined through individual experience, and through a more bio-politically oriented emphasis on populations or collectives" (Antebi and Jörgensen 2016, 3). An example of this individualized depiction appears when *ET* describes how both trans and disabled people invoke fundamental rights actions (tutela) [8] to access healthcare services after their providers deny them due to their high costs, as occurs in excerpts 7, 8, and 9.

(7) Pacientes con cáncer protestaron contra EPS en Armenia
Unas 50 personas piden que las EPS entreguen los tratamientos y los medicamentos a tiempo.
[ . . . ] Otro caso conmovedor es el del pequeño Luciano de casi tres años y a quien le diagnosticaron cáncer el pasado 15 de enero pero no ha podido iniciar su tratamiento de quimioterapia por las demoras de su EPS.

[Cancer patients protested against EPS in Armenia
About 50 people ask EPS to deliver treatments and medications on time.
[ . . . ] Another moving case is that of little Luciano, almost three years old, who was diagnosed with cancer on January 15th, but was unable to start his chemotherapy treatment due to delays in his EPS.] (*ET* 2017b).

(8) Clamor por niña afectada por enfermedad huérfana, en ladera de Cali
Una estudiante, de 9 años, espera tratamiento para que su movilidad mejore. La madre pide ayuda.

[Cry for girl affected by orphan disease, on Cali hillside
A 9-year-old student awaits treatment so that her mobility improves. Her mother is asking for help.] (*ET* 2015a).

(9) El "trans" que espera que su EPS le cambie de sexo
En octubre, el Tribunal Superior de Armenia falló a favor de Gina Vanesa.

[The "trans" waiting for his EPS to change his sex
In October, the Armenian High Court ruled in favor of Gina Vanesa.]
(*ET* 2017a).

Although *ET* occasionally addresses Colombia's legislation that specifically protects trans and disabled individuals' rights to access healthcare and non-discriminatory practices, this functions through what Dean Spade (2015) has named, in the case of trans communities, "equality law" (11). Anti-discrimination laws fail to address the real issues that create vulnerability for trans/disabled people since "legal equality goals threaten to provide nothing more than adjustments to the window-dressing of neoliberal violence that ultimately disserve and further marginalize the most vulnerable trans populations" (12). Furthermore, the rights-focused framework that *ET* uses to depict transness and disability serves to perpetuate the existing inequality since it creates an individualized and reductionist representation. The trans and disabled person is a victim of the (in)actions of a perpetrator, the health provider (*EPS*). This case-by-case approach negates the possibility to further understand ableism and transphobia within the healthcare system and its connections with, for example, neoliberalism and *Ley 100*. Individuals can achieve remediation without forcing the state to tackle and challenge the structural discrimination or deeper sociocultural and economic modifications needed to dismantle marginalization. The use of "passivization"—in which social actors "are represented as 'undergoing' the activity, or as being 'at the receiving end'" (van Leeuwen 2008, 33)—further reinforces the phenomenon. We observe this in examples 9 and 10 where trans and disabled social actors wait to receive benefits from a third party (the *EPS*).

(10) Esposa de exjugador de fútbol clama por atención en EPS por su hija
Alexandra Gómez, esposa del exjugador del América de Cali y del Santa Fe, Andrés Felipe González, dijo que hace más de un año vive el drama con una EPS para que a su hija, de 4 años, le den una silla de sedestación y así facilitar cargar a la menor que sufre parálisis cerebral.

[Wife of former football player cries out for EPS attention for his daughter
Alexandra Gómez, wife of the former player from América de Cali and Santa Fe, Andrés Felipe González, said that the drama has been going on for more than a year with an EPS so that her 4-year-

old daughter will be given a wheelchair and thus facilitate carrying the minor suffering from cerebral palsy.] (*ET* 2018).

Passivization often accompanies other linguistic mechanisms that serve to hide elements of the discriminatory acts being reported. On the one hand, passive constructions allow reporters to hide the perpetrators of discrimination and violence against trans and disabled people. We observe this in examples 11 and 12. In both cases, passive constructions hide the association between the negative actions and the majority group. On the other hand, journalists omit some elements of the social practice being represented through processes of nominalization that allow the actions to be objectivated (van Leeuwen 2008, 18). For instance, in examples 13 and 14, the reports elide the participant who discriminates through nominalization (bullying, discriminatory treatment/acts [las burlas, los tratos/actos discriminatorios]). Although representing discrimination through nominalization contributes to portraying oppression as a generalized practice, its extended use also creates the idea that there are no specific social actors responsible for such discrimination, a fact that further naturalizes this practice.

(11) El 99,68% de ellos expresan que han sido discriminadas o sus derechos vulnerados y limitados por cualquier razón . . .

[99.68% of them express that they have been discriminated against or their rights have been violated and limited for some reason . . . ] (Malaver 2014).

(12) En el caso de los homicidios, fueron 35 mujeres trans asesinadas en el 2017 frente a los tres hombres trans que sufrieron el mismo destino.

[In the case of homicides, 35 trans women were murdered in 2017 compared to three trans men who suffered the same fate.] (Barrientos 2018).

(13) Por las burlas y tratos discriminatorios de los que dicen ser víctimas cada vez que llegan a un centro de salud, transexuales de Cartagena reclamaron mayor atención al Distrito en este tema.

[Due to the bullying and discriminatory treatment of those who claim to be victims every time they arrive at a health center, transsexuals from Cartagena demanded more attention from the District on this issue.] (*ET* 2013).

(14) Ella, dijo Marrugo, fue víctima de actos discriminatorios en los centros asistenciales donde fue tratada en Cartagena.

[She, said Marrugo, was the victim of discriminatory acts in the healthcare centers where she was treated in Cartagena] (*ET* 2013)

The last element to briefly mention here has to do with how these news articles depict crip-time. As mentioned before, this concept refers to the "extra" time and energy needed by disabled people to carry out certain activities as well as the emotional burden experienced in ableist societies (Kafer 2013, 25–46). Baril (2015) argues that trans people experience "trans-crip-time," that is to say, additional time needed to find information on surgical procedures, educate doctors and society, and heal while at the same time finding ways to deal with financial costs that affect their lives and opportunities (72). However, *ET* tends to omit this element from its reports, perhaps in part because mentioning it would constitute a direct denouncement of the cis/able oppressive system in which trans and disabled individuals live. Additionally, omitting this time also allows the newspaper to hide the bureaucratic obstacles that the Colombian healthcare system has imposed on trans individuals. The reasons why this happens are difficult to determine. Ignorance from the reporter on the barriers that trans and disabled people face when accessing health services may be one explanation. The other possible reason is that the newspaper purposely conceals this element. In either case, *ET* fails to share the full story.

News articles tend to mention the additional time that disabled people require to face bureaucratic obstacles, but the articles discussed above represent trans women waiting for health service providers, underemployment rates, and cost of medical care less frequently. This avoidance of representing trans-crip-time also contributes to debilitating trans struggles, especially those related to healthcare services. It reduces the trans experience to a whim, a desire for physical modification. It ought not be forgotten that transness is a complex experience where ability, gender, and sexuality intersect. Trans communities are also diverse, and many trans individuals do not desire body modifications from the healthcare system. They possess other health needs that *ET* ignores as it reduces transness to a specific type of femininity, one that follows dominant ideas of gender and beauty. In other words, in the same way that dominant discourses tend to reduce disabled people to their disability, *ET* often reduces trans women's needs to a desire for "sex change." Such constructs ignore how trans people's interactions with the world may generate a whole range of health needs.

Finally, these articles portray trans women as obsessed with body modifications, while they cast disabled individuals as people who access healthcare in search of a cure. The newspaper does not mention the importance of accessing mental health services. Trans activists have noted that one of the main barriers to accessing healthcare is the lack of knowledge that medical professionals possess in regard to trans issues. They have also argued that health professionals only address issues of body modifications and omit other health conditions, especially those related to mental health. Similar observations can be made in relation to disabled people as their mental health is constantly undermined. There is no mention of which services are available to them and, on top of that, *ET* mainly addresses visible disabilities or rare diseases since other conditions may not be easily commodified within a voyeuristic approach. In other words, *ET*'s news articles uphold the current misrepresentation of trans and disabled individuals in the Colombian press that has led to negative stereotypes. In particular, *ET* focuses on body modifications/impairments and conceals how the Colombian state has implemented a neoliberal healthcare system that sets a series of barriers for minoritized groups.

**Closing Remarks**

We cannot conclude this chapter without reflecting on the effects of the COVID-19 pandemic on trans and disabled individuals. Trans and queer people, in particular, have relied on communal knowledge, novel forms of kinship and care, and experiences from the HIV pandemic to cope with COVID-19. As Susan Stryker noted in the webinar "COVID-19 Trans Lives and Trans Studies" (Stryker et al. 2020), queer folks have figured out different ways to be safe in a world that has not been designed for them. The pandemic has only worsened a situation where current healthcare systems do not serve trans people, especially those of color. Red Washburn in the same webinar, argued that this historical event is a moment to ask, following Judith Butler (1993): whose lives matter and who is human? Many trans health-related issues and everyday activities were on pause (for example, no surgeries and hormones, doctors denying evaluations for trans people, lawsuits on hold). This has increased mental and physical anxiety and violence for trans people. To support each other, organizations such as La Red Comunitaria Trans in Colombia have developed a series of strategies to protect trans women and men. Some strategies of mutual aid include webinars to share expertise, video tutorials on safer sexual practices for trans women working in prostitution, and fundraisers to help trans people afford permanent housing during quarantine. In this way, trans communities are helping each other at a time when systems of care mainly focus on cisheterosexual individuals.

Similarly, disabled people have been questioning ableist and ageist discourses during the pandemic. Trans disabled activist Elliot Kukla (2020) has reacted to messages of disposability—which have appeared in several media outlets and in discourse from able people—as a mechanism to cope with the pandemic. Disabled people have demonstrated that their lived experience can provide knowledge about social distancing, caring, and mental health; indeed, they are experts of these realities. In the same way, Alice Wong (2020) has discussed how the debates on healthcare rationing unveil the ways that society at large devalues vulnerable populations. Guidelines directed to hospitals on how to prepare during disastrous situations are examples of this necro-political approach, following Achille Mbembe (2003), where certain individuals (the elderly and disabled) are deemed disposable based on their (future) productivity. In Colombia, scholars and independent experts have made recommendations on how the state can guarantee safety and security for disabled people based on the United Nations Convention on the Rights of Persons with Disabilities. The Ministry of Health and Social Protection of Colombia has issued some guidelines on prevention and healthcare for disabled people and their families during COVID-19. Although this initiative has been well-received in the country, the pandemic has led (LGBTQI+/disabled) activists, scholars, politicians, and intellectuals to once again advocate for restructuring or abolishing *Ley 100*, which they identify as the main barrier that prevents minoritized social groups from truly accessing healthcare.

## Acknowledgments

We thank Kent Brintnall and the two editors for their valuable comments and for the style corrections. We also thank Anastasia Ramjag for the English translations as well as Laura Richiez Combas, research assistant at the Department of Languages and Culture Studies at UNC Charlotte, for her work on data collection. This work was supported, in part, by funds provided by The University of North Carolina, Charlotte.

## Notes

1. We use "trans/transgender" as an imperfect umbrella for transgender, transsexual, nonbinary, intersex, and gender-nonconforming people, and "cisgender" to mean non-trans.

2. Colombia's census does not include trans or gender non-conforming categories. Individuals must declare their sex/gender as it appears on legal documents such as the national identification card (*cédula*) or birth certificates.

3. Neoliberalism has been the dominant political economy since the 1980s. Specifically, President Gaviria (1990–1994) embraced neoliberal economics in Colombia through several reforms but especially by making land available to international companies.

4. Colombia's health system uses the term regime to refer to this two-tier scheme: *régimen contributivo* and *régimen subsidiado* [contributory and subsidized regimes, respectively].

5. Young adults (ages 18 to 25), regardless of their employment situation, can be co-insured by their parents. Insured adults can extend coverage to their parents if they meet the following criteria: 1) the former is single and has no children and 2) the latter is not retired and depends economically on the insured person.

6. Several articles of the Colombian Constitution aim to protect and promote special attention for disabled people. The country has also passed specific legislation to ensure the rights of disabled people. See Roth et al. (2019, 32–37).

7. Bonnin (2013; 2019) has explored doctor–patient communication in admission interviews at mental healthcare services in Argentina from a discourse studies perspective.

8. *Tutela* is a constitutional injunction meant to protect fundamental constitutional rights when any authority or institution violates them through action or omission.

## References

Agudelo Calderón, Carlos Alberto, Jaime Cardona Botero, Jesús Ortega Bolaños, and Rocio Robledo Martínez. 2011. "Sistema de salud en Colombia: 20 años de logros y problemas." *Ciencia e Saude Coletiva* 16 (6): 2817–27. https://doi.org/10.1590/S1413-81232011000600020.

Antebi, Susan, and Beth E. Jörgensen. 2016. "Introduction." In *Libre Acceso. Latin American Literature and Film through Disability Studies,* edited by Susan Antebi and Beth E. Jörgensen, 1–26. Albany: State University of New York Press.

Baril, Alexandre. 2015. "Transness as Debility: Rethinking Intersections between Trans and Disabled Embodiments." *Feminist Review* 111: 59–74. https://doi.org/doi:10.1057/fr.2015.21.

Barrientos, Julia. 2018. "Vulneración sistemática de derechos, realidad de los trans en el país." *El Tiempo,* July 14, 2018.

Benelli, Eva. 2003. "The Role of the Media in Steering Public Opinion on Healthcare Issues." *Health Policy* 63 (2): 179–86.

Biel Portero, Israel, and Tania G. Bolaños Enríquez. 2018. "Persons with Disabilities and the Colombian Armed Conflict." *Disability and Society* 33 (3): 487–91. https://doi.org/10.1080/09687599.2018.1423914.

Bonnin, Juan Eduardo. 2013. "The Public, the Private and the Intimate in Doctor–Patient Communication: Admission Interviews at an Outpatient Mental Health Care Service." *Discourse Studies* 15 (6): 687–711.

———. 2019. *Discourse and Mental Health. Voice, Inequality and Resistance in Medical Settings*. London: Routledge.

Briggs, Charles, and Clara Mantini-Briggs. 2003. *Stories in the Time of Cholera: Racial Profiling during a Medical Nightmare*. Berkeley: University of California Press.

Buitrago, Yudi. 2015. "Ideas, discurso y proceso de reforma en el sector salud. Colombia y Ecuador en perspectiva comparada." *Mundos Plurales. Revista Latinoamericana de Políticas y Acción Publica* 2 (2): 51–69. https://doi.org/https://doi.org/10.17141/mundosplurales.2.2015.1984.

Butler, Judith. 1993. *Bodies That Matter. On the Discursive Limits of "Sex."* New York: Routledge.

Caballero, Jorge. *Paciente*. 2016. Bogotá: Gusano Films and Señal Colombia.

Carrasco, José Miguel, Beatriz Gómez-Baceiredo, Alejandro Navas, Marian Krawczyk, Miriam García, and Carlos Centeno. 2019. "Social Representation of Palliative Care in the Spanish Printed Media: A Qualitative Analysis." *PLoS ONE* 14 (1): 1–12. https://doi.org/https://doi.org/10.1371/journal.pone.0211106.

Collins, Patricia, Julia Abelson, Heather Pyman, and John Lavis. 2006. "Are We Expecting too Much from Print Media? An Analysis of Newspaper Coverage of the 2002 Canadian Healthcare Reform Debate." *Social Science & Medicine* 63 (1): 89–102.

Correa-Montoya, Lucas, and Marta Catalina Castro Martínez. 2016. *Disability and Social Inclusion in Colombia. Saldarriaga-Concha Foundation. Alternative Report to the Committee on the Rights of Persons with Disabilities*. Bogota: Saldarriaga-Concha Foundation Press.

Departamento Administrativo Nacional de Estadística (DANE). 2018. *Censo nacional de población y vivienda 2018*. Gobierno de Colombia.

El Tiempo (ET). 2007. "Murió travesti tras inyectarse aceite de cocina en los glúteos y silicona para el pelo en el pecho." *El Tiempo*, August 15, 2007.

———. 2013. "Transexuales de Cartagena reclaman respeto en centros de salud." *El Tiempo*, February 19, 2013.

———. 2015a. "Clamor por niña afectada por enfermedad huérfana, en Ladera de Cali." *El Tiempo*, July 10, 2015.

———. 2015b. "'Mejor morir como mujer que vivir con el cuerpo de un hombre.'" *El Tiempo*, June 8, 2015.

———. 2017a. "El 'trans' que espera que su EPS le cambie de sexo." *El Tiempo*, January 23, 2017.

———. 2017b. "Pacientes con cáncer protestaron contra EPS en Armenia." *El Tiempo*, March 16, 2017.

———. 2018. "Esposa de exjugador de fútbol clama por atención en EPS por su hija." *El Tiempo*, January 17, 2018.

Escobar, María-Luisa, Ursula Giedion, Antonio Giuffrida, and Amanda L. Glassman. 2009. "Colombia: After a Decade of Health System Reform." In *From Few to Many*.

*Ten Years of Health Insurance Expansion in Colombia,* edited by Amanda L. Glassman, María-Luisa Escobar, Antonio Giuffrida, and Ursula Giedion, 1–13. Washington, DC: Inter-American Development Bank / The Brookings Institution.

Gallego, Juan Miguel, Manuela Ramírez, and Carlos Sepulveda. 2005. "The Determinants of the Health Status in a Developing Country: Results from the Colombian Case." *Lecturas de Economía* 63: 111–35.

García León, Javier E. 2019. "Documentando la producción audiovisual *transloca* colombiana. Apuntes críticos sobre la representación trans." *Canadian Journal of Latin American and Caribbean Studies* 44 (3): 261–80.

———. 2021. *Espectáculo, normalización y representaciones otras. Las personas transgénero en la prensa y el cine de Colombia y Venezuela.* Berlin: Peter Lang.

Garland-Thompson, Rosemarie. 1997. *Extraordinary Bodies. Figuring Physical Disability in American Culture and Literature.* New York: Columbia University Press.

Giedion, Ursula, and Manuela Villar. 2009. "Colombia's Universal Health Insurance System: The Results of Providing Health Insurance for All in a Middle-Income Country." *Health Affairs* 28 (2): 853–63.

Gómez Perea, Carlos Andres, Lina Marcela Pasos Revelo, Tatiana González Rojas, and Marcela Arrivillaga Quintero. 2018. "Acceso a servicios de salud de personas en situación de discapacidad física en Zarzal (Valle, Colombia)." *Revista Científica Salud Uninorte* 34 (2): 276–83.

Gossett, Reina, Eric Stanley, and Johanna Burton, eds. 2017. *Trap Door: Trans Cultural Production and the Politics of Visibility.* Cambridge: The MIT Press.

Grue, Jan. 2011. "Discourse Analysis and Disability: Some Topics and Issues." *Discourse & Society* 22 (5): 532–46. https://doi.org/10.1177/0957926511405572.

———. 2015. *Disability and Discourse Studies.* Farnhan: Ashgate Publishing Limited.

Gutiérrez-Coba, Liliana, Andrea Salgado-Cardona, Víctor García Perdomo, and Yahira Guzmán-Rossini. 2017. "Coverage of Mental Health in the Colombian Press, an Ongoing Contribution." *Revista Latina de Comunicación Social* 72: 114–28. http://www.revistalatinacs.org/072paper/1156/06en.html

Halberstam, Judith. 2005. *In a Queer Time and Place: Transgender Bodies, Subcultural Lives.* New York: New York University Press.

Homedes, Núria, and Antonio Ugalde. 2005. "Why Neoliberal Health Reforms Have Failed in Latin America." *Health Policy* 71 (1): 83–96.

Irving, Dan. 2013. "Normalized Transgressions: Legitimizing the Transsexual Body as Productive." In *The Transgender Studies Reader 2,* edited by Susan Stryker and Aren Aizura, 15–29. New York: Routledge.

Kafer, Alison. 2013. *Feminist Queer Crip.* Bloomington: Indiana University Press.

Kukla, Ellliot. 2020. "My Life is More 'Disposable' During This Pandemic." *The New York Times,* March 19, 2020.

Lasso Báez, Roberto. 2014. "Transexualidad y servicios de salud utilizados para transitar por los sexos-géneros." *Revista CES Psicología* 7 (2): 108–25.

Lewis, Sophie, Fran Collyer, Karen Willis, Kirsten Harley, Kanchan Marcus, Michael Calnan, and Jon Gabe. 2018. "Healthcare in the News Media: The Privileging of Private over Public." *Journal of Sociology* 54 (4): 574–90.

Lupton, Deborah. 1999. "Editorial: Health, Illness and Medicine in the Media." *Health* 3 (3): 259–62.
Malaver, Carol. 2014. "Las clínicas de garaje donde transgeneristas cambian su cuerpo." *El Tiempo*, October 3, 2014.
Mbembe, Achille. 2003. "Necropolitics." *Public Culture* 15 (1): 11–40.
Molina, Gloria, Julian Vargas, and Ivan Muñoz. 2010. "Dilemas en las decisiones en la atención en salud: Ética, derechos y deberes constitucionales frente a la rentabilidad financiera en el sistema de salud colombiano." *Revista Gerencia y Políticas de Salud* 9 (18): 103–17.
Panizza, Francisco. 2009. *Contemporary Latin America: Development and Democracy beyond the Washington Consensus*. New York: Zed Books.
Pinilla-Roncancio, Mónica. 2015. "Disability and Poverty: Two Related Conditions. A Review of the Literature." *Revista Facultad de Medicina* 63 (1): 113–23.
Prada, Clara, and Sonia Chaves. 2019. "Health System Structure and Transformations in Colombia between 1990 and 2013: A Socio-Historical Study." *Critical Public Health* 29 (3): 314–24. https://doi.org/10.1080/09581596.2018.1449943.
Puar, Jasbir K. 2017. *The Right to Maim: Debility, Capacity, Disability*. Durham, NC: Duke University Press.
Ritterbusch, Amy E, Catalina Correa Salazar, and Andrea Correa. 2018. "Stigma-Related Access Barriers and Violence against Trans Women in the Colombian Healthcare System." *Global Public Health* 13 (12): 1831–45.
Rivas Velarde, Minerva, Karim Garzon, and Tom Shakespeare. 2019. "Social Participation and Inclusion of Ex-Combatants with Disabilities in Colombia." *Disability and the Global South* 6 (2): 1736–55.
Roberts, Tiffany K., and Corinne R. Fantz. 2014. "Barriers to Quality Health Care for the Transgender Population." *Clinical Biochemistry* 47 (10–11): 983–87.
Rodríguez Moreno, Jaime, and Laura Vivas Martínez. 2017. *Primary Health Care Systems (PRIMASYS): Case Study from Colombia*. Geneva: World Health Organization.
Roth, André-Noël, Ángela Gordillo, Nancy González, and Eliana Suaréz. 2019. *Análisis de la política pública de discapacidad de Bogotá (2007–2017). La implementación vista desde los actores institucionales, las personas con discapacidad y sus cuidadores*. Bogotá: Universidad Nacional de Colombia.
Ryan Joelle. 2009. "Reel Gender: Examining the Politics of Trans Images in Film and Media." PhD diss., Bowling Green State University.
Sánchez Buitrago, Marcela, and Ana Alejandra Lichilín Piedrahita. 2005. *Periodismo para la diversidad*. Bogotá: Colombia Diversa/Centro de Investigación y Educación Popular.
Serano, Julia. 2007. *Whipping Girl. A Transsexual Woman on Sexism and the Scapegoating of Femininity*. Berkeley, CA: Seal Press.
———. 2013. "Why the Media Depicts the Trans Revolution in Lipstick and Heels." In *The Transgender Studies Reader 2*, edited by Susan Stryker and Aren Aizura, 226–33. New York: Routledge.
Silva-Santisteban, Alfonso, Shirley Eng, Gabriela de la Iglesia, Carlos Falistocco, and Rafael Mazin. 2016. "HIV Prevention among Transgender Women in Latin America:

Implementation, Gaps and Challenges." *Journal of the International AIDS Society* 19 (2): 1–10.

Spade, Dean. 2015. *Normal Life: Administrative Violence, Critical Trans Politics, and the Limits of Law*. 2nd ed. Durham: Duke University Press.

Stryker, Susan, Chanel Lopez, Amita Swadhin, Treva Ellison, Debanuj Dasgupta, and Red Washburn. 2020. "COVID-19 Trans Lives & Trans Studies." CLAGS: The Center for LGBTQ Studies.

Van Dijk, Teun, ed. 2009. *Racism and Discourse in Latin America*. Lanham, MD: Lexington Books.

van Leeuwen, Theo. 2008. *Discourse and Practice. New Tools for Critical Discourse Analysis*. New York: Oxford University Press.

Vargas, Ingrid, Luisa Vázquez, and Amparo Mogollón. 2010. "Acceso a la atención en salud en Colombia." *Revista de Salud Pública* 12 (5): 701–12. https://doi.org/doi:10.1590/S0124-00642010000500001.

Wong, Alice. 2020. "I'm Disabled and Need a Ventilator to Live. Am I Expendable during This Pandemic?" *Vox*, April 4, 2020.

World Health Organization (WHO). 2011. *World Report on Disability*. Malta.

Zottola, Angela. 2018. "Transgender Identity Labels in the British Press. A Corpus-Based Discourse Analysis." *Journal of Language and Sexuality* 7 (2): 237–62.

# 14

# Biomedicine and Ancestral Knowledges

*Vengo volviendo* and Healthcare Services in Ecuador

Manuel F. Medina

The social exclusion of the Ecuadorian lower classes, a direct consequence of the capitalist model, has occupied the inspiration of artists, writers, and intellectuals. For instance, in the 1930s the country saw the development of one of its most renowned literary periods led by writers whose work, based on denunciations of social inequality, became the trademark of Ecuadorian literature for readers around the world. We refer to the so-called Group of Guayaquil and Jorge Icaza's famous *Huasipungo* (1934), a novel about the plight of the Indigenous people of Ecuador who suffer the abuse of insensitive landowners. This social and political context changed minimally, if at all, over the next decades, and Ecuadorian writers mostly addressed topics associated with social realism. They experimented with literary form, but did not deviate from a social commitment to change and equality. During the 1970s and 1980s, authors such as Jorge Enrique Adoum published novels where narrative structure subverted traditional models, but, again, these texts retained a commitment to social change.

At the turn of the twenty-first century, with the advent of a booming film industry, Ecuadorian directors have often followed the nation's longstanding tendency of addressing social inequality. Unsurprisingly, many cultural productions of the new century—including art, literature and film—highlight flaws in the public health apparatus and the lack of access to care by those who belong to society's lower classes.[1] This dialogue has included an attempt to level social and economic discrepancies that cut across class, race, and gender. This chapter studies how the Ecuadorian film *Vengo volviendo* [Here and There] (2015), directed by Gabriel Páez Hernández and Isabel Rodas León, joins a discussion on healthcare within the context of the "good way of living," or *sumak kawsay*, and the role of establishing a new national identity that offers its citizens a place to live in harmony.[2] This chapter contends that *Vengo volviendo* intends to grant ancestral knowledges-based medicine a place alongside the practice of healthcare based on the established tradition of Western biomedicine. Along the way, the film comments as well on the persistence of colonialism and its legacy of discrimination based on race and class in granting access to public health to Ecuadorian citizens.

*Vengo volviendo*[3] narrates the story of Ismael and Luz, who find themselves on opposite sides of the spectrum. Luz has just relocated from an eight-year residence in the United States and plans to stay home. Ismael has only one goal in mind: migrate to the country up north by any means necessary. Ismael has a close relationship with his Abuela (or Grandmother) Mariana who raised him and who makes a living selling medicinal herbs. The plot develops its dramatic tension by showcasing Ismael's quest to flee to the modern world, leaving his birthplace behind. The film intertwines three stories that could stand as short films in their own right, with each depicting a mythical story associated with the region of Azuay, a province located approximately three hundred miles south of Quito, the country's capital.

Ecuador, like most Latin American countries, adopted a Eurocentric model of modernity, one based heavily on the exploitation of the non-European peoples of the Americas under the control of those who could trace their lineage back to the Empire (Quijano 2000, 289). This arrangement often resembled the colonial system centered on race and class brought over by the Spaniards, a colonial underpinning that eventually served as the basis for the capitalist system embraced by the region's national governments from Independence through the contemporary moment (Ayala Mora and Universidad Andina Simón Bolívar 2015, 31). Forging the concept of a nation and national identity throughout this period often resulted in the implementation of social structures that excluded or silenced Indigenous peasants and rural populations and placed the mestizo at a level slightly above them. Aníbal Quijano (2000) explains the interrelationships connecting coloniality, modernism, and capitalism: "The corresponding intersubjective relationships, which solidify into the colonialist and colonial experiences under the needs of capitalism, became a new universe of intersubjective relationships of control under a Eurocentric hegemony. This specific universe is what would later be labeled modernity." [Las relaciones intersubjetivas correspondientes, en las cuales se fueron fundiendo las experiencias del colonialismo y de la colonialidad con las necesidades del capitalismo, se fueron configurando como un nuevo universo de relaciones intersubjetivas de dominación bajo hegemonía eurocentrada. Ese específico universo es el que será después denominado como la modernidad] (342–43).[4]

Modernism adopts or perpetuates the hierarchical structure of power persistent through the colonial period in the country. The system brought over by the Spanish Empire resembles those of similar enterprises by European countries and their preferred means of colonization around the world: dominance, exploitation and abuse. Juan Ramos (2015), contextualizing the concept as it refers to the Ecuadorian coastal area, reiterates Quijano's argument: "While modernity is linked to a Eurocentric rhetoric and desire for progress and modernization, coloniality reveals the very limits of such a rhetoric and the impossibility of its fulfillment. The logic of coloniality shapes conceptions of race and gender, enables modes of control (social customs and laws), and creates hierarchies of domination" (63). However, Ramos demonstrates the impossibility and lack of logic of such an enterprise because of the close connection between coloniality, colonialism (the practice of colonial methods of subjugation), and modernity. The perpetual archetypes of power emanating from European colonialism remain embedded in a concept of modernity that is simply colonialism delivered under new assumptions or presumptions of power. Ramos reads issues concerning gender and social classification as an inherited flaw of Ecuadorian modernity derived from colonial systems. Ultimately, his goal is to unveil hidden forms of coloniality inherent in a presumed modern Ecuadorian society and how the short story that he analyzes ("La Tigra" by José de la Cuadra) destabilizes seemingly fixed and readily accepted categories of gender and social identity (64).

Ecuador's healthcare systems reflected the nation's ideologies favoring modern medicine, but making it accessible only to a select few—mostly city dwellers and mestizos—and excluding rural inhabitants. The Pan American Health Organization reported on this situation in 2004: "Ecuador's health protection system is highly fragmented, with a deficit of health care coverage of 20.7 percent, with 76 percent of the population lacking any type of insurance, with regressive household private expenditures, and with a weak steering role on the part of the Ministry of Health due to governance problems (weakness in coordination and in both strategic and operative consensus)" (Pan American Health Organization 2004). For some Ecuadorians, insurance could compensate for the lack of services provided by state-run and private healthcare centers in areas located away from urban centers.

However, in 1990, with the support of CONAIE (Confederación de Nacionalidades Indígenas del Ecuador or Confederation of Ecuadorian Indigenous Nations), Ecuador's autochthonous population organized one of Latin

America's strongest Indigenous movements (Yashar 2005, 85). As a direct result of these efforts, the 1998 constitution granted access to free universal healthcare without restrictions based on race and class (Asamblea Nacional Constituyente 1998, Art. 43). More importantly, Article 44 of this document commits the state to support and regulate the development of traditional and alternative medicines: "Art. 44. The State . . . will recognize, respect, and promote the development of traditional and alternative medicines, whose implementation will be regulated by law and will foment scientific and technological advances in health care, subject to bio-ethical principles." [Art. 44. El Estado . . . reconocerá, respetará y promoverá el desarrollo de las medicinas tradicional y alternativa, cuyo ejercicio será regulado por la ley, e impulsará el avance científico-tecnológico en el área de la salud, con sujeción a principios bioéticos.] (Asamblea Nacional Constituyente 1998).

Rochelle Dreyfuss and César Rodríguez-Garavito (2014) comment on the repercussion of the inclusion of these articles in the constitution. They maintain that it "consolidated and legitimized [the Ecuadorian Indigenous movement] as one of the main political powers in the country" (202). Henry Tarco Carrera (2020) studies *Vengo volviendo* as an example of a decolonizing trend in contemporary Ecuadorian film. He shows how the film works within an intercultural paradigm that showcases members of the Indigenous universe, mestizo subjects, and white Ecuadorians. Thus, he affirms Ecuador as a pluricultural space that seeks the interest of all its citizens, regardless of race, social class, or status (349).

*Vengo volviendo* takes on the postulates of Article 44 of the 1998 Constitution, later confirmed in the 2008 Constitution: "Article 360. The system shall guarantee, through the institutions that comprise it, the promotion of family and community health, prevention and integral care, on the basis of primary healthcare; it shall articulate various levels of care; and it shall promote complementariness with ancestral and alternative medicines" (National Assembly 2008). The updated version, written and approved when the CONAIE had less influence than ten years earlier, emphasizes the complementary nature of traditional medicine, labeled as "ancestral and alternative" in the document currently in effect (National Assembly 2008, Art. 360). The omission, deletion, or replacement of the phrase "recognize, respect, and promote" removes the inclusiveness associated with the previous constitution (National Assembly 2008, Art. 360).

*Vengo volviendo* traces its origin to a project initiated by Filmarte, an organization funded by a group of socially minded filmmakers who set out to empower underrepresented Ecuadorian communities, as indicated in its mission statement: "Share cinema to people in areas with limited access to this tool, encouraging the production of their own quality films" (Filmarte 2019). Filmarte expands this raison d'être by declaring its desire to provide a means for those who lack the opportunity to voice their own narratives: "Promoting visibility of communities through their own voice and identity. Providing high quality training, production and dissemination of feature films with social and cultural relevance. We seek to showcase the diverse communities, transcending cultural and social barriers, creating bonds among people from different socio-cultural backgrounds, finding historical commonalities, and forming one cohesive narrative that can speak for more than one person" (Filmarte 2019).

The directors and producers Gabriel Páez and Isabel Rodas traveled to the Province of Azuay, located in the southern Andean area of Ecuador. They visited the fifteen cantons composing the province where they conducted two hundred and twenty-two interviews, eventually selecting twenty-one individuals to form the novice cast and crew (Páez 2015). They aimed to have a true sample of the whole region and avoid having Cuenca, the city with the largest population, overrepresented. Most inhabitants of the province identify as mestizos, a grouping that accounts for 89.6 percent of the total population of Azuay according to the 2010 census (INEC 2010, 2). The label "mestizo" denotes a person of mixed heritage, Spanish and Indigenous, whose origin dates back to colonial times. Traditionally, the Spanish or European and those who accumulated wealth have operated under the privilege granted them by a social and political system based on race and class (Quijano 2000, 342–43). Páez and Rodas set out to be more inclusive and, while selecting cast members, they ensured the participation of the underrepresented mestizo "other," providing these individuals with a platform from which they could tell the tales of their own ancestors. And they set out to collect alternative stories passed down through generations: "The first task asked of the young group was to talk to their grandparents and to bring back to the workshop an oral tradition autochthonous to their hometowns." [El primer deber de los jóvenes era hablar con sus abuelos y traer al taller una historia que venga de la tradición oral de sus pueblos] (Páez 2015, n.p.). All of the storylines included in the film originated from the group's first homework assignment: "From 21 stories, workshop attendees and instructors democratically selected three to make them into one tale that would be acted out by the group." [De 21 historias se seleccionaron democráticamente entre talleristas e instructores, tres para convertirlas en un relato a partir de la re-interpretación de las mismas por parte de los jóvenes] (Páez 2015, n.p.). Each story follows the plot structure of a tale where all ends well. They share the common thread of narrating how locals overcome the colonial system

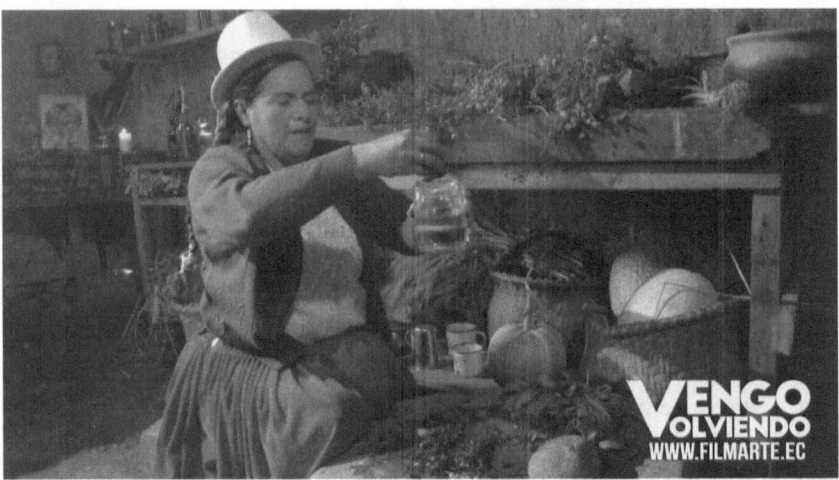

Figure 14.1. Abuela Mariana mixes medicinal herbs. ©*Vengo volviendo*, Filmarte, 2015. Used with permission.

and the unjust exercise of power by landowners acting with the complicity of the authorities, both civil and military.

These embedded stories are framed by a larger narrative that explores the role of traditional and ancestral knowledges within the practice of medicine and, as such, respond to Ecuador's most recent constitutions (1998 and 2008) that have granted alternative medicine a role within the nation's attempt to provide healthcare to its citizens. Article 360 of the 2008 Constitution, for example, emphasizes how ancient medical traditions can supplement the widely trusted and efficient practice of modern Western medicine. In that same spirit, *Vengo volviendo* explores the value of traditional medical as represented by Abuela Mariana who runs a medicinal herbs home business.

Ismael grew up watching his grandmother, Abuela Mariana, prepare herbal medicines based on the ancestral knowledges of natural remedies transmitted through generations. In one important scene, the camera pans from left to right to show Abuela Mariana in the act of preparing a recipe to relieve stomach pain: grinding, chopping, and mixing herbs. In a voiceover narration, the aged woman sounds out each step of the process: "For stomach ache, chamomile with onion. A bunch of chamomiles and half an onion." [Para la pancita, manzanilla con cebolla. Media cebolla, y un atado de manzanilla.] (04:20:00). In the background, Ismael, as a young boy, appears fully engaged writing in a notebook. At the end of the scene, the camera zooms in to capture his final product: a rendering of the recipe, complete with a drawing of Abuela in the act of preparing infusions, a compound of medicinal herbs. Ismael refers to the process as "curando;" the term appears in the caption of his drawing: "Mi abuelita curando," which, in Ismael's context, more closely translates to "My Abuela healing." Abuela Mariana practices *curanderismo*, a tradition inherited from her ancestors. She falls within the most common definition of this practice as seen in Brett Hendrickson (2015): "For *curanderos/as*, the hybrid nature of their tradition often can mean treating an illness with herbal remedies native to the Americas along with recitations of Catholic prayers and within an Iberian Muslim understanding of the body's humors. Religious healing traditions generally gain authority from claims of ancient wisdom and authenticity . . ." (27).

As a post-2008 Constitution production, *Vengo volviendo* advocates for the use of *curanderismo* as a complement rather than a replacement to Western modern medical practices. The film carefully avoids traversing into the realm of the more controversial shamanism and its customary practices (see Hendrickson 2015, 27).[5] Much of the action of the film's primary storyline—with Ismael traveling to deliver his grandmother's home remedies—takes place inside a vehicle, a 1962 Ford Anglia, still running after more than fifty years because it has adopted and embraced new technology to remain in circulation. The body and engine have been repaired and rebuilt with parts from myriad automobiles from assorted makers. The vehicle stands as a tribute to how the past and the present can complement each other, and it becomes a clear metaphor for the role of time-honored, herbal-based natural medicines within modern healthcare. Both forms can coexist by allowing each to serve its own purposes.

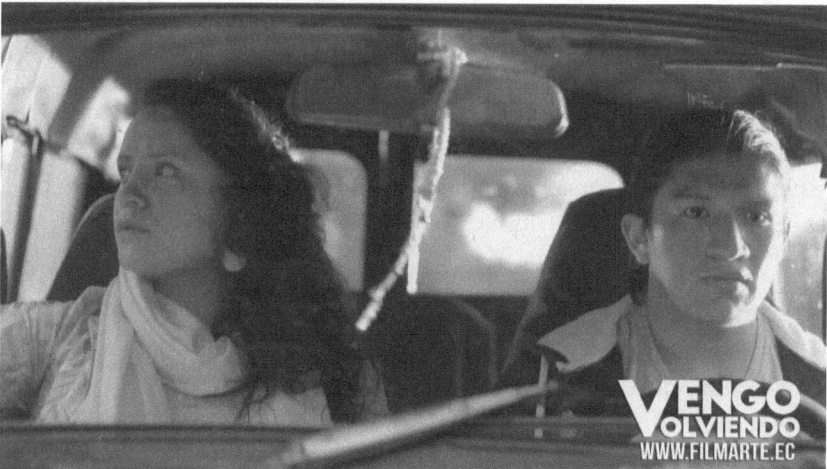

Figure 14.2. Ismael and Luz driving to distribute Abuela's product in a Ford Anglia vehicle. ©*Vengo volviendo*, Filmarte, 2015. Used with permission.

Nonetheless, Ismael, who grew up watching his grandmother harvest her plants and prepare infusions, echoes the skepticism of those who consider the use and distribution of medicinal herbs to be fraudulent. Abuela Mariana's husband has passed away, and she needs help distributing the product. Ismael has no desire to pursue this family tradition, but reluctantly and out of economic need, he agrees to temporarily aid his grandmother. As such, he literally and symbolically replaces his grandfather who distributed Abuela Mariana's herbs by driving the Ford Anglia and becoming associated with the car's metaphoric significance. However, Ismael seems uneasy with his new role, and he imagines the vehicle as a space that confines him rather than allowing him to roam free in the beautiful Andean setting. He lacks faith in the curative properties of his grandmother's herbs. Indeed, he regrets having any part of a fraudulent process, as we gather from this exchange with Luz:

>   —Isma don't be mad. There are people who don't have money and need your grandma's medicine.
>   —Medicine, you say. It is a lie. It is just water with herbs.[6]
>   [—Isma no estés bravo. Hay gente que no tiene dinero y necesita la medicina de tu abue.
>   —Medicina dices. Es pura mentira. Agua con yerbas es lo que es.]
>   (01:07:37)

Ismael's disbelief is challenged when a young woman requests his help with her sister who is suffering from severe headaches and a lack of appetite. At first, Ismael refuses to intervene: "I don't know." [Es que yo no sé.] (01:08:38). He changes his mind and lends a hand, however, when he recalls having heard his Abuela Mariana reciting the list of herbs for a certain infusion. His actions while working with the young woman resemble the work of *curanderos* performing *limpias* [cleansings] with alcohol, water, and herbs. The sister recovers, but Ismael plays down the ramifications of his performance, as seen in this exchange with Luz:

>   —How did you do that?
>   —What?
>   —Cure the child?
>   —I didn't cure her. She wasn't that sick.
>   [—Oye.
>   —¿Cómo hiciste eso?
>   —¿Qué cosa?

—Curar a la guagua.
—No la curé. No estaba tan grave.] (01:11:40)

The meaning of Ismael's disavowal of having helped the young woman is not immediately clear. It could be interpreted, as Luz seems to suggest, as a sign of humility or a feeling of inadequacy that the protagonist feels at having performed the work of a healer. A reading more consistent with his attitude of skepticism toward ancestral practices, however, suggests, at this moment, that Ismael still questions the value of his efforts: they worked, but only as a complement to modern medicine. In other words, Ismael had employed medicinal herbs in the same way that he had seen his Abuela Mariana do, using a healing knowledge passed down from generations, but he imagines that his patient simply "wasn't that sick."

Later, when Ismael finds Abuela Mariana collapsed on the floor of her home, he rushes her to the hospital. In the waiting room, Luz inquires: "And her medicine, why don't you use it to try to cure her?" [¿Y sus medicinas, por qué no tratas tú de curarla?] (01:13:15). Ismael does not reply. His immediate reliance on a hospital reaffirms the value of Western medicine over traditional and alternative healing practices. Abuela Mariana recovers thanks to the work of modernity, or modern medicine. The film closes with her finding the proper space for her medicinal herbs in a store strategically located in a commercial area of Cuenca, the province's most prominent urban center. The store advertises the sale of natural products which supports the premise that ancestral and traditional knowledges complement modern Western medicine. María Constanza Torri (2013), in an investigation that looked at alternative medical options in Ecuador, explains how biomedical and traditional midwifery stand as an example of modern and ancestral knowledge working together: "While there are still issues with the inequality between indigenous and non-indigenous patients, the complementarity of the services offered by the *partera* [midwife] and the obstetrician at Jambi Huasi represents an interesting example of intercultural behavior of the patients. The patients' use of both types of prenatal service at the clinic demonstrates the need to revitalize and revalue health care options that act as alternatives and enhance the dominant occidental health care system" (210). Similarly, in *Vengo volviendo* the medicinal herbs grown, prepared and distributed by Abuela Mariana do not intend to replace biomedicine, but to enhance it.

Nonetheless, the film seems to suggest the need for *curanderas,* like Abuela Mariana, due to a lack of access to modern medical centers, hospitals, or doctors' offices. The two most recent constitutions adopted in Ecuador clearly guarantee free healthcare to everyone based on universal principles of equity (Asamblea Nacional Constituyente 1998, Art. 42 and 43; National Assembly 2008, Art. 362.). Despite these advances, the healthcare system has not yet proven successful in overcoming the lack of access experienced by the underprivileged and underrepresented, such as those characters portrayed in the film. Modernity moves forward, but carries with it the heavy weight of long-standing colonial ways where members of privileged races and classes benefit first. Some of Abuela Mariana's customers live far removed from biomedical healthcare centers that are located more frequently in the nation's main urban centers. Abuela Mariana's herbal treatments stand as their sole option to anything resembling medicine because she can get herbs and infusions to them using her private distribution system. Her customers, who often lack monetary funds, even have the option of paying in-kind with guinea pigs or chickens, for instance. Hendrickson (2015) finds a similar trend among Mexican Americans who turn to the services of *curanderos* and healers: "In the twentieth century, the spread of biomedicine, hospitals and clinics in the region often were unavailable to Mexican Americans. *Curanderismo* became either the only healthcare option for poor Mexican Americans, or the first resort for healing that at times could result in a referral to costly biomedical services" (29). In Ecuador, in places marked by poverty and lack of public services, people have more difficulty getting to centers that provide biomedical treatment, as demonstrated in the analysis of social and economic determinants of healthcare utilization conducted by Daniel Lopez-Cevallos and Chunhuei Chi (2012): "We found that various layers of social inequalities persist in the Ecuadorian society. Indigenous, low-income, and rural households are particularly limited in their ability to access health care services in Ecuador" (1).

Beyond its concern for questions of healthcare, *Vengo volviendo* also places itself in the ongoing conversation about the meaning of the phrase "good way of living system" institutionalized in the current Ecuadorian constitution (National Assembly 2008, Sect. 7). In its traditional meaning, the term alludes to the "Sumak kawsay," which translates from Quechua as "Living well" or "The Good Life," or *El buen vivir* in Spanish. It refers to "a way of living in harmony within communities, ourselves, and most importantly, nature" ("Sumak Kawsay"). As it is connected to healthcare, the concept mandates advancing the following goal described in Article 358 of the 2008 constitution: "The national health system shall be aimed at ensuring the development, protection, and recovery of capacities and potential for a healthy and integral life, both individual and collective, and shall recognize social and cultural diversity. The system shall be governed by the general principles of the national system of social inclusion and equity and by those of bioethics, adequacy and interculturalism, with a gender and generation approach" (National Assembly 2008, Art. 358).

Incidentally, *Vengo volviendo* stands as a great example of a film that portrays characters who stand on opposite sides of the argument about the implementation of the good way of life system. Luz's attitude lines up with those who prefer life in Ecuador. "Ecuador loves life" [Ecuador ama la vida], she states, affirming the official slogan of the administration of former president Rafael Correa (2007–17). Luz's perception carries weight because she spent eight years living in the United States and chose to return to her home country. Luz approaches the experience of traveling through Ecuador as an emancipating act, and she revels in the green and lush mountainous backdrop. She views it as a welcome change to the cement-covered US metropolitan setting from which she has escaped. Her joy is demonstrated through a gregarious attitude and a use of space that places her, inside the vehicle, in a higher vertical position than Ismael, even when he is noticeably taller than she when they stand next to each other. Luz feels accomplished and sits tall to symbolize her mood. In terms of quality of life, she describes Ecuador as a "little jewel" [una joyita]. She focuses on her birthplace through a filter of nostalgia and longing for the country she was forced to abandon by a decision of her parents. Luz compares life in Azuay to what she experienced in the United States, and she accepts the ideals of the officially promoted doctrines of *El buen vivir* and *sumak kawsay*. In her opinion, life in Ecuador far surpasses what the United States offered, and she happily adopts an Ecuadorian lifestyle.

In contrast, Ismael plans to leave Ecuador and migrate to the United States in search of a better quality of life. He endures the task of distributing Abuela Mariana's medicine—fraudulent in his mind—only because he is making money that will allow him to pay the coyote who will get him into the United States. Ismael shows his frustration in a conversation with Luz after a customer pays him with a hen rather than with hard currency:

Ismael—This way, I am never going to leave.
Luz—Where are you going to go? You, as well? If this country is a treasure.
Ismael—A treasure, you say. It is pure fantasy. (00:35:37)
[Ismael—Así no me voy nunca.
Luz—¿Y a dónde te vas a ir? Tú también? Si este país es una joyita.
Ismael—Una joyita, dices. Si es pura fantasía.]

While Luz enthusiastically embraces the benefits of the good life in Ecuador. Ismael decisively counters: "It's pure fantasy." Gioconda Coello (2020), who outlines the use of storytelling strategies in the construction of the "good life" narrative pushed by President Correa, would agree with Ismael when she argues that the official position of romanticizing the Indian way of living has a fictional foundation. In its preamble, the 2008 Constitution emphasizes Ecuador's commitment to the "good way of living," or *sumak kawsay*, where all citizens can live in communal harmony: "A new form of public co-existence, in diversity and in harmony with nature, to achieve the good way of living, the *sumak kawsay*: A society that respects, in all its dimensions, the dignity of individuals and community groups" (National Assembly 2008, Preamble). Coello (2020) suggests that the Correa administration exaggerated its work for the underprivileged, while, in practice, it simply validated the social and economic gap separating the non-Indigenous "us" from the Indigenous "other":

> The way in which the government, during the past decade, mobilized sumac kawsay as a guide for the construction of the "society of good living" can be dangerous given that it uses such resonances in a selective way, erasing the historical references to suffering and struggle and re-establishing both categories of alterity and a dichotomy between a "we" tacitly normalized and the Indigenous as the other.
>
> [Al mismo tiempo [este ensayo] ha sugerido que la forma en la que el gobierno, durante la década pasada, movilizó el sumak kawsay como una guía para la construcción de la 'sociedad del buen vivir' puede ser peligrosa dado que usa esas resonancias de manera selectiva, borra las referencias de sufrimiento y de lucha en la historia y restablece tanto categorías de alteridad como una dicotomía entre un 'nosotros' tácito y normalizado y lo indio como lo otro.] (416)

Interestingly, Ismael abandons his plan to relocate to the United States because of the difficulties associated with this odyssey-like journey. He chooses instead to stay and make it in Cuenca helping Abuela Mariana set up her herbal business. *Vengo volviendo* reiterates the message that life in Ecuador transcends residing anywhere else. And the sentiment has begun to spread to the point that the coyotes have gone out of business. They sell their storefront to Abuela Mariana; the Ecuadorian traditional business replaces that of selling the American Dream.

*Vengo volviendo* operates within the ideological proposals of the governments that ruled Ecuador from 1998 until 2017. The last two constitutions reveal the active role played by local Indigenous movements that have inserted themselves within the sectors that write legislation. The film places Indigenous peoples' ancestral knowledges within the role warranted by the 2008 constitution to serve as a complement to widely used biomedicine. It reflects the spirit of the law, of not neglecting the value of ancestral knowledges passed down through generations of Indigenous peoples who have inhabited the limits of present-day Ecuador for centuries. The film similarly attempts to depict the country as a harmonious place to live within a community of those who share similar goals of reaching the good living system (*el buen vivir*) modeled after the *sumak kawsay* system of the Indigenous nations. The Ecuador depicted in the film resembles a bucolic setting that no one would consider abandoning or trading for a life in the United States or Europe. Ecuador loves life, as the Correa administration slogan advertised. But similarly, the film reveals the inconsistencies of a system that could be labeled, at best, a work-in-progress. In particular, those living in or near urban centers have easier access to biomedicine. The advantages of a better quality of life provided by modernity excludes those who live in the periphery of society who usually belong to underrepresented and underprivileged groups placed toward the lower strata of the economic spectrum based on race and class.

## Notes

1. The term "cultural productions" refers to postulates of Marxist and cultural studies critics who see an artistic product such as a literary work or film as part of the social context in which an artist or writer created it, encompassing the social, historical, economic, and political moment. For more information, see Pierre Bourdieu and Randal Johnson (1993), especially the "Editors Introduction" and chapter 1 (9, 36).

2. *Sumak kawsay*, or "good life," refers to a way of living based on the Indigenous idea of harmony across society, individual, and nature as an alternative to a capitalist economic system. Philipp Altmann (2017) describes it as the main ideology behind an Indigenous movement attempting to decolonize the current system (749). Gioconda Coello (2020) sees the system as a failure, and the critic places the blame on the administration of former President Rafael Correa (2007–2017) who, according to Coello, took control of the movement for propagandist reasons, revising the philosophy to the point that it lost its original intent and meaning (415).

3. For distribution information, contact the Filmarte bilingual website at https://www.filmarte.ec. The DVD has English subtitles. Streaming versions are available.

4. Translations are mine, except when otherwise indicated.

5. For a list of documentary films dealing with *curanderismo* using methods beyond herbal medicines, such as eggs, guinea pigs, and holy water, please refer to the review of five documentaries written by Stephen D. Glazier (1987, 776–78).

6. All English translations of the film's dialogue are taken from the film's official subtitles.

## References

Altmann, Philipp. 2017. "Sumak Kawsay as an Element of Local Decolonization in Ecuador." *Latin American Research Review* 52 (5): 749–59. https://doi.org/10.25222/larr.242.

Asamblea Nacional Constituyente. 1998. "Constitución política de la República del Ecuador." In *Registro oficial*. Asamblea Nacional Constituyente.

Ayala Mora, Enrique, and Universidad Andina Simón Bolívar. 2015. *Resumen de historia del Ecuador*. Quito: Universidad Andina Simón Bolívar/Corporación Editora Nacional. https://public.ebookcentral.proquest.com/choice/publicfullrecord.aspx?p=5102868.

Bourdieu, Pierre, and Randal Johnson. 1993. *The Field of Cultural Production: Essays on Art and Literature. European Perspectives*. New York: Columbia University Press.

Coello, Gioconda. 2020. "Producciones narrativas, tesis culturales y ficciones: Una historia del presente del Sumak Kawsay." In *Convergencias sobre la cultura ecuatoriana*, edited by Manuel Medina and Norman Gonzalez, 405–18. Loja, Ecuador: Ediloja, Universidad Técnica Particular de Loja.

Dreyfuss, Rochelle Cooper, and César A. Rodríguez-Garavito. 2014. *Balancing Wealth and Health: The Battle over Intellectual Property and Access to Medicines in Latin America*. First edition. *Law and Global Governance Series*. Oxford, United Kingdom: Oxford University Press.

Filmarte. 2019. "About Us." *Filmarte.ec*. https://www.filmarte.ec/nosotros?lang=en.

Glazier, Stephen D. 1987. "Andean Ethnomedicine: Birth and Childhood Illnesses in Six Ecuadorian Communities." *American Anthropologist* 89 (3): 776–78.

Hendrickson, Brett. 2015. "Neo-shamans, *Curanderismo* and Scholars: Metaphysical Blending in Contemporary Mexican American Folk Healing." *Nova Religio: The Journal of Alternative and Emergent Religions* 19 (1): 25–44. www.jstor.org/stable/10.1525/nr.2015.19.1.25

INEC. 2010. *Resultados del Censo 2010 de población y vivienda en el Ecuador. Fascículo Provincial Azuay*. INEC, Instituto Nacional de Estadísticas y Censos (Instituto Nacional de Estadísticas y Censos INEC). https://www.ecuadorencifras.gob.ec/wp-content/descargas/Manu-lateral/Resultados-provinciales/azuay.pdf.

Lopez-Cevallos, Daniel, and Chunhuei Chi. 2012. "Inequity in Health Care Utilization in Ecuador: An Analysis of Current Issues and Potential Solutions." *International Journal for Equity in Health* 11 (Suppl. 1). https://doi.org/10.1186/1475-9276-11-S1-A6.

National Assembly Legislative and Oversight Committee. 2008. *Constitution of the Republic of Ecuador*. In *Official Register*. National Assembly: Legislative and Oversight Committee.

Ocho y Medio, editors. 2015. "Entrevista a Gabriel Páez (Director de la película ecuatoriana 'Vengo volviendo')." *Ocho y Medio: El cine de La Floresta*. https://www.ochoymedio.net/entrevista-a-gabriel-paez-director-de-la-pelicula-ecuatoriana-vengo-volviendo/.

Páez Hernández, Gabriel, and Isabel Rodas León, directors. 2015. *Vengo volviendo* [Here and There]. Ecuador: Filmarte.

Pan American Health Organization. 2004. *Exclusion in Health in Latin America and the Caribbean.* Pan-American Health Organisation. http://www.myilibrary.com?id =163783.

Quijano, Aníbal. 2000. "Colonialidad del poder y clasificación social." *Journal of World-Systems Research* Special Issue: *Festchrift for Immanuel Wallerstein–Part I* 6 (2): 342–86.

Ramos, Juan G. 2015. "Contesting Domination: Modernity, Coloniality of Gender, and Decolonial Feminism in José De La Cuadra's 'La Tigra.'" *Romance Notes* 55 (1): 61–75.

Pachamama Alliance. 2019. "Sumak Kawsay: Ancient Teachings of Indigenous Peoples." *Pachamama Alliance.* https://www.pachamama.org/sumak-kawsay.

Tarco Carrera, Henry. 2020. "Descolonizando el texto visual: Bases para interpretar cuatro estéticas cinematográficas indigenistas ecuatorianas del siglo XXI." In *Convergencias sobre la cultura ecuatoriana,* edited by Manuel Medina and Norman Gonzalez, 349–60. Loja, Ecuador: Ediloja, Universidad Técnica Particular de Loja.

Torri, María Constanza. 2013. "Choosing between Traditional Medicine and Allopathy during Pregnancy: Health Practices in Prenatal and Reproductive Health Care in Ecuador." *Journal of Health Management* 15 (3): 397–413. https://doi.org/10.1177 /0972063413492036.

Yashar, Deborah J. 2005. *Contesting Citizenship in Latin America: The Rise of Indigenous Movements and the Postliberal Challenge.* Cambridge Studies in Contentious Politics. Cambridge: Cambridge University Press.

# PART V

## Healthcare in the Southern Cone

# 15

## Health Systems in Argentina and Chile
### A Comparative History

Eric D. Carter

This chapter compares the historical development of health systems in Argentina and Chile from the early 1900s to the present. Comparison of national health systems requires not only analysis of the systems' constituent elements (for example, personnel, funding, administrative structure, organization of medical services, and so forth) but also attentiveness to how distinctive political, economic, and cultural histories shape those systems (Birn, Pillay, and Holtz 2009). There has been little effort to compare the experiences of Chile and Argentina, despite each nation having its own rich historiography of medicine and public health, not to mention their long history as neighbors in the Southern Cone. While both countries have fragmented and stratified health systems, they have taken different paths to get there.

Comparing Chile and Argentina may help shed light on a classic problem in development studies: the relationship between economic development and improvement in population health. Common sense and historical experience suggest that rising affluence or modernization translates into health progress; people in wealthier countries, by and large, tend to lead longer and healthier lives than those in poorer countries. However, as Nobel laureate Amartya Sen (2001) notes, countries with similar levels of affluence may have radically divergent health outcomes; likewise, countries with low incomes may outperform wealthier countries in indicators of social development, such as health, literacy, and women and girls' access to education. To make sense of this pattern, Sen (2001) distinguished between two general development pathways: "growth-mediated" and "support-led" progress. Nations along the first pathway prioritize economic development, with the expansion of social services coming later, as, in theory, economic growth creates the resources necessary to pay for a "welfare state." On the "support-led" pathway, countries invest early in welfare-promoting institutions that "reduce mortality and improve the quality of life" (Sen 2001, 339). Consistent with Sen's model, Michael Marmot (2015) and the WHO Commission on the Social Determinants of Health have argued that reliance on free markets may lead to economic growth, but solid and sustainable structures of state support are necessary to produce equitable health conditions.

Sen, and others, have pointed to countries of Latin America and the Caribbean, in comparative and in-depth case studies, to further unpack this relationship between economic development and public health progress, and, more importantly, to explain why some countries manage the support-led pathway despite economic disadvantages and predictable domestic political opposition from conservative forces. James McGuire (2001, 2010), in historical-comparative studies of Latin American and East Asian states, has argued that democratization processes help to produce a national ruling class that is more disposed to react to the demands of organized popular sectors and also interested in expanding the state to maintain basic, rights-based guarantees to adequate health services. Similarly, Anne-Emanuelle Birn (2009), among others, emphasizes the importance of "political will," meaning that, through deliberative and (usually) democratic processes, some nations have made a "historical commitment to health as a social goal" (175).

This still raises the question of where such political will comes from (and why it is directed toward health improvement, as opposed to other worthwhile policy goals). Once a country has developed an adequate and broad-based social safety net, a strong sense of social solidarity is vital to maintaining those gains; universal health systems (like that of Costa Rica) can easily disintegrate if this sense of social solidarity—notably hard to quantify, nurture, and sustain—breaks down (Martínez Franzoni and Sánchez-Ancochea 2016). More broadly, health systems convey—in a manner that is sometimes hard to pin down analytically—the prevailing values of a society. One key indicator is "the extent to which health is viewed as a public good and human right as opposed to a commodity or privilege" (Birn, Pillay, and Holtz 2009, 585). Countries like Cuba, Jamaica, or Costa Rica have emphasized a primary healthcare model, with cost-effective interventions that reach a broad swath of the population, layered onto achievements in areas like nutrition, sanitation, and education (Cueto and Palmer 2015, 65–73; Palmer 2003; Riley 2005).

A juxtaposition of Argentina and Chile to answer these big-picture questions can only reveal so much, since these are just two countries out of many. Despite their many differences, it is important to recognize that both

Argentina and Chile are middle- to high-income countries with good to excellent population health conditions and, importantly, very high societal expectations about the government's role in ensuring broad access to, and high quality of, health services. Neither country is a perfect exemplar of a theoretical model or typology of a healthcare system. This chapter demonstrates—as Birn, Pillay, and Holtz (2009) have done elsewhere—that the "organization of health care systems is also the fruition of historical processes and political and economic structures" with specific variables, including "class-based political parties, civil society organizations, trade unions, big business, economic elites, and social movements" as well as "the state's power vis-à-vis international business interests and global economic policy" (585). The development of the Argentine and Chilean healthcare systems took place within often-tumultuous historical circumstances, but with a high degree of path dependency, as the institutional innovations of a given historical moment have considerable inertia and help to shape future health policy choices.

## Argentina: The Construction of a Fragmented Health System

Today, Argentina is considered an archetype of a country that suffers the burden of a "fragmented and segmented" health system, typified by complexity, inefficiency, inequity, and resistance to change (Kreplak 2017, 4). In terms of public health progress, however, Argentina was once a leader in Latin America, going back to the late nineteenth century. At that time, Argentina's liberal ruling class tied improvements in health to a modernizing or "civilizing" project of national development (Rodriguez 2006; Zimmermann 1995). Investments in hygiene and sanitation were especially visible in the nation's capital, Buenos Aires. A devastating yellow fever epidemic in 1871, which killed about 10 percent of the city's population, sparked a transformation of the city's layout, social geography, and sanitation infrastructure. Drawing inspiration from dynamic European capital cities such as London, Paris, and Berlin, the Argentine government and private investors installed a system of potable piped water by the middle of the 1880s, and these efforts were accompanied by the construction of sanitary sewers, an impressive system of parks and plazas, and broad, monumental avenues to permit the entry of sunlight and circulation of air. The newest advances of the bacteriological revolution were incorporated into disease control programs, even though the spread of contagious diseases, most notably tuberculosis, continued to be a major problem in the densely populated and rapidly growing city (Armus 2011). Nevertheless, in 1914, the year of

Argentina's third national census, Buenos Aires reported population health conditions—as measured, for example, by infant mortality rates—on par with Europe's capital cities and better than anywhere else in Latin America (Carter 2012).

In this same era, Argentina's medical profession reached the apex of its cultural and political influence. In this "liberal" era, with power vested in a tightly knit oligarchy dominated by large landowners, bankers, and professionals, so-called *médicos políticos*—political doctors—were commonplace. Through their networks, and sometimes in individual career trajectories, they connected the arenas of legislative politics, government ministries, universities, and scientific institutions to advance public health objectives (Cueto and Palmer 2015, 65–73). For instance, the national campaign against malaria in northwest Argentina was instigated by political doctors from the provincial oligarchy of Tucumán, where the disease was especially intense. Their involvement with the National Department of Hygiene helped to spread the largesse of the federal government and the expertise of internationally trained experts to the interior provinces, which were usually lacking in resources (Carter 2012).

Beyond these state-centered spheres of action, the medical profession had outsized cultural influence. Many Argentine hygienists were associated with a Pan-American eugenics movement and thus believed they had a transcendental role in fashioning a racialized national identity (Armus 2016; Miranda and Vallejo 2012). Increasingly, the language and values of medical science and hygiene penetrated heretofore private realms (of procreation, childbirth, and motherhood) and shaped persistent elements of national culture, such as diet, cuisine, and an emphasis on physical exercise as part of a healthy lifestyle (Biernat and Ramacciotti 2008; Ledesma Prietto 2016; Scharagrodsky 2016). A broader point here is that these values and attendant practices are hard to separate from the rise of and the broadening of a consumerist middle class; not all of the gains in health and well being can be attributed to medicine and public health alone.

The first or "classic" Perón era (1945–1955) intensified government intervention to improve living conditions for the working class, with emphasis on investing in public health (Ramacciotti 2009). For all the public health achievements of Argentina's government in the fifty years preceding Perón's vertiginous rise to power, there was a sense that more could be done with the country's great wealth to provide a better standard of healthcare and social security to a broader contingent of the country's citizens. Only Perón, and just for a short time, was able to overcome political roadblocks to institutionalize some semblance of a modern welfare state. Early on, Perón turned the National Department of Hygiene into the Ministry of Public Health. With this elevated administrative status, under the direction of the neurosurgeon Ramón Carrillo, the ministry launched an energetic and detailed plan to transform national health. With Perón's encouragement, Carrillo directed funds and human resources into the malaria eradication campaign, which achieved dramatic results in just a few short years under the direction of malariologist Carlos Alberto Alvarado (Carter 2012). Carrillo also launched a plan to build a comprehensive, national network of hospitals and clinics, which would provide better coverage, higher standards of care, and centralized control over healthcare in one government agency. These efforts were accompanied by other disease control and vaccination campaigns, along with accompanying social policy efforts (such as salary increases and construction of public housing) that also improved population health conditions.

The ambitious Peronist public health agenda was never fully realized, due not only to powerful external opposition but also to contradictions within Perón's regime. The corporatist structure of Perón's political machine hinged on the patronage of trade unions that he had empowered. The Ministry of Health was largely disconnected from this center of power, and, instead, the unions focused their support on the Eva Perón Foundation, run by the president's charismatic wife, which started taking on visible health-related projects, such as building hospitals. In addition, the logic of corporatism permanently undermined the possibilities for a fully national, centralized, and universal healthcare system. Instead, by way of strengthening the labor unions, Perón's government embedded their largely independent health insurance programs and medical care systems (which came to be known as the *obras sociales* [health insurance funds]). These sprang from an even longer tradition of mutual-aid societies built by immigrant or professional groups starting in the 1800s (Arce 2010; Belmartino 2005). An emblematic example is the Hospital Ferroviario, an enormous (and now defunct) hospital built for the powerful railroad workers' union near the central train station of Retiro in Buenos Aires (Belmartino 2005; Biernat, Cerdá, and Ramacciotti 2015, 29–30). The unions and their *obras sociales* typify what social security expert Carmelo Mesa-Lago (1991) called the "labor aristocracy," one sector with special privileges in a stratified Latin American welfare state model (359). The Peronist state (and its successors) "offered very heterogeneous social benefits to different occupational groups, depending on their powers of negotiation or proximity to the government" (Biernat,

Cerdá, and Ramacciotti 2015, 34); this left out domestic workers, rural laborers, and others in the informal economy (which was small during the 1940s and 1950s, in comparison to today).

Peronism and its aftermath—a sometimes chaotic succession of alternating military and civilian governments from 1955 to 1983—set the conditions for the fragmented and stratified health system that persists to this day. The very wealthy are able to purchase insurance or healthcare directly in a private market; most of these individuals receive health insurance benefits through *obras sociales*, connected to their conditions of formal employment. They also have privileged access to well-run private hospitals and clinics. Care in public hospitals continues to be free of charge, funded by national and provincial governments. Not surprisingly, over time, the quality of care has fluctuated with economic conditions and political priorities. Similarly, the Ministry of Health has been persistently weak within the national government bureaucracy, save for ephemeral efforts of especially energetic ministers, such as Carrillo or Arturo Oñativia, who, while serving under President Arturo Illia from 1963–66, attempted to lower prescription drug prices (Arce 2010; Biernat, Cerdá, and Ramacciotti 2015; Ramacciotti and Romero 2017). Funding for disease control, vaccination, school nutrition, and other standard health programs has been unstable at best. On a more positive note, Argentina enjoys the highest doctor-to-population ratio of any country in Latin America (other than Cuba): approximately 3.9 doctors per 1,000 people. This is mostly a consequence of a commitment to free medical school education at large public universities. Whatever might trouble Argentina's health system, a lack of human resources is not the principal problem, although medical personnel tend to be distributed unevenly, concentrated in major cities.

It is difficult to separate the changing fortunes of Argentina's public health conditions from its broader macroeconomic and political circumstances. Over the last several decades, the country's economy has lurched from crisis to crisis, some of them quite profound and with lasting social impacts. After a severe debt crisis and a destabilizing bout of hyperinflation from 1989 to 1990, the government of Carlos Menem agreed to the International Monetary Fund (IMF) and the World Bank Group's terms for "structural adjustment," which meant, among other things, budget cuts for public health programs and public hospitals. In addition, the health insurance sector was liberalized, meaning the creation of something like a market, and the entry of private firms (including multinational corporations and investors) into the ownership of *obras sociales* as well as other types of insurance and healthcare businesses (Iriart, Merhy, and Waitzkin 2001). Unsurprisingly, this kind of public disinvestment and market liberalization exacerbated the existing stratification or inequalities of the health system (Biernat, Cerdá, and Ramacciotti 2015, 237–40). Following the cataclysmic financial crisis of 2001–02, Argentina shifted course, embracing the neo-populism of the Kirchners (both Néstor and Cristina), who occupied the presidency from 2003 to 2015. Rejecting the prescriptions of the international financial institutions, this neo-Peronist regime multiplied investment in the public health sector, accompanied by progressive and welfare-oriented social policies, and opened political spaces for participatory and community-oriented health projects. The succeeding presidency of Mauricio Macri, marked by a sluggish economy, represented a retrenchment of sorts, with severe cuts in the government health budget and the relegation of the Ministry of Health to the inferior status of a "secretariat" in 2018 (Ramacciotti 2018). New president Alberto Fernández, a Peronist who soundly defeated Macri in the October 2019 general election, will undoubtedly move to restore the state health sector while navigating the challenging economic circumstances that four years of *macrismo* left behind.

## Chile: From Welfare State to Neoliberalism and Back Again

Compared to Argentina, Chile experienced dismal social, economic, and public health conditions at the turn of the twentieth century. For example, just one indicator, the national infant mortality rate, oscillated between 200 to 300 per 1,000 live births during the early 1900s, an almost unimaginable figure today. Epidemics of communicable diseases—cholera, typhus, tuberculosis—occurred with regularity, and malnutrition was rampant. During the 1920s, an increasingly well-organized labor sector, along with a passionate group of mostly left-wing physicians, would begin to construct a national health system, aimed at addressing the massive health crisis (Illanes 1993).

Arguably, Chile started on the path of developing a modern welfare state before Argentina. As early as 1924, a national health insurance system was introduced, partly in response to rising social turmoil. This government also created the national Ministry of Hygiene, progressive labor laws, and an updated national health code (the original, from 1918, was the first of its kind in Latin America). The new insurance system was based on the *cajas* or insurance funds, the largest of which was the Caja del Seguro Obrero Obligatorio (CSO). Chile was thus an early adopter of a model with origins in Bismarck's Germany promoted by the International Labour Organization, whereby "social insurance" (for healthcare, disability, unemployment, and other worker's needs) was funded by payroll contributions in three parts: employee, employer, and the state (Carter 2019). This funding model offered the *cajas* some autonomy from the central government and its budgetary priorities, and their capital grew quite large. The CSO used its income to establish its own network of clinics, promote preventive care, establish other services for workers and their families, and even lend money to the national government for other development projects.

Although a large part of the Chilean population was covered by the various *cajas*, many were left out of the system: urban lower-class workers, domestic servants, and almost everyone in the countryside. These groups continued to rely on a charity model of care (historically, public hospitals were run by religious orders, but by the 1920s these functions were taken over by the Chilean state). Thus, Chile was also saddled with a stratified and fragmented healthcare system for several decades (Molina Bustos 2010). Still, it is worth noting that Chile's CSO was the direct inspiration for Costa Rica's state-run health insurance system, starting in the 1940s, which eventually provided near universal coverage and high-quality care at low cost (Martínez Franzoni and Sánchez-Ancochea 2016)—but that is another story.

In Chile during the 1920s through to the 1940s, there was an active and vibrant "social medicine" movement of politically engaged medical professionals, mostly from the political left wing (Labra 2004). Embodied in groups such as the Sindicato de Médicos, the Vanguardia Médica, and Asociación Médica de Chile [Chilean Medical Association] (AMECH), these activists had a multifaceted and sometimes contradictory agenda: agitation for the continued improvement of the public health system, expansion of insurance coverage to meet the needs of the whole population, a broadly progressive political economic model and social policy agenda, and the protection of doctors and their autonomy in the government's health system (Waitzkin et al. 2001). A young Salvador Allende rose through the ranks of university student activists to become one of the leaders of the social medicine movement, and, in 1939, he was installed as Minister of Health under the center-left Popular Front government. After the fracturing of this political coalition, Allende continued his political career as a legislator representing the Socialist Party, a position he used to advocate for a single, universal healthcare system (Birn and Nervi 2015).

By 1952, Allende and his allies from many political parties had succeeded in establishing the Servicio Nacional de Salud (SNS, National Health Service). It was inspired, as the name suggests, by the British National Health Service created in the aftermath of World War II. Due to political compromises, however, Chile's new system was quite different from its British counterpart. Although the SNS consolidated most of the state's health-related institutions, some of the old *cajas* persisted independently, and there was a clear distinction between services for professional and government employees on the one hand and rank-and-file laborers on the other (Molina Bustos 2010). The funding of the system continued to depend on the tripartite payroll contribution system, rather than income from general taxation as in Britain. Nevertheless, the SNS was viewed across Latin America as a model, especially with respect to preventive medicine, public health programs, and health economics and planning. Santiago's School of Public Health, established with the support of the Rockefeller Foundation in the late 1940s, was staffed by a gifted generation of *salubristas* [public health experts] affiliated with the SNS, including Benjamin Viel, Hernán Romero, Abraham Horwitz, and Hugo Behm. Modeled on the school of public health at Johns Hopkins University, it became an influential training ground for public health workers from across Latin America, and Chile's renown in this arena was solidified with Horwitz's appointment as Director of the Pan American Health Organization in 1958, a post he occupied until 1975.

Domestic political divisions, however, began to trouble the foundations of the health system. For one, the solidarity of the country's medical professionals with the project of socialized medicine—a commitment toward a single, universal healthcare system—disintegrated in the 1960s. The AMECH, one of the driving forces behind the SNS, radically reoriented its political mission, defending the rights of doctors to private practice, a successful effort that culminated in 1968 with the Ley de Medicina Curativa (Molina Bustos 2010). As Chilean politics became increasingly polarized in the late 1960s and early 1970s, the medical profession became a conservative political force. When the Unidad Popular coalition took power in 1970, with Allende as the first democratically elected socialist leader in Latin America, it sought to improve population health conditions by changing the political economic structure of the country, creating spaces for community participation in health policy, and moving toward a single public healthcare system. Despite the vigorous commitment of Allende's allies in the health sector, doctors' organizations impeded programmatic change and condoned Allende's overthrow in the 1973 coup d'état (Navarro 1974).

The conservative counter-reaction was fierce and introduced radical reforms to the health sector and the welfare state. Pinochet's government became a laboratory for neoliberal (free-market-oriented) reforms under the direction of "the Chicago Boys," a group of Chilean economists trained at the University of Chicago. Although there were some public health achievements during the Pinochet regime, including a notable decline in childhood malnutrition, the overall effect was to undo the health system that had been crafted over the previous six decades (Labra 2002). State investment in the health sector dropped precipitously, and most significantly, with a series of reform decrees between 1979 and 1985, a free-market orientation was imposed on the health system. With these changes, Chileans could elect to have their mandatory payroll contributions for health insurance go either to the public system or to private insurance companies called Instituciones de Salud Previsional [Health Insurance Institutions] (ISAPREs) (Missoni and Solimano 2010). Somewhat predictably (and probably by design), this innovation led to rampant inequality in healthcare, with the wealthier (and healthier) segments of the population migrating to the ISAPREs and the poorer remaining in the deteriorating public system. By 2005, while only 22 percent of Chile's population was enrolled in the ISAPREs, they accounted for 43 percent of all health expenditures (Homedes and Ugalde 2005). This imbalance was exacerbated by geographical inequalities in health introduced by another neoliberal strategy, the decentralization of government health services to the level of the municipality. Quality of health services and health outcomes began to vary widely, according to the economic status of the municipalities. In all, these neoliberal reforms did not produce the kind of free-market competition that would supposedly reduce costs to consumers; instead, as health expenditures rose, quality declined and inequality increased (Molina Bustos 2010).

Subsequent reforms in the early 2000s under the *Concertación* government have tempered these inequalities to some extent. The Universal Access to Explicit Guarantees [Acceso Universal a Garantías Explícitas](AUGE) plan guarantees a standard package of health services for all citizens, regardless of ability to pay. Other policies regulate the private healthcare sector by placing limits on out-of-pocket expenses and restricting the ability of ISAPREs to offload high-risk clients onto the public system (Homedes and Ugalde 2005; Missoni and Solimano 2010). Such reforms improved the public system, which now serves about 85 percent of the population. The country's impressive overall economic growth and poverty reduction might also help explain why public health conditions have improved. In terms of life expectancy at birth, at 80.7 years, Chile is second only to Canada among countries in the Americas.

With its strong guarantees of basic protections, effective delivery of services, improvements in equity, and mix of private and public actors, the Chilean system has been held up as an exemplar of the potential of the Universal Health Coverage approach currently favored by the WHO (Missoni and Solimano 2010). However, in 2018, the center-right president, Sebastian

Piñera, admitted that "more than three-quarters of [Chilean] citizens are not satisfied with the government's management of health, and with good reason" (Paúl 2019). Violent protests and widespread demonstrations across Chile in late 2019 laid bare this latent discontent and exposed the fragility of Chile's social and economic policy consensus.

## Discussion

Evidently, Chile and Argentina have taken distinctive paths in the evolution of their health systems. Where do the countries stand now (or at least recently) in terms of their social and economic development and key health indicators? Table 15.1 presents a selection of key indicators, between approximately 1990 and 2018, that help us make some preliminary comparisons. One pivotal fact is that Chile's economic performance over this period has been much stronger than Argentina's. In 1990, Argentina's national income per capita was 65 percent higher than Chile's, and today it is around 22 percent lower. Average income statistics can be misleading, so it is worth noting that the two countries have similar levels of extreme poverty (less than 1 percent), although poverty reduction has been much more impressive in Chile over the last few decades. The relatively grim economic situation of Argentina impacts population health in at least two ways: first, poverty and scarcity can lead directly to illness and premature death (per the social determinants of health framework), and second, public and private expenditures on healthcare are reduced, perhaps especially in the area of preventive care. It is noteworthy that health spending in Argentina, as a percentage of GDP, has fallen over this timespan, while in Chile, it has increased. Of course, a reduction in health spending could plausibly be a sign of a healthier population with diminishing needs for medical care, but that does not seem to be the case; on every important health outcome measure (life expectancy, child mortality, maternal mortality), Chile has shown better results than Argentina throughout this period. These data also raise an interesting question about the impact of the density of medical personnel on population health outcomes. Argentina has a much higher—and even rising—physician-to-population ratio compared with Chile, but with worse population health outcomes.

National averages can be misleading. If we were to drill down in the statistical data, we would likely find that Argentina has much greater variation geographically in population health conditions. More research is necessary, but to give one example, we can compare sub-national variation in infant mortality rates, using similar time periods (2010–2015 for Chile and

Table 15.1. Demographic, economic, and health indicators for Argentina and Chile

|  | Argentina | | Chile | |
| --- | --- | --- | --- | --- |
|  | 1990 | 2018 | 1990 | 2018 |
| Population, total (millions) | 32.62 | 44.49 | 13.27 | 18.73 |
| Life expectancy at birth, years | 72 | 77 | 74 | 80 |
| Mortality rate, under 5 (per 1,000 live births) | 29 | 10 | 19 | 7 |
| Maternal mortality rate (per 100,000 live births) | 71 | 52[h] | 55 | 22[h] |
| Gross national income per capita, US$[a] | 7,060 | 19,820 | 4,270 | 24,250 |
| Poverty headcount ratio (percent of population below US$1.90 per day)[b] | 1.1 | 0.4 | 8.1 | 0.7 |
| Total expenditure on health per capita, US$[c] | n/a | 1,137 | n/a | 1,749 |
| Total expenditure on health as percent of GDP | 8.31[d] | 4.8[e] | 6.71[d] | 7.8[e] |
| Medical doctors (per 1,000 people) | 2.68 | 3.91[f] | 1.1 | 1.08[g] |

*Notes*:
[a] Inflation-adjusted, using 2018 PPP international $
[b] Inflation-adjusted, using 2011 PPP international $
[c] Inflation-adjusted, using 2014 PPP international $
[d] Data for 1995
[e] Data for 2014
[f] Data for 2017
[g] Data for 2016
[h] Data for 2015
*Sources*: World Bank Country Profiles, World Health Organization Global Health Observatory, Gapminder.org.

2012–2016 for Argentina). In Argentina, the worst-off province (Formosa: 14.65 per 1,000 live births) has an infant mortality rate almost twice that of the best-off province (Tierra del Fuego: 7.51 per 1,000) (INDEC Argentina 2019). Meanwhile, in Chile, the worst-off region (Magallanes: 8.15 per 1,000 live births) has an infant mortality rate just 21 percent higher than that of the best-off region (Tarapacá: 6.71 per 1,000 live births) (Instituto Nacional de Estadísticas Chile 2017). Arguably, the Chilean government has made a more concerted and effective effort to reduce interregional inequities in health over the last few decades.

This simple quantitative analysis points to some underlying issues that complicate any comparison between the two countries. Argentina is larger in both area and population, with widely dispersed population centers. Chile has a heterogeneous geography and isolated regions (e.g., in Patagonia, or the Atacama Desert), but the vast majority of the population is concentrated in a relatively small area—its Central Valley—which includes the capital of Santiago. Similarly, in its political structure, Argentina is a federation of provinces, while Chile has always had a unitary system of government. In Argentina, similar to the United States, the provinces have considerable autonomy, uneven socioeconomic conditions, and distinctive public policy priorities—that is, some prioritize health policy more than others. Decisions made by Argentina's national health leadership are parsed, filtered, and interpreted through provincial governments. By contrast, in Chile, the Ministry of Health centralizes decision-making and the execution of health policy; though it has local administrative units, these do not have real autonomy. Possibly, then, national-level policy decisions, once made, reverberate more rapidly and evenly throughout the system. In Argentina, Ramón Carrillo himself recognized this issue in the 1940s, and he pushed (unsuccessfully) for more radical constitutional reforms to give the national Ministry of Health the authority he thought it deserved (Arce 2010, 57). On the other hand, federalism in Argentina may promote local-level experimentation in health policy, for example the organization of innovative primary healthcare programs in Rosario, Argentina under socialist mayor (and physician) Hermes Binner starting in the late 1990s (Báscolo and Yavich 2010). Still, more research is needed to analyze how macro-level political structure (e.g., federal versus unitary systems) influences health policy and outcomes.

Possibly, there is a stronger political consensus around health policy in Chile, which leads to more consistency and stability in the design and implementation of such policies. The legacy of the *Concertación*, a coalition of center-left governments that held the presidency from 1990 to 2010, means that the current mixed model in the health system—with room for both private initiative and investment and government action to promote equity and regulate the quality and cost of healthcare—has broad political ownership. No one party can claim to have created this system—and the same has been said of the SNS, created in 1952 with support and input from multiple parties. In contrast, in Argentina, the political left, including, currently, most of the neo-Peronist parties, appears to "own" the health issue as part of their social justice platform. What could be a consensus-building issue area, instead, is subject to the same forces of polarization that have characterized Argentine politics for a long time, and more conservative governments (like Macri's) play their part by cutting back or eliminating government health programs. Such sudden and unexpected political shifts in Argentina undermine the stability of the health system and lead to much wasted effort, a problem that has been recognized for a long time (Arce 2010, 242). Then again, it must be conceded that the consensus around health policy in Chile only congealed after the abrupt reforms introduced by a military government, and that a small, unelected minority promoted the intrusion of capitalist logic into the health sector.

My analysis also suggests that the medical profession should be considered an autonomous and powerful force in the shaping of the health system. Although neither country has anything like the American Medical Association, which, since the early 1900s, has exercised its considerable leverage to maintain a mostly private healthcare regime in the United States (Barr 2016), in both Chile and Argentina the development of health systems has been accompanied by the labor organizing of medical professionals. Until midcentury, hygienists, social medicine advocates, public health experts, and health planners represented a socially progressive wing of the ruling class that took special interest in raising the levels of health and well being among the poor, even though their attitudes could be quite paternalistic. As social, economic, and health policies became more responsive to the demands of the working class in both Chile and Argentina, doctors became more conservative, fearful of the rise of socialism, skeptical of the state's ability to administer the health system, and convinced that socialized medicine would diminish their own earnings and erode their social status. Nevertheless, perhaps especially in Argentina where medical education is still largely free and state-supported, there is a normalized sense of *compromiso social*—social commitment—among doctors, demonstrated through typical part-time work in public hospitals to complement their private practices.

The comparison of Argentina and Chile offers ambiguous signals about the respective role of the private sector and the government in the regulation and ownership of the health system. Until the 1970s, Chile would seem to illustrate Sen's (2001) concept of the "support-led" process, in which the state takes the leading role in building the health system prior to sustained and broad-based economic growth. The problem, however, is that the system of socialized medicine under the SNS was never that universal, and evidence that the system improved population health is hard to find. Free-market oriented reforms to the health system starting in the 1970s exacerbated health inequalities, but in the early years of Chile's post-dictatorship politics, a consensus around a mixed private-public model was achieved. Sustained economic growth in itself has had a positive impact on population health. Although controversial, neoliberal reforms in some parts of the economy have created favorable economic conditions, but the state continues to play a strong part in the health sector. Argentina, meanwhile, has been diminished by one economic crisis after another. Not only does this directly impact population health, but political instability and polarization probably impede a move toward universal health coverage. The fragmented, segmented, and widely variable quality of the Argentine health system is only partly a product of conservative opposition; it also comes from the internal contradictions of earlier rounds of social policy reform dating back to the Perón period. Jonathan Hagood (2008) argues that "the true legacy of Perón's vision of Argentine citizenship was its articulation as membership in an autonomous social group—either ethnically-, labor-, or municipally-based—rather than citizenship in a social welfare state where such services are delivered by an autonomous nation-state itself" (190). Membership in one of the *obras sociales* is a sign of middle-class status, a hard-won right that is not easily parted with.

## Conclusion

The health systems of Argentina and Chile, in their present states, are products of distinctive political, economic, and social histories, which seldom followed a predictable trajectory. Instead, the health systems of both countries are marked by moments of rapid shifts that introduce new institutional frameworks and policy innovations, followed by long periods of relative inertia and resistance to change. The complexity of these health systems, with their mix of public and private actors (including for-profit and nonprofit, domestic and multinational) in the functions of funding, insurance, and provision of healthcare, is an outcome of layers of history, all of which complicates generalizations from this comparative analysis. Still, I would argue that Chile's post-dictatorship governments have managed to improve its health system, making it more efficient, transparent, and effective, while Argentina's health system is marked by instability and a much higher degree of complexity. In Chile, a strong Ministry of Health lays down a regulatory regime that guarantees access—either via the public or the private route—to adequate services. The gap in quality between the private and public sectors is not quite so marked as in Argentina, where the quality of the public system has varied significantly between regions and over time, with political changes determining budgetary priorities.

In Argentina and Chile, we see the merit of both of Amartya Sen's models: the growth-mediated and support-led processes. Over the long run, the governments of both countries made large investments in public health, particularly during periods of influence of leftist and populist politics around midcentury. In more recent years, since the 1990s at least, even opponents of free-market capitalism might grudgingly admit that Chile's steady economic growth has helped to produce political stability and facilitated the creation of more generous social policies, including in the health sector. In contrast, Argentina's economic performance has been erratic and often dismal. When the economic pie is growing, as in Chile, political conflicts over welfare state expansion are reduced; when the pie appears to shrink or stay the same, as in Argentina, politics becomes more of a zero-sum game where the gain of one group seems to come at the expense of another, and conflict is a predictable result. Both countries represent, to varying degrees, the notion that "segmentation in the realm of medicine and public health was part and parcel of the great problematic tangle of Latin American societies—dysfunctional attempts at integration, the existence of undemocratic privileges, and the hypermarginalization of the poor" (Cueto and Palmer 2015, 4).

Thus, this comparison between Chile and Argentina demonstrates that the problems of economic development, effective governance, and public health are intertwined. But beyond this fairly obvious conclusion, we can also assert that historical analysis is essential to understanding why national health systems have particular institutional arrangements, political structures, and values. Historical understanding is not antithetical to innovation and change, but rather, can serve as a foundation for carrying out the difficult and continuous work of making a right to health a concrete reality for all.

## Acknowledgments

The author wishes to thank Karina Ramacciotti and Marcelo López Campillay for their thoughtful comments on drafts of this chapter.

## References

Arce, Hugo E. 2010. *El sistema de salud: De dónde viene y hacia dónde va: que pasó en el mundo, en el país y en los hospitales durante el siglo XX: por qué estamos como estamos.* Buenos Aires: Prometeo Libros.

Armus, Diego. 2011. *The Ailing City: Health, Tuberculosis, and Culture in Buenos Aires, 1870–1950.* Durham, NC: Duke University Press.

———. 2016. "Eugenesia en Buenos Aires: Discursos, prácticas, historiografía." *História, Ciências, Saúde-Manguinhos* 23: 149–70.

Barr, Donald A. 2016. *Introduction to US Health Policy: The Organization, Financing and Delivery of Health Care in America*. Baltimore, MD: Johns Hopkins University Press.

Báscolo, Ernesto, and Natalia Yavich. 2010. "Gobernanza del desarrollo de la APS en Rosario, Argentina." *Revista de Salud Pública* 12: 89–104.

Belmartino, Susana. 2005. *La atención médica argentina en el siglo XX: Instituciones y procesos*. Buenos Aires: Siglo Veintiuno Editores Argentina.

Biernat, Carolina, Juan Manuel Cerdá, and Karina Ramacciotti. 2015. *La salud pública y la enfermería en la Argentina*. Bernal: Universidad Nacional de Quilmes.

Biernat, Carolina, and Karina Ramacciotti. 2008. "Las madres y sus hijos en foco." In *La Fundación Eva Perón y Las Mujeres: Entre la Provocación y La Inclusión*, edited by Carolina Barry, Karina Ramacciotti, and Adriana Valobra, 51–75. Buenos Aires: Biblos.

Birn, A. E. (2009). "Making it Politic(al): Closing the gap in a Generation: Health Equity through Action on the Social Determinants of Health." *Social Medicine* 4 (3): 166–182.

Birn, Anne-Emanuelle, and Laura Nervi. 2015. "Political Roots of the Struggle for Health Justice in Latin America." *The Lancet* 385 (9974): 1174–75. DOI: 10.1016/s0140-6736(14)61844-4.

Birn, Anne-Emanuelle, Yogan Pillay, and Timothy H Holtz. 2009. *Textbook of International Health: Global Health in a Dynamic World*: Oxford: Oxford University Press.

Carter, Eric D. 2012. *Enemy in the Blood: Malaria, Environment, and Development in Argentina*. Tuscaloosa, AL: University of Alabama Press.

———. 2019. "Social Medicine and International Expert Networks in Latin America, 1930–1945." *Global Public Health* 14 (6–7): 791–802.

Cueto, Marcos, and Steven Palmer. 2015. *Medicine and Public Health in Latin America: A History*. New York: Cambridge University Press.

Gapminder. n.d. *Gapminder.org*. https://www.gapminder.org/tools/#$chart-type=bubbles&url=v1.

Hagood, Jonathan David. 2008. "Cells in the Body Politic: Physicians, Social Medicine, and Public Health in Peronist Argentina." PhD Diss., University of California, Davis.

Homedes, Núria, and Antonio Ugalde. 2005. "Why Neoliberal Health Reforms Have Failed in Latin America." *Health Policy* 71 (1): 83–96.

Illanes, María Angélica. 1993. *En el nombre del pueblo, del estado y de la ciencia': Historia social de la salud pública, Chile 1880–1973: Hacia una historia social del siglo XX*. Santiago de Chile: Colectivo de Atención Primaria.

INDEC Argentina. 2019. *Tasa de mortalidad infantil por 1.000 nacidos vivos*. Buenos Aires: INDEC. https://www.indec.gob.ar/ftp/cuadros/sociedad/030306_2019.xls.

Instituto Nacional de Estadísticas Chile. 2017. *Estadísticas Vitales Anuario 2015* (table 1.2.2.2.5-01). https://www.ine.cl/docs/default-source/publicaciones/2017/anuario-de-estadisticas-vitales-2015.pdf.

Iriart, Celia, Emerson Elías Merhy, and Howard Waitzkin. 2001. "Managed Care in Latin America: The New Common Sense in Health Policy Reform." *Social Science & Medicine* 52 (8): 1243–53.

Kreplak, Nicolás. 2017. "Política sanitaria." *Soberanía Sanitaria* 1 (0): 4–5.

Labra, Maria Eliana. 2002. "La reinvención neoliberal de la inequidad en Chile. El caso de la salud." *Cadernos de Saúde Pública* 18 (4): 1041–52.

———. 2004. "Medicina social en Chile: Propuestas y debates (1920–1950)." *Cuad Méd Soc* 44 (4): 207–19.
Ledesma Prietto, Nadia Florencia. 2016. *"La revolución sexual de nuestro tiempo." El discurso médico anarquista sobre el control de la natalidad, la maternidad y el placer sexual. Argentina, 1931–1951*. Buenos Aires: Biblos.
Marmot, Michael. 2015. "The Health Gap: The Challenge of an Unequal World." *The Lancet* 386 (10011): 2442–44.
Martínez Franzoni, Juliana, and Diego Sánchez-Ancochea. 2016. *The Quest for Universal Social Policy in the South: Actors, Ideas and Architectures*. Cambridge: Cambridge University Press.
McGuire, James W. 2001. "Social Policy and Mortality Decline in East Asia and Latin America." *World Development* 29 (10): 1673–97.
———. 2010. *Wealth, Health, and Democracy in East Asia and Latin America*. Cambridge: Cambridge University Press.
Mesa-Lago, Carmelo. 1991. "Social Security in Latin America and the Caribbean: A Comparative Assessment." In *Social Security in Developing Countries*, edited by Ehtisham Ahmad, Jean Drèze, John Hills, and Amartya Sen, 356–94. Oxford, England: Clarendon Press.
Miranda, Marisa, and Gustavo Vallejo. 2012. *Una historia de la eugenesia argentina y las redes biopolíticas internacionales, 1912–1945*. Buenos Aires: Editorial Biblos.
Missoni, Eduardo, and Giorgio Solimano. 2010. "Towards Universal Health Coverage: The Chilean Experience." In *World Health Report (2010) Background Paper*. Geneva: WHO.
Molina Bustos, Carlos Antonio. 2010. *Institucionalidad sanitaria chilena, 1889–1989*. Santiago, Chile: LOM Ediciones.
Navarro, Vicente. 1974. "What Does Chile Mean: An Analysis of Events in the Health Sector before, during, and after Allende's Administration." *Milbank Memorial Fund Quarterly* 52 (2): 93–130.
Palmer, Steven Paul. 2003. *From Popular Medicine to Medical Populism: Doctors, Healers, and Public Power in Costa Rica, 1800–1940*. Durham, NC: Duke University Press.
Paúl, Fernanda. 2019. "Protestas en Chile: Las 6 grandes deudas sociales por las que muchos chilenos dicen sentirse 'abusados.'" *BBC News Mundo*, October 21. https://www.bbc.com/mundo/noticias-america-latina-50124583
Ramacciotti, Karina. 2009. *La política sanitaria del peronismo*. Buenos Aires: Biblos.
———. 2018. "Sentidos de los recortes en salud pública en tiempos democráticos." *Boletín de la Asociación Argentina para la Investigación en Historia de las Mujeres y Estudios de Género* 2 (3): 7–8.
Ramacciotti, Karina, and Lucia Ana Romero. 2017. "La regulación de medicamentos en la Argentina (1946–2014)." *Revista Iberoamericana de Ciencia, Tecnología y Salud* 35 (12): 153–74.
Riley, James C. 2005. *Poverty and Life Expectancy: The Jamaica Paradox*. Cambridge: Cambridge University Press.
Rodriguez, Julia. 2006. *Civilizing Argentina: Science, Medicine, and the Modern State*. Chapel Hill: University of North Carolina Press.

Scharagrodsky, Pablo. 2016. *Mujeres en movimiento: Deporte, cultura física y feminidades: Argentina, 1870–1980*. Buenos Aires: Prometeo Libros.
Sen, Amartya. 2001. "Economic Progress and Health." In *Poverty, Inequality, and Health: An International Perspective*, edited by David A. Leon and Gill Walt, 333–45. Oxford: Oxford University Press.
Waitzkin, Howard, Celia Iriart, Alfredo Estrada, and Silvia Lamadrid. 2001. "Social Medicine Then and Now: Lessons from Latin America." *American Journal of Public Health* 91 (10): 1592–1601.
World Bank. n.d. *World Bank Country Profiles*. https://data.worldbank.org/country.
World Health Organization. n.d. *Global Health Observatory*. https://www.who.int/data/gho.
Zimmermann, Eduardo A. 1995. *Los liberales reformistas: La cuestión social en la Argentina 1890–1916*. Buenos Aires: Editorial Sudamericana Universidad de San Andrés.

# 16

## Health as a Right in Brazil and Argentina

Carlos S. Dimas

In the opening quarter of the twenty-first century, the economies of Brazil and Argentina have witnessed a cycle of booms and busts. For instance, during the presidency of Lula da Silva (2003–2010), the Brazilian government's increase in petroleum, iron, and soybean exports to China helped finance the elimination of its foreign debt, fueled a steady yearly growth of 4 percent to its GDP (Gross Domestic Product), and facilitated Brazil's shift to an international creditor (Brooks 2010). This led reporters, economists, and international observers to declare Brazil a "Sleeping Giant." The cover of the November 2009 issue of *The Economist* went as far as to depict the statue of Christ that sits atop Sugarloaf Mountain overlooking Rio de Janeiro as a rocket taking off. By 2015, however, the dream was over, the economy had collapsed, and the Brazilian state had started working to restructure its budget through changes to national healthcare management, among others.

In contrast, Argentina opened the century with a recession, a massive economic crash in 2001, and a US$95 billion debt. Beginning in 2003, the administrations of Néstor Kirchner and Cristina Fernández de Kirchner (2003–2015) took on rebuilding the economy following Néstor's successful restructuring of Argentina's debt to the IMF (International Monetary Fund). On the domestic side, the Kirchner Era increased investments in social programs intended to reduce poverty rates, increase wages, and improved accessibility to healthcare. However, these plans also increased the national debt to the extent that the national inflation rate rose to 40 percent, a fact that the government denied. Other indices revealed the true state of the Argentine economy. For example, a clandestine market emerged for currency exchange of the Peso to Euros, British Pounds, and US Dollars known as the *Dólar blue* (Informal Dollar);[1] there were many general strikes from the nation's largest union, the General Confederation of Workers [Confederación

General del Trabajo] (CGT), and there was widespread looting. In 2015, Argentine voters responded by electing Mauricio Macri to the presidency, a businessman and former mayor of Buenos Aires. Macri's platform centered on stabilizing the economy, opening the nation to foreign investment, repairing the relationship with the IMF, and reducing public expenditures by cutting public spending. Given the economic instability, both the Brazilian and Argentine states have seen public health programs and healthcare as an area to reduce government expenses.

Nevertheless, local society has responded against austerity measures because of the important place of universal health coverage (UHC) in Brazil and Argentina. Throughout August of 2017, for instance, citizens and doctors in the northern Brazilian city of Recife gathered in the streets to protest the government's proposed plan to privatize the nation's public healthcare system, Sistema Único de Saúde, [Sole System of Health] (SUS). The following year, Argentines took to the streets to protest similar proposals within their own government to privatize the state-run healthcare system.

This chapter has three primary objectives: first, to demonstrate the history of universal health coverage in Argentina and Brazil and the social, political, and cultural contexts that established healthcare as a right and not a privilege; second, to show how the governments of Argentina and Brazil see reductions to public health as a response to improve the state of a national debt and increased inflation; last, to show the historical and cultural factors that push Argentines and Brazilians to protest for the protection of universal health coverage.

## Central Argument(s)

This chapter is an overview of the history of public health in Argentina and Brazil from the nineteenth century to the present that begins by detailing the mutual rise of doctors as political-medical actors whose work interjected the importance of public health through the discourse of *higienismo* [hygiene], into the building of the nation-state over the course of the nineteenth century. Indeed, by the closing half of the 1800s, medical professionals in Latin America rose to prominent political positions on platforms of medical and social reform. This was fundamental in the convergence of political, economic, and public health concerns that formed the Medical State. For state builders of the era, public health was one way to advance economic progress and social order; as such, it made public health a concern of the state that extended into the twentieth century. The second portion of this chapter examines the early development of universal health coverage in Argentina and Brazil within the development of these nations' respective modern welfare states and populist governments of the 1930s and 1940s.

Scholars have long debated the defining aspects of populism. Studies have proposed the ideology as the promotion of an anti-elite narrative, a feeling of how politics should function, and incorporating areas of the social fabric believed to have been excluded from the political process. Ultimately, the goal of populism is to create a centralized and intervening state. According to Kirk A. Hawkins and Cristóbal Rovira Kaltwasser (2017), earlier definitions of populism centered on left-leaning charismatic leaders who passed short-lived social and economic policies, such as import substitute industrialization, that appeased the masses in exchange for support. The newer literature, however, has pulled away from condensing populism to a set of policies or an exclusive practice of the Left. Instead, populism is the formulation of ideas, a form of rhetoric, and a part of a political cosmology alongside pluralism and elitism that political actors from the Right or Left can employ in what is referred to as the "ideational approach" (Hawkins and Rovira Kaltwasser 2017). The study of the presidencies of Juan Domingo Perón (1946–1955 and 1973–1974) and Peronism embodies the changes in the literature on populism. For example, historians and political scientists have used fascism, populism, nationalism, socialism, and authoritarianism to classify his presidency (Buchrucker 1998). More recently, Argentine historians have used "democratic-authoritarianism" to define *Peronismo* (Romero and Brennan 2013).

This chapter places the expansion of healthcare at the center of an ideational approach to populism. For Argentina, UHC was born in the Peronist era, but was maintained even during governments opposed to Peronism, such as the military dictatorship of 1976–1983. Indeed, healthcare was a valuable avenue for the expansion of the state, since public health institutions went through a process of centralization/verticalization. Healthcare served to initiate sweeping social welfare programs, such as universal health coverage, social security, public housing, and pension programs, to name a few (see Aboy 2005; James 2001; Karush and Chamosa 2010; Ramacciotti 2009). Similarly, in Brazil, the populist government of Getúlio Vargas (1930–1945, 1951–1954) laid the foundation for UHC, but the current SUS stems from the government of José Sarney (1985–1990) and the 1988 Constitutional Reform. Thus, the expansion of healthcare gained momentum under populist governments, but continued past their eras further emphasizing the central place of healthcare in local society. Nevertheless, in Argentina and Brazil, public health is repeatedly under fiscal threat.

The chapter concludes with a discussion of the current state of universal healthcare in both countries, in particular, the place of healthcare since the Return to Democracy and the Neoliberal Era (1990 to today). Faced in the 1990s with expanding debt and inflation, Latin American governments proposed privatization of state-controlled programs to reduce the government's subsidization. Advocates for market-oriented restructuring claim that access to coverage and services will improve as companies will compete for business. Opponents counter that millions of people will lose access to the healthcare that they have depended on for decades. Since then, public mobilization has been a common occurrence to protect healthcare in both countries.

## The Medical State

During the nineteenth century, Argentina and Brazil witnessed significant changes. By the mid-1800s, each country became a popular destination for immigration. Population centers on the coast and the interior grew from small communities to bustling towns. For instance, between the 1890s and 1940s, the population of Buenos Aires increased from roughly 700,000 to just under 3 million (Pirez 1998). Under the famous Argentine totem, "to govern is to populate" [*gobernar es poblar*], open lands were forcibly appropriated from Indigenous communities to make way for medium- and large-scale settler farms that, through the production of important agrocommodities, could meet the needs of the global market. These factors contributed to the generation of a level of wealth that was concentrated among national elites.

But this era of growth had its problems: larger populations resulted in cities that were crowded and dirty, and shantytowns became part of nineteenth-century urban life. Increased trade also connected southern South America to global epidemic chains. The absence of basic provisions like potable water, private plumbing, or municipal services created a breeding ground for contagious disease. Between the 1860s and 1910s, cholera, bubonic plague, and yellow fever were just some of the epidemics that broke out in the region. Ailments such as tuberculosis, beriberi, malnutrition, and malaria became endemic. Meanwhile, in rural regions little medical infrastructure existed well into the opening decades of the twentieth century. For state builders, disease became synonymous with underdevelopment.

## Positivism and Medical Crises as Social Problems

In nineteenth-century Latin America, the social theory of Positivism became popular among elites and government officials. Positivism held that social order and economic progress were predicated on certain coefficients, like a strong centralized government, imitation of European social and cultural ideals and immigration, industrialization, and investment in the sciences.[2] In the mid-1800s, hygiene and public health became one way for government officials to advance national economic progress and social order. An important development was the emergence of the hygienist as a political-medical actor. Part politician, part medical professional, hygienists throughout Latin America advocated for broad sweeping medical and social reforms that responded to the civic problems of the era: urbanization, poverty, endemic and epidemic diseases, and high mortality rates.

Through their political positions, hygienists transformed public health into an area of government oversight. This shift stood in contrast to previous decades in which religious and philanthropic associations managed healthcare. In Argentina, for instance, Guillermo Rawson and Eduardo Wilde embodied the late-nineteenth century hygienist. Both taught at the University of Buenos Aires's School of Medicine and wrote extensively on the negative impact of urbanization on personal and collective health. In addition, they each served as Ministers of the Interior.[3] As one of the most important cabinet positions, the ministry served as a liaison between the federal government and the provinces. Because of its expansive governmental responsibilities it housed numerous departments, such as the National Department of Hygiene [Departamento Nacional de Higiene] which was founded in 1880, and later responded to national epidemics.

One of the most important aspects of the nineteenth-century medical community was that hygienists discussed medical concerns as social problems that mandated coordinated responses between doctors and the government. Writing on Afro-Brazilian maternity and infant mortality in post-abolition Brazil, the historian Okezi T. Otovo (2016) remarks that "physicians helped establish a widely shared consensus that Brazilian development absolutely depended on social reform guided by scientific interventions" (3). Thus, over the course of the nineteenth and early twentieth centuries, the state merged governance and public health.

The increased association between the governments of Brazil and Argentina, as well as medical actors, facilitated the growth and professionalization of the medical field. During the era, physicians in the two nations founded medical associations, medical journals, and undertook medical and scientific missions to North America and Europe to expand their training. In Argentina and Brazil, these programs served as foundations for challenging European ideas of Social Darwinism that held the region as inferior and underdeveloped (Peard 1999; Stepan 1991). In Brazil, the internationally recognized physician Oswaldo Cruz worked with the government to establish compulsory vaccination programs, local production of bubonic plague serums, national hygienic measures to reduce yellow fever and malaria rates, and a bacteriological institute, the Oswaldo Cruz Institute [Instituto Oswaldo Cruz].

The development of public health as a national concern continued the medicalization of society, meaning that medical actors became more interwoven into society and extended their influence with varying degrees of success. For instance, the French-Argentine writer Gabriela Laperrière was active in the Argentine League Against Tuberculosis [Liga Argentina Contra La Tuberculosis] (ALAT), a private-publicly funded organization tasked with creating public awareness of a disease that was extremely common throughout Buenos Aires. The ALAT also became a jumping-off point for many doctors into government positions. Once they got these positions, they would continue the ALAT's campaign in their new roles. Others, like the women-led Society of Beneficence [Sociedad de Beneficencia] of Argentina helped form a national child welfare policy. Indeed, this organization's work established an administrative apparatus and a social link during the Medical State era that would later be utilized with the emergence of the Argentine welfare state (Guy 2009).

The development of the Medical State in post-independence Latin America is central to understanding the formation of UHC in the mid-twentieth century. The most important point to understand is that governance and public health merged to such an extent that the standardization of medical practice, investment in medical research, public health campaigns, and social services became part of everyday culture.

However, the era also had its problems. Optimal healthcare was reserved for the upper and middle classes, which, until the 1950s, constituted the minority. In addition, the best services were confined to the most urbanized regions. Rural areas in Argentina and Brazil had little to no medical infrastructure. It was during the early twentieth century that steps were taken to expand medical services to all regions and sectors of society. In Argentina, this occurred during the opening quarter of the twentieth century with the development of the "National Question." Under this model, state and medical officials balanced the health of the nation with conditions beyond the metropole (Carter 2012; Hochman, Di Liscia, and Palmer 2012).

## Populism and the Welfare State

Latin America's transition to the twentieth century was tumultuous. The wealth that agro-exports generated concentrated capital in the hands of national elites who worked to safeguard their position. The widening socioeconomic gap generated sociopolitical responses. At the turn of the twentieth century, labor unions, political movements—such as anarchism, communism, socialism, and populism—and middle-class-oriented political parties emerged. Although all very different, the common denominator of these institutions and movements was their advocacy for improved social conditions, such as public health.

Between 1900 and 1950, most of Latin America went through an era of political instability. Throughout the region, conservative, liberal, and military governments all vied for control to initiate programs with the intention of transforming their nations or maintaining the status quo.[4] Populism in Argentina and Brazil grew out of this era under the presidencies of Juan D. Perón and Getúlio Vargas. Building upon the definition of populism given earlier, the Peronist and Vargas movements advocated for a new political process that departed from the oligarchic and conservative governments that had been in power before.[5] Each advanced an anti-elite narrative that intermixed nationalist as well as anti-imperialist, anti-socialist, and anti-communist sentiments. Similarly, the political base of both governments was grounded in labor unions, the working class, and sectors of the middle class in an effort to "take back" power from the elites (Hawkins and Rovira Kaltwasser 2017; see also Debowicz and Segal 2014; Hawkins et al. 2019). Through their charismatic leadership styles, Perón and Vargas promoted centralizing politics, culture, and society under the state, often oscillating between democracy and authoritarianism.

## Peronism

Juan Domingo Perón entered political life through the military coup of 1943 headed by a nationalist cohort within the army known as the Group of United Officers [Grupo de Oficiales Unidos] (GOU). Under the new military government, Perón became Secretary of Labor. In this position, he worked closely with labor unions as the base for his support (Romero and Brennan 2013). Eventually, Perón became so popular among the unions that on October 9, 1945 he was forced to resign his position and was then arrested. Eight days later, thousands of *descamisados* (the "shirtless," but referring to impoverished laborers) marched into the main plaza of Buenos

Aires demanding Perón's release. He was freed and soon announced his presidential candidacy.

In 1946, Perón became president. His approach to governing centered around the political ideology of *Justicialismo* [justicialism] (Plotkin 2003). This ideology went beyond politics into social, economic, and cultural practices. Perón himself described *Justicialismo* as "Christian and humanist," taking the best parts of "collectivism and individualism, idealism and materialism" to foment national stability through guaranteed work, global economic independence, social welfare, and the protection of citizens (Rock 2006, 28). Fueling classic definitions of populism, Perón funneled the dissemination of *Justicialismo* through the national Five-Year Plan (1947–1951, FYP). The FYP tasked the government with reducing the national debt, nationalizing foreign controlled industries to reduce costs for consumers, establishing full national employment, creating unions in all industries, increasing agricultural output, supporting local industrialists to produce goods that were formerly imported (import substitute industrialization), and expanding workers' rights.

Public health was one aspect of the FYP. In 1946, Perón formed the Secretariat of Public Health [Secretaría de Salud Pública]. In 1949, this organization was promoted to the Ministry of Public Health [Ministerio de Salud Pública] (MSP), under the helm of the neurosurgeon, Ramón Carrillo, who served in the Peronist administration until the coup of 1955. Prior to the secretariat and MPH, the National Department of Hygiene [Departamento Nacional de Higiene] was the closest equivalent to a national public institution. However, matters were often delegated to provincial assistance commissions, and the level of services fluctuated across the provinces (Bohoslavsky and Di Liscia 2008).

In line with the form of governance Perón championed, Carrillo focused on centralizing and expanding medical assistance at the national and provincial levels. Improvements centered on reforming Argentina's nineteenth-century horizontal public health structure into a vertical format with the government at the top. The MSP created more clinics and representation in the Argentine countryside (Bohoslavsky and Di Liscia 2008). In addition, the MSP invested in programs meant to address long-standing medical problems, such as tuberculosis, infant mortality, malaria, and Chagas disease. The state also invested in increasing the number of medical graduates. Between 1934 and 1954, the number of doctors in Argentina almost tripled from about 8,000 to 22,000. In a short amount of time, thousands of Argentines gained access to healthcare (Hirschegger 2007; Ramacotti 2009).

The state also improved access to healthcare through the founding of the *Obra Social*[6] program that coincided with the developing relationship between the Peronist government and labor unions. Since the beginning of the twentieth century, Argentine employers had deducted a portion of workers' salaries to fund private medical insurance. By the early 1940s, the state matched contributions to improve medical coverage. In 1944, the Peronist government passed a law that established the Commission of Social Services [Comisión de Servicio Social] (CSS). The CSS was responsible for ensuring that all workers had access to subsidized medication and medical care. Following the CSS, the state created the National Institute of Social Prevention [Instituto Nacional de Previsión Social], which enforced annual physical exams for all citizens and extended healthcare to preventive care (Garay 2017). Thus, the state, alongside labor unions, created a UHC system.

In contrast to movements from previous generations, Peronism established healthcare as a right and not a privilege, thus embedding it within populist definitions of social welfare and social justice. Beyond healthcare, the government built public housing [*viviendas*] for laborers, which included schools, markets, churches, parks, and clinics. In addition, other social welfare reforms created affordable vacation resorts, mandated paid vacations, introduced sick and maternity leave, and established the *aguinaldo* program, which provided everyone with a year-end extra month of income. Peronism, as a political, cultural, and social movement, exists to this day. The continued support of this program is based on a generation of Argentines that witnessed social mobility and public health as a part of everyday culture.

### Getúlio Vargas

In Brazil, the development of public health as a centralized government program took place under the government of Getúlio Vargas. Peronism and Vargasismo shared similarities, but they also had key differences. Like Perón, Vargas consolidated the Brazilian state and society under a strong executive branch. Referred to as "Father of the Poor" [O Pai dos Pobres], it should come as no surprise that public health provided a space for the government to engage with the Social Question to build mass appeal among the lower classes that had been marginalized in previous decades.[7] As in Argentina, regional medical concerns, such as initiatives to fight malaria in the northeast and tuberculosis in the cities, were "nationalized." Moreover, unlike Perón, Vargas worked more closely with foreign governments. The Rockefeller Foundation's International Health Division assisted in eradicating yellow fever and hookworm disease in Brazil, for example.

Following the coup of 1930, Vargas created the Ministry of Education and Public Health [Ministério da Educação e Saúde Pública] (MESP). However, in its first four years the ministry accomplished very little due to limited government investment, lackluster leadership, and minimal jurisdiction. In 1934, lawyer Gustavo Capanema and the hygienist João Barros Barreto were placed in the MESP.[8] Capanema spearheaded a complete restructuring of the MESP to align the ministry with Vargas's plans for a more vertical organization of Brazilian government institutions through removing local impediments—department and state officials, or elites—that stymied the expansion of the state in handling public health. For instance, Vargas routinely removed state governors that rejected his policies and appointed loyalists instead.

The first area of restructuring the public health system consisted of the creation of a program called the Federal Delegations of Health [Delegações Federais de Saúde] (DFS). In doing so, Vargas elevated healthcare from state-level management to a national concern. The DFS placed federal representatives in each Brazilian state to handle daily public health concerns. In addition, Capanema created the National Services [Serviços Nacionais] (SN) in 1941 to oversee the eradication of all large-scale endemic diseases, such as yellow fever. Thus, the SN worked closely with the Rockefeller Foundation and the Oswaldo Cruz Center in responding to infectious diseases.

The MESP also worked to strengthen the relationship between the state and physicians. Under Capanema, the federal government initiated yearly National Medical Conferences [Conferências Nacionais de Saúde], which were interrupted during the military dictatorship (1964–1985). Scholars show that the reforms the MESP initiated, as a whole, expanded the spatial reach, the bureaucratic organization, and the professionalization of the Brazilian medical community (Cueto and Palmer 2015; Hochman 2005).

At the end of the populist eras that defined Peronism and Vargasism, only Argentina had established universal healthcare. Yet, under Vargas, the scope of the Medical State expanded at both the regional and national levels. For Brazil, UHC would not be established until 1988. Several factors need to be taken into consideration to explain this phenomenon. For example, we must account for population and country size and the socioeconomic, political, and cultural divisions between the various regions of Brazil: Rio de Janeiro and São Paulo, Northern and Southern Brazil, and the coastal urban and rural interior. Last, many aspects of the healthcare program were undone during the Military Era. In the 1970s, even in the midst of "the Brazilian (economic) Miracle" many areas of the country had no health infrastructure whatsoever. The next section explores the place of public health in both nations during the 1990s.

## Neoliberalism and Pressures on Universal Healthcare

As societies change over time, so does their definition of what constitutes health. In 1978, the Alma-Ata Conference (Kazakhstan) convened doctors from around the world. There, under the slogan of "Health for All," the international medical community shifted toward preventive approaches and primary healthcare in contrast to previous decades of responding to disease.

In the twentieth and twenty-first centuries, populations are living longer. As a result, non-communicable diseases, such as heart disease, cancer, and diabetes, have provided new challenges—both medical and bureaucratic—to an aging population. In contrast to previous generations, the current climate sees health as a combination of lifestyle, environmental, and biological factors. Faced with growing and aging populations and mounting socioeconomic and health disparities, governments have had to adapt. Faced with these challenges, states and societies are grappling with the obligation to provide medical services for citizens, even as they often must face the reality of dwindling economic resources. In response, many Latin American governments have initiated neoliberal market reforms in which state-controlled entities, like public health, are sold to private companies. The logic of these actions is to reduce public expenditures. In Argentina, for instance, the increase in national subsidies and investment in social welfare programs pushed citizens to vote-in the center-right candidate Mauricio Macri (2015–19) who campaigned on a platform of fixing a beleaguered economy.

Supporters of neoliberalism hold that a privately managed and market-driven system will extend coverage while simultaneously reducing costs for medical consumers and will adapt more readily to local needs as companies compete for business. In addition, proponents have argued that state-run systems are riddled with lapses in coverage—especially in the most geographically distant and socioeconomically disadvantaged areas—that they are a bureaucratic turmoil, and that they have resulted in increased medical costs (Massuda et al. 2018). These critiques extend to countries where public and private systems coexist, since blended systems, it is argued, do not promote a true free-market (Machado 2018).

Nevertheless, support for state-run systems remains strong. Opponents of privatization note countries where governments removed universal public healthcare produced disastrous results. In Colombia, for example, privatization led to increased medical costs for citizens, many hospitals declared bankruptcy, and the accessible public health gap increased (Vargas Bustamante and Méndez 2014). In Argentina, where coverage is compulsory, supporters for the continuation of a state-run system note that the broad market-driven reforms of the early 1990s that privatized many state utility companies did initially reduce consumer prices and improve services. However, it also opened the door for monopolies and the eventual increase in the price of services. Moreover, it paved the way for the reliance on foreign loans and deregulation that formed the economic collapse of 2001 (Rodríguez-Boetsch 2005). Similar occurrences took place under President Macri who reduced subsidies on utilities, thereby increasing prices for Argentines as part of a general shift toward free-market reforms.[9] As a result, advocates for the state-run system argue that privatization will increase the price of medication and cause thousands to lose their insurance. Elections in October 2019 demonstrated that Macri's policies were not enough to convince voters to give him a second term; instead, they opted for the ticket of Alberto Fernández and Cristina Fernández de Kirchner and their populist approaches to fixing the economy.

The following section explores the state of universal healthcare in Argentina and Brazil in the twenty-first century. I show that at the end of the twentieth century, Latin America went through a significant moment of transition from the end of the military dictatorships, the rebuilding of economies, and the rise of neoliberalism. Due to a collection of factors, pressure has mounted for Latin American states to divest from managing healthcare and to allow market-oriented changes to take place with the hope that this will improve medical services.

### Argentina

The 1980s were a return to democracy for many regions of Latin America.[10] The new civilian governments that replaced military dictatorships inherited divided societies, massive debts, unprecedented inflation, high unemployment, and economies teetering on collapse. Since the 1990s, Argentina's public expenditures have been targets for fiscal reform or immediate privatization.

Currently, Argentina is in the midst of an increasing financial crisis. The average Argentine has witnessed prices in common goods increase, while their wages have remained stagnant. In hopes of deterring a repeat of the 2001 Economic Crash or rampant inflation, the Argentine government has sought assistance from the IMF. Under the presidency of Macri, Argentina received loans nearing $28.09 billion. Nevertheless, the IMF's loans come with the requirement that the nation undertake Structural Adjustments Programs (SAP). Central to the SAP is the initiation of austerity plans, where the national deficit is reduced by cutting public spending through privatization. Macri's bold reforms looked to change a system that has remained almost intact since it was inaugurated in 1946 under Juan Domingo Perón.

In Argentina, private and public medical insurance coexist. All citizens have access to public hospitals, but only private insurers can go to private hospitals without paying out of pocket. All Argentines form part of an insurance system, known as *Obra Social* that is half-funded through their representative union, and the other half through the federal government. Critics of the system have noted the closed nature of the *Obra Social*. Until 2000, for example, an individual was mandated to stay within their system with no option of leaving, even if their plan did not cover certain treatments. The only option was private insurance. Now, citizens can join an *Obra Social* from another union that meets their health needs. As a result, in the twenty-first century, the state has had to balance improving healthcare with cutting public spending.

During his tenure, Macri unveiled the Universal Medical Coverage plan [Cobertura Universal de Salud] (CUS) for individuals who did not have private insurance or coverage through their employer and union (*Obra Social*). According to government calculations, the CUS was poised to benefit roughly 15 million people. The plan was launched in the western Argentine province of Mendoza in October of 2017, with similar programs already in place in other provinces.[11] The CUS connected each person to a specific doctor. Patient medical history was uploaded to a national database, Telesalud, that would allow Argentines to receive medical care beyond their general practitioner anywhere in the county. The program also worked to end long waits that are common in all Argentine state services offices.[12] Thus, Macri's plan was grounded on persistent problems the Argentine healthcare system has faced.

Nevertheless, the *Obra Social* has wide-ranging support in Argentina. Proponents of the state-run system argue that neoliberal reforms to public health in fellow Latin American countries like Chile, Colombia, and Mexico have generated greater inequality without improving services (Homedes and Ugalde 2005; Vargas Bustamante and Méndez 2014). In reference to the CUS, critics hold that Argentina already has universal healthcare since those without insurance are still guaranteed free admittance to public hospitals. Rather, problems in the healthcare systems stem from underfunding.

Argentines worry that an overhaul of the health system will establish a trend of the state prioritizing fiscal management over health as a right, which may further accelerate health inequalities and socioeconomic disparities (Sakellariou and Rotarou 2017). In short, under neoliberal models, those who can afford healthcare out-of-pocket are not negatively impacted, and they often prosper. On the other hand, the marginalized sectors of society are further ostracized.

## Brazil

In 1988, the new democratic Brazilian state enacted a revised constitution to annul changes made under the military government. Under Brazil's return to democracy, the Brazilian state emphasized the notion of "social protection policy" and health as a right of citizens as the bedrock for a new democratic social order (de Faria Baptista, Vieria Machado, and de Lima 2009). The Speaker of the Assembly at the time, Ulysses Guimares, proclaimed: "This constitution will protect the weak and punish those who abuse power" (Associated Press 1988). The SUS emerged from the constitution under the moniker of universality and equity (Barbara 2018).

Since 1988, the SUS has gone through a series of changes in relation to the shifting political landscape of Brazil. Some of the challenges it faces are the continual hurdle of Brazilian conservatism, social inequality evident in the *favelas,* and inflation that coalesced with the presidency of Fernando Collor de Mello (1990–92), who resigned to stave off impeachment. Brazil's large population and the concentration of services in key urban areas have created bottlenecks where patients have died in medical corridors (Barbara 2018). Yet, for three-quarters of Brazil's 190 million population, the SUS is the sole source of medical coverage.

Under the SUS, immunization percentages hover around 95 percent for all children, and vaccines themselves are quite inexpensive because they are produced nationally. Brazil is second to the United States in the size of its transplant network and the number of transplants completed in the world. In the 1990s, the SUS served as the frontline of the HIV/AIDS epidemic where the state provided free antiretroviral therapy (Barbara 2018). In addition, state-run hospitals have expanded into the poorest areas of Brazil. Despite serious problems, the World Health Organization (WHO) considered the SUS "an outstanding success" (WHO 2008).

## Conclusion

Brazil and Argentina are at a crossroads over the future of public health. As this chapter shows, the convergence of public health and government forces dates back to the nineteenth century. During the populist era, the ideal of health as a right of all citizens emerged. Nevertheless, straggling economies of the late twentieth and early twenty-first centuries have put a strain on national resources. In response, governments have looked for ways to cut medical coverage without losing key public support. In Brazil and Argentina, citizens continue to rely on state-run systems, while medical figures and observers relay their concerns that privatization will worsen an already precarious situation. It is unclear what will happen next.

## Notes

1. For example, on August 25, 2015, the official exchange rate of USD to ARS was 1 to 9.28. The informal dollar was 1 to 15.97.

2. Positivism was a philosophical theory credited to the French philosopher Auguste Comte that championed a more scientific approach to form society, which in turn shapes the individual. Believing this approach to be more objective and reliant on quantitative data, proponents of Positivism held that certain coefficients—railroads, institutions of higher learning, free trade, urban beautification, and imitation of North American and Western European culture—would result in the attainment of progress and pull Latin American nations from a colonial and Iberian past believed to be backwards. In Latin America, prominent positivist figures were Domingo F. Sarmiento and Porfirio Diaz.

3. Guillermo Rawson (1821–1890), served as Minister of the Interior from 1862 to 1868. Eduardo Wilde (1844–1913) followed in the same capacity from 1886 to 1890.

4. Some examples include the Mexican Revolution and subsequent postrevolutionary actions (1910–1940); the 1928 United Fruit Banana Massacre in Colombia; the 1932 Peasant Massacre in El Salvador; the Jacobo Árbenz government in Guatemala (1951–1954); the 1952 Bolivian National Revolution; and the dictatorship of Rafael Trujillo in the Dominican Republic (1930–1938, 1942–1952).

5. For Brazil, this was the República Velha (Old Republic) that ruled from 1889 to 1930, and in Argentina the 1928 military coup that ousted Hipólito Yrigoyen (1916–22, 1928–1930) and initiated the Década Infame (Infamous Decade, 1930–1943).

6. I do not include an English translation of this phrase since the term "social work" is limiting. In reality, the term "obra social" would be much closer to universal healthcare, public health insurance, or something like the US version of medicare.

7. The Social Question is a nineteenth-century idea that looked at the social and cultural problems, such as inequality, that industrial society generated.

8. In 1953, it was promoted to the Ministry of Public Health [Ministério da Saúde Pública].

9. On May 31, 2018, Macri vetoed a bill that would have frozen water and electricity prices.

10. In Argentina, the military government collapsed and, in Brazil, there was an organized transition.

11. Public health in Argentina is decentralized to the provincial level. Thus, the UMC can be tested in Mendoza or a county in Mendoza with no changes to any other province. Other healthcare systems exist in Jujuy, Buenos Aires, Corrientes, and Santiago del Estero.

12. For the long waits that Argentines are accustomed to whenever going to a state office, see Javier Auyero's 2012 book *The Patients of the State: The Politics of Waiting in Argentina*. (Durham: Duke University Press)

## References

Aboy, Rosa. 2005. *Viviendas para el pueblo: Espacio urbano y sociabilidad en el barrio de Los Perales, 1946–1955*. Buenos Aires: Fondo de Cultura Económica.

Associated Press. 1988. "Brazil Completes New Constitution." *The New York Times*. September 3, 1988. https://www.nytimes.com/1988/09/03/world/brazil-complete-new-constitution.html.

Auyero, Javier. 2012. *The Patients of the State: The Politics of Waiting in Argentina*. Durham: Duke University Press.

Barbara, Vanessa. 2018. "Brazil's New President Isn't Even in Office Yet and He's Already Damaged Our Health Care" *New York Times* December 11, 2018.

Bohoslavsky, Ernesto, and María Silvia Di Liscia. 2008. "The Wind Prophylaxis. Repressive and Sanitary Institutions in Argentina's Patagonia, 1880–1940." *Asclepio: Revista de Historia de la Medicina y de la Ciencia* 60 (2): 187–206.

Brooks, Sarah. 2010. "South America's 'Sleeping Giant' Wakes: Brazil's 2010 Election." *Origins: Current Events in Historical Perspective* 4 (3). https://origins.osu.edu/users/sarah-brooks

Buchrucker, Cristián. 1998. "Interpretations of Peronism: Old Frameworks and New Perspectives." In *Peronism and Argentina*, edited by James P. Brennan, 3–15. Wilmingtin, DE: SR Books.

Carter, Eric. 2012. *Enemy in the Blood: Malaria, Environment, and Development in Argentina*. Tuscaloosa: University of Alabama Press.

Cueto, Marcos, and Steven Palmer. 2015. *Medicine and Public Health in Latin America: A History*. New York: Cambridge University Press.

Debowicz, Dario, and Paul Segal. 2014. "Structural Change in Argentina, 1935–1960: The Role of Import Substitution and Factor Endowments." *Journal of Economic History*. 74 (1): 230–58.

de Faria Baptista, Tatiana Wargas, Cristina Vieria Machado, and Luciana Dias de Lima. 2009. "State Responsibility and Right to Health in Brazil: A Balance of the Branches' Actions." *Ciencia & Saude Coletiva* 14 (3): 829–39.

Garay, Oscar Ernesto. 2017. "Obras sociales: Antecedents." *Ministerio de Salud*. http://www.salud.gob.ar/dels/printpdf/150

Guy, Donna J. 2009. *Women Build the Welfare State: Performing Charity and Creating Rights in Argentina, 1880–1955*. Durham: Duke University Press.
Hawkins, Kirk Andrew, Ryan E. Carlin, Levente Littvay, and Cristóbal Rovira Kaltwasser. 2019. *The Ideational Approach to Populism: Concept, Theory, and Analysis*. New York: Routledge.
Hawkins, Kirk A., and Cristóbal Rovira Kaltwasser. 2017. "The Ideational Approach to Populism." *Latin American Research Review* 52 (4): 513–28.
Hirschegger, Ivana. 2007. "La medicina asistencial, sanitaria y social peronista: Discurso, acciones y logros. El caso de San Rafael, Mendoza (1949–1952)." *Revista de Historia Americana y Argentina*. 42: 57–90.
Hochman, Gilberto. 2005. "Cambio político y reformas de la salud pública en Brasil. El primer gobierno Vargas (1930–1945)." *Dynamis* 25: 199–226.
Hochman, Gilberto, María Silvia Di Liscia, and Steven Paul Palmer. 2012. *Patologías de la patria: Enfermedades, enfermos y nación en América Latina*. Buenos Aires: Lugar Editorial.
Homedes, Núria, and Ugalde, Antonio. 2005. "Why Neoliberal Health Reforms have failed in Latin America." *Health Policy* 71: 83–96.
James, Daniel. 2001. *Resistance and Integration: Peronism and the Argentine Working Class, 1946–1976*. Cambridge: Cambridge University Press.
Karush, Matthew B., and Oscar Chamosa, eds. 2010. *The New Cultural History of Peronism: Power and Identity in Mid-Twentieth-Century Argentina*. Durham: Duke University Press.
Machado, Cristiani Vieira. 2018. "Health Policies in Argentina, Brazil and Mexico: Different Paths, Many Challenges." *Ciência & Saúde Coletiva* 23 (7): 2197–212.
Massuda, Adriano, Thomas Hone, Fernando Antonio Gomes Leles, Marcia C de Castro, and Rifat Atun. 2018. "The Brazilian Health System at Crossroads: Progress, Crisis and Resilience." *BMJ Global Health* 3 (4): 1–8.
Otovo, Okezi T. 2016. *Progressive Mothers, Better Babies: Race, Public Health, and the State in Brazil, 1850–1945*. Austin: University of Texas Press.
Peard, Julyan G. 1999. *Race, Place, and Medicine: The Idea of the Tropics in Nineteenth-Century Brazilian Medicine*. Durham: Duke University Press.
Pirez, Pedro. 1998. "The Management of Urban Services in the City of Buenos Aires." *Environment and Urbanization* 10 (2) 209–22.
Plotkin, Mariano Ben. 2003. *Mañana es San Perón: A Cultural History of Perón's Argentina*. Wilmington, DE: SR Books.
Ramacciotti, Karina. 2009. *La política sanitaria del Peronismo*. Buenos Aires: Editorial Biblos.
Rock, David. 2006. *Argentina 1516–1987: From Spanish Colonization to Alfonsín*. Berkeley: University of California Press.
Rodríguez-Boetsch, Leopoldo. 2005. "Public Service Privatisation and Crisis in Argentina." *Development in Practice* 15 (3–4): 302–15.
Romero, Luis Alberto, and James P. Brennan. 2013. *A History of Argentina in the Twentieth Century*. University Park: Pennsylvania State University Press.
Sakellariou, Dikaios, and Elena S. Rotarou. 2017. "The Effects of Neoliberal Policies on

Access to Healthcare for People with Disabilities." *International Journal of Equity Health* 16 (1): 1–8.

Stepan, Nancy Leys. 1991. *The Hour of Eugenics: Race, Gender, and Nation in Latin America*. Ithaca, NY: Cornell University Press.

Vargas Bustamante, Arturo, and Claudio A. Méndez. 2014. "Health Care Privatization in Latin America: Comparing Divergent Privatization Approaches in Chile, Colombia, and Mexico." *Journal of Health Politics, Policy and Law* 39 (4): 841–86.

World Health Organization (WHO). 2008. "Flawed but Fair: Brazil's Health System Reaches Out to the Poor." *Bulletin of the World Health Organization* 86 (4): 248–49.

# 17

## The Politics and Medical Discourse of Intersexuality in Argentina through Film

Lucía Puenzo's *XXY*

JAVIER BARROSO

For years, Argentina has distinguished itself as a country that has made important advances in constitutional amendments and other legal protections for members of the LGBTQ+ community. For instance, in 2010, it became the first Latin American country to legalize same-sex marriage, in 2012, the Ley de Identidad de Género [Gender Identity Law] removed many bureaucratic and medical barriers for individuals to change their legal gender, and, since 2013, non-normative couples have had equal access to in vitro fertilization procedures. However, as in most of the world, the Argentine LGBTQ+ community continues to face tremendous challenges, including prejudice, exclusion, and lack of dignified representation in media and entertainment. Intersex individuals, often and antiquatedly referred to as hermaphrodites in common vernacular and medical settings, face particular challenges that highlight the work that is still needed to continue promoting inclusion and equality, even in countries as constitutionally progressive as Argentina. The Argentine National Institute Against Discrimination, Xenophobia and Racism [Instituto Nacional contra la Discriminación, la Xenofobia y el Racismo] (INADI) (2016) notes that intersexuality is not constrained to just one sex variation, but a wide spectrum (22). Intersex persons are those who are "born with 'atypical' sex anatomies and reproductive organs," including ambiguous genitalia, atypical hormone producing organs, or atypical genetic make-up, according to the International Intersex Human Rights NGO (Bauer et al. 2016, 39).[1] The specificity of the challenges faced by intersex individuals—and what differentiates them from the rest of the LGBTQ+ community—relies mainly on the "corrective" operations (often referred as

Intersex Genital Mutilations [IGM] by human rights advocates) that are normally performed shortly after birth. The perceived purpose of these often-compulsory operations is to assign non-ambiguous sex physiology and identity. However, since these interventions are often performed during infancy, many patients are never informed of their original genital configuration or genetic make-up. These pediatric clinical interventions bring to the fore intersex individuals' unique medical, legal, and social challenges. Furthermore, since intersexuality is considered a broad spectrum of atypical genital and endocrinal conditions, intersex individuals challenge the rigid binaries that are normally associated with sex and gender—perhaps even more acutely than other members of the LGBTQ+ community.

Lucía Puenzo's film *XXY* (2007) highlights some of the unique challenges facing the intersex community.[2] Given that one of *XXY*'s subplots is a dispute between two scientists—a marine biologist and a plastic surgeon—regarding the treatment of the main character's atypical genital composition, it can be interpreted as a simultaneous denunciation and challenging of the practice of "sex confirmation" operations that many intersex people receive. The opposing views of these two characters, both also father figures in the film, are representative of the conflicting positions between international intersex advocacy groups and established medical procedures in infants with atypical genital and hormonal composition.[3] However, an analysis of the representation of these two characters and key scenes in the film will demonstrate that *XXY* is challenging these medical procedures at the same time that it is, perhaps unintentionally, reinforcing and perpetuating binaries that continue to permeate societal views and understandings of sex and gender. These same binaries are the ones that lead both medical doctors and parents (in Argentina and elsewhere) to elect to perform these problematic procedures when presented with a newborn intersex child.

*XXY* tells the story of Alex, a troubled intersex teenager who was raised as a girl and is now trying to establish her identity as she comes of age.[4] The film was released to major critical acclaim at the 2007 Cannes Film Festival, and it won the Grand Prize during *La Semaine de la Critique*. It won several other international prizes in competitions like Spain's *Premios Goya*, Mexico's *Premios Ariel*, and Argentina's *Premios Clarín*. Loosely based on "Cinismo" ("Cynical"), a short story written by Puenzo's husband Sergio Bizzio, *XXY* gained notoriety not only for being a strong showcase by a first-time director but also for tackling a social issue that few films had previously portrayed, especially in Latin America. Puenzo explains in the press materials for the US DVD release of the film that, before *XXY*, there was a "strange cultural silence" regarding intersexuality, and even when "the subject is explored, it's in the language of testimony, of medical diagnosis, but with almost no fictions, as if the subject would be a taboo for any kind of poetry and fiction around it" (Puenzo 2008). Not surprisingly, *XXY* is now a canonical film in queer and gender studies programs and is part of a select group of Argentine films that are regularly included in undergraduate and graduate Spanish courses in North American universities.

*XXY*'s plot centers on intersex teenager Alex (Inés Efron) who lives with her parents in a small and secluded coastal town in Uruguay, far from their native Buenos Aires. The family left the Argentine capital a few years back, "to avoid all the idiots in the world giving their opinion"[5] [*para evitar que todos los idiotas del mundo se pusieran a opinar*], as Alex's mother, Suli (Valeria Bertuccelli) bluntly puts it. As the film opens, an old friend of Suli, Erika (Carolina Peleritti), arrives with her husband Ramiro (Germán Palacios) and his son Álvaro (Martín Piroyanski) for a visit. At first unbeknownst to Alex and her father, Néstor Kraken (Ricardo Darín), Suli invited her old friend and her family to Uruguay because Ramiro is considered one of the best corrective plastic surgeons in the country. During the visitors' stay, the two teenagers begin a romantic relationship, which culminates with them having sexual relations. Meanwhile, tensions between the guests and Alex's parents build as the former try to convince the latter that it is in their daughter's best interest to have a corrective operation. Ramiro and his family leave the coastal town at the end of the film, as Alex and her parents decide it will be better for her not to choose between being a man or a woman through surgery but simply to remain an intersex individual.

Academics have predominantly analyzed *XXY* within a wide range of theoretical frameworks grounded mainly in queer, gender, and women's studies. For example, Zoila Clark (2012) focuses on the fluidity of gender boundaries through her analysis of Alex, and on the interconnectedness of these boundaries with race, class, and age. Viera Cherro (2011) analyzes the film from a feminist standpoint, focusing on the stigmatization of sex and sexuality. She also examines how the film portrays the social and cultural construction of sexual bodies. Margaret Frohlich (2012) studies the relationship between discourses of nature, gender, and sexuality, with particular emphasis on how the film challenges binaries such as natural/unnatural. Deborah Martin (2013) views Alex as the personification of "the intersex body as a site of embodied becoming, largely through the connections which it establishes with the animal" (37). Charlotte E. Gleghorn (2011) focuses on the film's strategies to underscore Alex's otherness in contrast to what is considered normal. She also explores how most critics before her used the term "hermaphrodite" (which originated in Greek mythology) to describe the protagonist, something that is endemic to the tension in the binary myth/reality, which she argues is part of *XXY*'s narrative structure. Through this approach, most critics have generally focused on the images, themes, and plot conflicts that deal with the film's apparent juxtaposition and problematization of binaries such as man/woman, natural/unnatural, and otherness/normality. Some other academics interpret the film's representation of its intersex protagonist as an example of the limits of our expectations of what can be considered human. For instance, Debra A. Castillo (2015) argues that "traditional understandings of human sexuality are insufficient to account for Alex's situation since Alex is outside the binaries of male/female, gay/straight, and Alex's conundrum exposes the limits of our imagination in defining the human" (159). Given the emphasis of these analyses, it is not surprising that a few of these critics have also focused their research on the importance of the sea shore in the film as an allegory of a third space, between ocean and land, that challenges clear-cut binaries imposed by society.

Many of these studies have successfully illuminated the manner in which *XXY* challenges common notions of gender identity and sexuality. However, it is important also to note that Puenzo's work contains implicit oppositional binaries that paradoxically contradict what most critics identify as the film's main expression: the promotion of otherness, transgression of borders, and inclusion. These contradicting elements are mainly represented by the film's two father figures, both of whom are scientists with strikingly different worldviews that leave no room for a middle ground, ultimately betraying *XXY*'s apparent challenge to binaries that negate a space for intersex individuals. The conflict between these two can also be interpreted as representations of the film's criticism of genital "corrective" operations that are still informed by medical discourses more than half a century old, which in turn were based on a rigid, binary understanding of sex and gender. According to INADI (2016), the medical practices on intersex individuals in Argentina and most of the world continue to be anchored in ideas first posited in the 1950s by New Zealand sexologist John Money (23). He maintained that gender identity was established during the first two years of life, after which it remains constant, and he also posited that genitals perceived as normal were essential to the formation of a gender identity, so those that were deemed ambiguous needed to be corrected surgically (INADI 2016, 24). INADI argues that through his posits, Money "reinforced the knowledge-power of medics and the idea of 'normal bodies'" [afianza el saber-poder del equipo medico y la idea de "cuerpos normales"] (25). Although more progressive ways of treating intersex individuals have emerged since the 1950s, Money's theorizations continue to permeate most medical decisions after birth. Furthermore, current medical assessments of intersex bodies are anchored to a desire to normalize them in order for these individuals to satisfy societal and clinical norms. Even medical teams that acknowledge that Money's methods are now antiquated continue to favor operations based on the perceived emotional impact on parents, and not necessarily due to a patient's medical need. For instance, Piró Biosca et al. (2014) argue that corrective surgical decisions should no longer be based solely on phenotype observations as first posited by Money, but that they should also include molecular studies to analyze androgens (70). However, their report also notes that "these surgical interventions should be performed early, and if possible before 18 months of age, due to psychological and social reasons pertaining to the patient's family as well as the patient" [Estas intervenciones quirúrgicas deben ser realizadas de forma precoz, y a ser posible antes de los 18 meses de vida, por motivos psicológicos y sociales tanto de la familia, como del propio paciente] (71). Similarly, Marcela Bailez (2010) notes that the general medical position in Argentina regarding gonadectomies (the removal of testicles or ovaries) is that it should be performed as early as possible in patients identified with DSD (disorders of sex development), which is a medical term often used to refer to intersex individuals that emphasizes a binary understanding of sex and gender. The three main arguments for performing these early pediatric operations in Argentina are listed in the following order: "the risk (although very low) of neoplasia; the psychological benefit for parents in knowing that any foreign nascent sexual tissue has been removed; and to avoid re-operation" [*el riesgo (aunque muy bajo) de neoplasia; el beneficio psicológico para los padres de saber que cualquier tejido extraño al sexo de crianza ha sido extirpado; y evitar la reoperación*] (Bailez 2010, 212). The importance placed on the peace of mind of the intersex patient's parents, and by extension society in general, as one of the main reasons to perform "corrective surgery" is represented in Puenzo's *XXY* through the interactions and discussions among Alex's and Álvaro's parents, particularly Kraken and Ramiro, the two scientists.

The personalities and even physical characteristics of these two characters, and what they represent, are so different that they create a polarizing opposition that paradoxically subverts the film's apparent criticism of a world ruled by binaries. Ironically, therefore, the film leaves no space for doubts or gray areas within the Ramiro/Kraken binary. On the surface, both parents share several similarities. They are both scientists (Kraken is a marine biologist, while Ramiro is a surgeon), they are both married with teenage children, and they seem to be of about the same social class. At first glance, they are similar enough that—in a scene in which the two teenage protagonists are watching Kraken operate on a turtle—Alex points out to Álvaro that "in reality your father and mine are the same person" [al final tu papá y el mío son lo mismo]. However, as the film progresses, the divide between Kraken and Ramiro widens so much that they essentially become each other's opposite. Kraken is presented as a concerned parent who is open to allowing Alex to continue her life as an intersex individual, without the need to continue taking hormone treatments or going through a corrective surgery. In contrast, Ramiro is a renowned plastic surgeon who, throughout the film, tries to convince Alex's family that she needs to at least continue her hormonal treatments. The sharp variance between the two parents is visually represented through their physical appearance, their vehicles, and even their demeanor. Kraken, the more open of the two parents to change and understanding, has wild salt-and-pepper hair, and he sports a beard that matches his weathered-but-sensible and earthly look. On the other hand, the short-tempered Ramiro has a very clean-cut look that goes well with his strong facial features, short hair, and perfect shave. While the Buenos Aires surgeon drives a clean, late-model sedan, Kraken gets around in an old, rugged mini pickup truck that sports on the rear windshield a sticker of the Beatles that is predominantly displayed in several key scenes. The film's limited dialogue greatly accentuates the differences between the two fathers. So few words are spoken, particularly by these two characters, that when they do speak, their lines emphasize their differences. For instance, the following dialogue highlights Ramiro's reluctance to accept a person who transgresses normative definitions of gender or sex. This exchange occurs when Alex's mother complains to Erika and Ramiro about society's obsession with labels and classifications as they stand on the sea shore, near the place where Alex was conceived:

> SULI: You get questioned all the time: Are you pregnant? Is it male or female? You go to the clinic and that is the first thing they ask you. Is it a boy or a girl?
> RAMIRO: How long has it been since she took her corticoids?
> SULI: I don't know. Two weeks, more or less.
> RAMIRO: You know what's going to happen if she doesn't take them anymore, right?
> ERIKA: What's going to happen?
> RAMIRO: She is going to virilize. Everything will change for her. Her body and cycles. She is going to stop developing as a woman.

[SULI: Todo el tiempo te preguntan: ¿Estás embarazada? ¿Es varón o mujer? Vas a la clínica y es lo primero que preguntan. ¿Es nena o nene?
RAMIRO: ¿Hace cuánto que no toma los corticoides?
SULI: No sé. Dos semanas, más o menos.
RAMIRO: Vos sabés lo que le va a pasar si no las toma más, ¿no?
ERIKA: ¿Qué le va a pasar?
RAMIRO: Se va a virilizar. Le va a cambiar todo. El cuerpo y los ciclos. Va a dejar de desarrollarse como mujer.]

Instead of offering some kind of support to Suli, or at least keeping quiet, Ramiro perpetuates the same stance that Alex's mother was complaining about. He speaks about Alex's changes as something undesirable and wrong. As the surgeon talks, Suli walks away and Erika asks her husband to stop. Ramiro looks away, indignant.

Another scene that emphasizes Ramiro's aversion to any kind of dissonance or anomaly that threatens his rigid worldview occurs when Álvaro and Alex are talking about his medical profession, and Álvaro explains his father's true passion. In this scene, Alex asks Álvaro if he has ever witnessed how his father "butchers bodies." The question offends the teen: "He doesn't butcher bodies, he fixes them. My dad does tits and noses for money, but what really interests him are other things" [No rebana cuerpos, los arregla. Mi papá hace tetas y narices por plata, pero a él en realidad le interesan otras cosas.] Álvaro is clearly upset as he responds, and he adds that what Ramiro is really interested in is correcting deformities such as those found on individuals who are born with eleven fingers. This exchange illustrates Ramiro's representation as a surgeon who not only opposes anything that distorts his notion of bodily normalcy but that he is bent on correcting these "deformities." This depiction of Ramiro's medical profile can be interpreted as a reference to the medical discourses that inform decisions made regarding corrective surgeries on underage intersex people.

Kraken, on the other hand, is presented as more understanding than Ramiro. Throughout the film, he challenges Ramiro's stance on correcting Alex's body, and the differences between the two are also exacerbated by the way in which Kraken's open-mindedness permeates most of the scenes in which he appears. For example, after Alex is verbally and sexually attacked by a group of teenagers, Kraken and Ramiro go looking for the assailants. When they find them at the fishing dock, Kraken suffers an uncharacteristic fit of rage and violently threatens the young men. Accentuating the confrontational relationship between the two, Ramiro comes between Kraken and the teenagers, and Alex's father berates the plastic surgeon, telling him he is just as bad as the assailants. He then drives to the police station with the intention of reporting the assault, but remains in his truck, pensive, until he decides to leave. In another example of the film's depiction of Kraken as more wholesome than Ramiro, Alex's father does not file a police report and instead searches for his child to consult her about the possibility of denouncing the attack. Another key scene highlighting Kraken's and Ramiro's antagonistic stances occurs when the two families are shown eating dinner during which the surgeon bullies his son Álvaro into drinking wine. Álvaro is offered the drink along with the rest of the adults at the table, but he is hesitant to partake. The father pressures his son, which clearly upsets Kraken, who angrily says: "We left Buenos Aires to be away from a certain type of people. Do you remember? Now it turns out that we are all sitting at the same table." [Nos fuimos de Buenos Aires para estar lejos de cierta clase de gente. ¿Te acordás? Ahora resulta que todos estamos sentados en la misma mesa.] A storm rages outside during this argument, and the quarrel ends because the lights go out following a clap of thunder, signaling that there is no possible resolution to the conflict between the two fathers.

The constant struggle between the two characters can be interpreted as the film's way of highlighting the disruption caused by the presence of an element—in this case Alex—that challenges notions of normalcy in society. But the sharp differences between Kraken and Ramiro become so evident that they leave no room for a middle ground. These two central characters are either understanding to a fault or grossly closed-minded, ultimately betraying the film's challenging of the binaries that rule our understanding of the world, particularly sex and gender. Even Kraken's character fails to accept Alex's body as a space that negates these binary understandings of gender and sex. For instance, Jeffrey Zamostny (2012) notes that throughout the film Kraken goes through a transformation that culminates in his total acceptance of Alex's condition: "Symbolically charged speech and images gauge the degree of Kraken's evolution. While he inaugurates the film's dialogue by identifying [a] turtle as an hembra, by the end he calls Alex both hijo and hija" (197–98). Ultimately, Kraken's acceptance of Alex's intersexuality is still grounded in the male/female binary as noted by his decision to call the teenager *hijo* and *hija*.

This worldview centered on binaries negates the broad spectrum represented by individuals such as Alex. Even the film's description of Alex's genitals, which are never shown on screen, fall into the male/female binary that intersex individuals' bodies normally challenge. Instead of portraying intersexuality's wide-ranging diversity, Alex's body is described in the film as having fully developed both reproductive organs, effectively negating her uniqueness as an individual beyond these rigid male/female binaries. These binaries that permeate the film should not necessarily be considered Puenzo's failure to create a work that truly challenges the lack of inclusion and understanding in society. Instead, the presence of such clear-cut binaries could be interpreted as the way in which social, political, and medical subtexts inherent to early twenty-first-century Argentina filtered into the film. For instance, although Buenos Aires had very progressive laws that guaranteed some civil rights to the LGBTQ+ community—for example, civil unions between same-sex couples were approved in 2002 despite strong opposition from the Catholic Church and evangelical organizations—the rest of the country lagged behind. Several years had to pass before a nationwide mandate that guaranteed those rights to all Argentines could be approved. The film's apparently unintentional use of binaries to tell the story of an intersex individual is itself a representation of the contradictory nature of the treatment of Argentina's LGBTQ+ community by the rest of society, particularly when comparing the country's progressive constitutional rights against the reality of living in a society that often continues to challenge inclusivity. For example, an analysis of media coverage of the 2010 law that guaranteed equal marriage rights nationwide showed that some of the news not only reported incorrect information regarding the law but also that the stories were reported with "a mocking tone" (Centeno, Cornejo, and Gil 2011, 72; see also J. García León and D. García León's chapter in this book). Similar contradictory occurrences in language regarding the LBGTQ+ community's rights are also evident in medical discourses that relate to intersexuality.

According to a report by Justicia Intersex (Cabral Grinspan 2017), an Argentine human rights non-profit organization, "Argentine doctors have an ambivalent position on human rights" (13). The report notes, on the one hand, that some doctors recognize the need to reassess the current methods and protocols to treat intersex individuals. On the other, doctors often disregard the testimonies of those who went through surgeries and hormonal treatments as children as they consider them to be "based on resentment and radical perspectives" (13). Despite the small advances in an acknowledgment by the medical community that protocols need to be revised, according to the report, Argentine doctors continue to routinely perform gonadectomies, sterilizing procedures, and "arbitrary imposition of hormone" therapy to intersex individuals (Cabral Grinspan 2017, 9). These instances of contradictions in the medical discourses regarding intersexuality, coupled with clinical articles that continue to promote early corrective operations, show that it is hard to imagine substantial changes occurring in the near future regarding medical practices and treatment for individuals born as intersex humans.

Argentina is often considered a country that, through political reforms, has advanced to the forefront of civil rights laws to protect the LGBTQ+ community. Nonetheless, it has not advanced much socially in that respect given the strong reaction from several sectors of society against the reforms. These contradictory components of Argentine reality have inevitably filtered into artistic expressions such as Puenzo's *XXY*. Perhaps those particular subtexts and incongruencies present in the film have been mostly overlooked by some critics precisely because of the film's subject matter, which has been considered a universal topic that transcends the Argentine context. While the film's themes definitely lend themselves to a universal reading—particularly because the same unresolved issues that create tensions in Argentina are occurring in different regions of the world—the film's historical temporality and its local social context should not be overlooked. Many academics have identified the film as an artistic celebration of intersex bodies as a space of otherness where binaries are challenged. For example, Martin (2013) concludes that "*XXY* makes the intersex body the site of a post-gender, 'no-choice-to-make' utopianism, and defies the prescription in place on everybody to grow up to sameness" (44). Also, while Gleghorn (2011) acknowledges that the film underlines "Alex's otherness in a society that seeks to monitor discrete categories of sex and gender" (168), she also concludes that "*XXY* suggests that in recognizing difference, the post- of post-gender is not only possible but is already a reality for many, dislocating the myth from reality once and for all" (169). However, by focusing on *XXY*'s implicit championing of otherness, these readings tend to overlook very clear-cut binaries that could be working against the film's intended message. In turn, by overseeing these binary tensions in the film, exemplified by the Kraken/Ramiro dichotomy and even the representation of Alex's genital composition, most readings of *XXY* tend not to consider the local social tensions and medical discourses that have filtered into Puenzo's film. Considering these discourses in Puenzo's work has evidenced the ways in which the film inadvertently could be working against what other critics have identified as its main message: the promotion of Alex's otherness through her challenging of medical and social understanding of gender and sex normality that are informed by notions of rigid binaries.

## Notes

1. The Intersex Society of North America notes that intersexuality is "a socially constructed category that reflects real biological variation" covering a wide spectrum of genital and hormonal conditions. It also notes that "doctors' opinions about what should count as 'intersex' vary substantially" ("What is intersex?").

2. Lucía Puenzo is an Argentine filmmaker and writer. She has published several novels and short stories, and some of her films have received international accolades and awards. *XXY* was her first film.

3. The Intersex Society of America, for instance, lists one of their main missions as the objection to "elective surgeries done on people (usually children) without their informed consent" ("What's ISNA's position on surgery?"). Likewise, the Intersex Justice Project demands that these "surgeries should be delayed and only done with the full informed consent of the intersex patient" ("The End Intersex Surgery Campaign").

4. The protagonist was raised as a woman, and throughout the film, Alex is referred to with female pronouns. In this chapter, I will use female pronouns to refer to Alex with an understanding that this difficulty in nomenclature highlights the binaries that constrain our perceptions of sex and gender.

5. All dialogue translations are my own.

## References

Argentine National Institute Against Discrimination, Xenophobia and Racism (INADI). 2016. *Intersexualidad*. Buenos Aires: INADI.

Bailez, Marcela. 2010. "Rol de la cirugía en pacientes con anomalías de la diferenciación sexual (DSD)." *Medicina Infantil* 17 (2): 212–16.

Bauer, Markus, Nadine Coquete, Vincent Guillot, and Daniela Truffer. 2016. *Intersex Genital Mutilations: Human Rights Violations of Persons with Variations of Sex Anatomy*. Zurich: Human Rights for Hermaphrodites Too!

Cabral Grinspan, Mauro. 2017. *Intersex Genital Mutilations: Human Rights Violations of Persons with Variations of Sex Anatomy*. Buenos Aires: Justicia Intersex.

Castillo, Debra A. 2015. "Haunted: XXY (Lucía Puenzo 2007)." In *Despite All Adversities: Spanish-American Adversities Queer Cinema*, edited by. Andrés Lema-Hincapié, Debra A. Castillo, and Daniel Balderston, 155–71. Albany: State University of New York Press.

Centeno, Matías E., Lucía Cornejo, and Mariela Quiroga Gil. 2011. "La ley del matrimonio igualitario en los medios." *Revistas Metavoces* 8 (11): 71–75.

Clark, Zoila. 2012. "Our Monstrous Humanimality in Lucía Puenzo's *XXY* and *The Fish Child*." *Hispanet Journal* 5: 1–24.

Frohlich, Margaret. 2012. "What of Unnatural Bodies? The Discourse of Nature in Lucía Puenzo's *XXY* and *El niño pez/The Fish Child*." *Studies in Hispanic Cinema* 8 (2): 159–74.

Gleghorn, Charlotte E. 2011. "Myth and the Monster of Intersex: Narrative Strategies of Otherness in Lucía Puenzo's *XXY*." In *Latin American Cinemas: Local Views and*

*Transnational Connections,* edited by Nayibe Bermúdez Barrios, 141–74. Calgary, AB: University of Calgary Press.
Intersex Society of North America. "What is Intersex?" https://isna.org/faq/what_is_intersex/
———. "What's ISNA's Position on Surgery?" https://isna.org/faq/surgery/.
Intersex Justice Project. "The End Intersex Surgery Campaign." http://www.intersexjusticeproject.org/.
Martin, Deborah. 2013. "Growing Sideways in Argentine Cinema: Lucía Puenzo's *XXY* and Julia Solomonoff's *El último verano de la boyita.*" *Journal of Romance Studies* 13 (1): 34–48.
Piró Biosca, C., L. Audi Parera, M. Fernández Cancio, J.A. Martín Osorio, N. Toran Fuentes, M. Asensio Llorente, and A. Carrascosa lezcano. 2014. "Diagnóstico y tratamiento quirúrgico del pseudohermafroditismo masculino en una unidad multidisciplinaria de estados intersexuales." *Cirugía Pediátrica* 17: 70–75.
Puenzo, Lucía, dir. *XXY.* 2007. New York: Film Movement, 2008. DVD.
———. "Director's Statement." 2008. *XXY Press Kit.* New York: Film Movement.
Viera Cherro, Mariana. 2011. "Que se enteren: Cuerpo y sexualidad en el zoom social. Sobre *XXY.*" *Revista Estudos Feministas* 19 (2): 351–69.
Zamostny, Jeffrey. 2012. "Constructing Ethical Attention in Lucía Puenzo's *XXY*: Cinematic Strategy, Intersubjectivity, and Intersexuality." In *Representing History, Class, and Gender in Spain and Latin America,* edited by Carolina Rocha and Georgia Seminet, 189–204. New York: Palgrave Macmillan.

# Contributors

Benny J. Andrés Jr. is associate professor of history and Latin American studies at the University of North Carolina at Charlotte. He is the author of *Power and Control in the Imperial Valley: Nature, Agribusiness, and Workers on the California Borderland, 1900–1940*, which *Choice* selected as an Outstanding Academic Title in 2015.

Javier Barroso is lecturer in Spanish at the Massachusetts Institute of Technology. His research focuses on the intersection of Latin American fictional narratives, history, and politics. His main fields of study include twentieth and twenty-first century Latin American fiction, with an emphasis on Mexican and Argentine narrative, contemporary Mexican and Southern Cone film, and language instruction. His most recent research projects focus on representations of World War II and Nazism in the literature of Argentina and Mexico.

Katherine E. Bliss is senior fellow and director of immunizations and health systems resilience at the CSIS Global Health Policy Center. She is also adjunct professor at Georgetown University's School of Foreign Service. She is the author of *Compromised Positions: Prostitution, Public Health and Gender Politics in Revolutionary Mexico City* and editor, with William E. French, of *Gender and Sexuality in Post-Independence Latin America*. Her current research focuses on US-Mexico cooperation on health, development, and national security during the Cold War.

Eric D. Carter is the Edens Professor of Geography and Global Health at Macalester College in Saint Paul, Minnesota. His interdisciplinary research lies at the nexus of medical geography, environmental history, and the history of public health, with a regional focus on Latin America. He has published the book, *Enemy in the Blood: Malaria, Environment, and Development in Argentina*, and articles in such journals as *Social Science and Medicine*, *História, Ciências, Saúde–Manguinhos*, *Journal of Historical Geography*, and *Health and Place*.

David S. Dalton is associate professor of Spanish and Latin American studies at the University of North Carolina at Charlotte. His research theorizes the interface of science, technology, and the body and how this contributes to racial and gender hierarchies in Mexico and throughout Latin America. He is the author of *Mestizo Modernity: Race, Technology, and the Body in Postrevolutionary Mexico*, and he is finishing a book called *Robo Sacer: Necroliberalism and Cyborg Resistance in Mexican and Chicanx Dystopias*. He has also edited several books and special editions in journals: *The Transatlantic Undead: Zombies in Hispanic and Luso-Brazilian Literatures*; *El cine de luchadores*; *Imagining Latinidad: Digital Diasporas and Public Engagement Among Latin American Migrants*. He has written around thirty articles and book chapters on different aspects of Mexican and Latin American studies.

Carlos S. Dimas is assistant professor of history at the University of Nevada, Las Vegas. His research centers on Science and Technology Studies in Latin America has appeared in the *Journal of Latin American Studies*, *Bulletin of Latin American Research*, and *Agricultural History* in topics ranging from epidemics and agriculture, rural health, and the history of meteorology. His first book, *Poisoned Eden: Cholera Epidemics, State-Building, and the Problem of Public Health in Tucumán, Argentina, 1865–1908*, is published through the University of Nebraska Press. His next work will be a technological and social history of electricity, power outages, and culture in Argentina from the 1890s to 1990s.

Sophie Esch is associate professor of Mexican and Central American literature and culture at Rice University. She studies the intersection of literature, politics, and war in modern Latin America and Africa. She is the author of *Modernity at Gunpoint: Firearms, Politics, and Culture in Mexico and Central America* (winner of the 2019 Best Book in the Humanities Award of the Mexico section of the Latin American Studies Association) and numerous articles on Central American and Mexican literature.

Renata Forste is international vice president at Brigham Young University. She received her PhD in Sociology from the University of Chicago, with an emphasis in demography. Her research interests focus on maternal and child health, as well as patterns of family formation in Latin America, and include publications in journals such as *Social Science & Medicine*, and *Journal of Family Violence*.

David L. García León is assistant professor in Spanish and Intercultural studies at the School of Modern Languages, Literatures, and Cultures at Maynooth University. He has extensively studied issues of sociolinguistics, critical discourse analysis, queer linguistics, and Latin American cultural and media studies with a focus on masculinities and queer/crip theory. His work has been published in journals such as the *Canadian Journal of Latin American* and *Caribbean Studies, Bulletin of Hispanic Studies, Latin American Research Review, Lingüística y Literatura, Cuadernos de Lingüística Hispánica, Forma y Función, Boletín de Filología*, and *Revista de Estudios Hispánicos*. His most current research project explores the depiction of male disability in the Colombian media industry.

Javier E. García León is assistant professor of Spanish linguistics at the Department of Languages and Culture Studies at the University of North Carolina at Charlotte. He conducts interdisciplinary research on sociolinguistics, critical discourse analysis, queer linguistics, and Latin American (LGBTQI+) media studies. In particular, he has examined the representation of transgender people in Latin American newspapers and audiovisual journalism of the last decades. His latest publications include his monograph *Espectáculo, normalización y representaciones otras. Las personas transgénero en la prensa y el cine de Colombia y Venezuela*.

Jethro Hernández Berrones is associate professor of history at Southwestern University. Hernández Berrones has published research articles in the journals *Medical History* and *História, Ciências, Saúde-Manguinhos*. His book manuscript titled *A Revolution in Small Doses: Homeopathy, the Medical Profession, and the State in Mexico, 1893–1942* is under contract with the University of North Carolina Press. He is interested in the history of science, medicine, medical pluralism, and public health in Mexico and Latin America.

Katherine Hirschfeld, professor of anthropology at the University of Oklahoma, is a medical anthropologist interested in structural determinants of health. She received her PhD from Emory University in 2001. Her first book, *Health, Politics and Revolution in Cuba since 1898*, was published by Transaction Books in 2007. Her current research focuses on modeling post-Soviet health transitions and theorizing the political economy of organized crime, corruption, and population health declines.

Emily J. Kirk, postdoctoral fellow at Dalhousie University, focuses her research on global health, Latin American development issues, and south-south cooperation. Much of her work focuses on Cuba, where she has carried out extensive research. She is currently writing about the different aspects of the Cuban Development Model, particularly regarding healthcare and education. Her investigations also more broadly examine south-south cooperation and its impact on developing countries. She is author of *Cuba's Gay Revolution: Normalizing Sexual Diversity Through a Health-Based Approach*.

Gabriela León-Pérez is assistant professor of sociology at Virginia Commonwealth University. Her research interests include internal and international migration, the health and well-being of Latino immigrants in the United States, and health disparities. Her most recent project examined work and parenting stress among Mexican immigrant mothers. Other ongoing projects include research on the relationship between legal status and health, and the incorporation of Latinos in a new immigrant destination. The underlying goal of León-Pérez's research agenda is to clarify the role of social, structural, and contextual factors in creating health and social inequalities, as well as to identify resources that improve the outcomes of immigrants and other marginalized populations. Gabriela received a PhD in Sociology from Vanderbilt University, an MA in Sociology from Texas A&M International University, and a BA in International Studies from Universidad de Monterrey in Mexico.

Manuel F. Medina is professor of Spanish at the University of Louisville. He has received that institution's President's Exemplary Multicultural Teaching Award (2012), and he has been named Outstanding MA Mentor (2014) and Diversity Champion (2011). Medina has published extensively in the areas of Latin American literature and film, with special emphasis on Mexico, Ecuador, Brazil, and US Latino. His monographic study, *Archivo y discurso en la nueva novela histórica mexicana (1980–1994)*, reveals a long-standing interest in the Latin American historical novel. Medina serves as the current president of the Asociación de Ecuatorianistas.

Christopher D. Mellinger is associate professor in the Department of Languages and Culture Studies and is affiliate faculty for the Latin American Studies program at the University of North Carolina at Charlotte. Mellinger is the coeditor of the journal *Translation and Interpreting Studies*, coauthor with Thomas A. Hanson of *Quantitative Research Methods in Translation and Interpreting Studies*, and coeditor with Brian Baer of *Translating Texts: An Introductory Coursebook on Translation and Text Formation*. His research interests include translation and interpreting studies, language access, and translation and interpreting process research.

Alicia Z. Miklos is assistant professor of Spanish in the Department of Classical and Modern Languages and Literatures at Texas Tech University. Her main research areas include Contemporary Central American literature, Gender and Sexuality Studies, and Media studies. Within these fields, she focuses on contemporary Central American chronicles, documentary film, and digital media about women, migrants, and youth.

Nicole L. Pacino is associate professor of history at the University of Alabama in Huntsville. Her research interests include twentieth-century Andean history, the history of public health, revolutions and social movements, and gender. Her work has been published in journals based in the United States, Europe, and Latin America, including *Diplomatic History*, the *Journal of Women's History*, the *Bulletin of Latin American Research*, and *História, Ciências, Saúde–Manguinhos*.

Douglas J. Weatherford is professor of Hispanic literature and film at Brigham Young University. Much of his recent scholarship examines Mexican author Juan Rulfo's connection to the visual image. Weatherford published the first English-language translation of Rulfo's second novel, *El gallo de oro* (*The Golden Cockerel and Other Writings*) and a transcription and study of the screenplays used to film that author's two novels (*Juan Rulfo y el cine: Los guiones de* Pedro Páramo *y* El gallo de oro). Currently, Weatherford is working on a long-term project that examines US and Mexican filmmakers who cross the border to make movies.

# Index

Page numbers in *italics* indicate illustrations.

Abortion laws, 169, 172
American Eugenics Society, 102, 104
Andean region, 4, 9–10; care, 214; contraception, 208; enrollment, 212–13; fertility, *208t*; health, 214, *204t*; prenatal care, 206; women, 204
Andrés, Benny J., Jr., 7
Argentina: care, 11, 283, 285, 289, 215; changes, 281; collapse, 293n10; economy, 278; film, 298; insurance, 279, 290; LGBTQ+, 296; malaria, 4; programs, 283; public, 293n11, 288
Asexualization procedure, 106–7, 108, 110
Association for Voluntary Sterilization, The, 132
Authoritarian, 146, 148, 153
Aztec, 21–22
Azuela, Mariano, 73

Barreda, Gabino, 27
Barroso, Javier, 11
Batista, Fulgencio, 146, 147, 148
Belli, Gioconda, 169, 172; personal, 174
Beltrán, Gonzalo Aguirre, 25
Bernard, Claude, 26
Berrones, Jethro Hernández, 5
Bliss, Katherine E., 6
Bolivia, 9–10, 207; marriage rates, *209t*; mortality rates, 205–6
Bolsonaro, Jair, 1
Bracero Program, 100
Brazil, 1, 215; care, 283, 289; changes, 281; economy, 278; health insurance, 279; programs, 283; public, 288
Brunner, D. F., 144, 153n3
Burgos, Elizabeth, 169

Caribbean, 4, 8
Carillo, Ramón, 285

Carter, Eric D., 11
Castro, Fidel, 152; authoritarian, 146, 148; death, 153; healthcare, 8; speeches, 154n9
Castro, Raúl: authoritarian, 146, 148, 152; healthcare, 8; power, 153
Catholic, 23–24, 107
Central America, 4, 8, 9; childbirth, 169, 170
Chávez, Hugo, 10, 152, 203
Chicano: movement, 134–35, 137; sterilization, 130, 131, 136; use, 138n2
Chile: disaster preparation, 157, 158; healthcare, 11; management system, 161, 166; natural disaster, 160, 162, 163, 165
Colonial: demographic, 25; institution, 24; medicine, 93, 98, 108
Comte, Auguste, 36n3, 292n3
Contraception: advocate, 106; birth control, 45, 101, 104; fertility, 44
Costa Rica, 9, 171
*Country under My Skin: A Memoir of Love and War, The*, 169, 172–73
COVID-19 pandemic, 1, 2; climate change, 164; disparities, 146; government, 151, 153n2, 165; leadership, 152; Ministry of Health, 148; programs, 146, 159
Cruz, Oswaldo, 283
Cuba, 8; economy, 150; healthcare, 143, 144, 153n1; malpractice, 149; services, 151; workers, 152
Cuban 1959 Revolution, 8, 143, 147

Dalton, David S., 7–8
Davenport, Charles, 102
*de Abajo, Los*, 73, 80
Department of Public Health, 29, 31, 32, 41, 42, 44. *See also* Secretariat of Public Health and Social Welfare
Depression symptoms, 57, 58, 62, *63t*, 64. *See also* Mexican Family Life Survey
de Seguier, Ulises, 28
de Silva, Lula, 278

316 · Index

Diaz, Porfirio, 29. *See also* Porfiriato
Díaz-Canel, Miguel, 8, 153
Dictatorship, 29, 143, 287
Dimas, Carlos S., 11; military, 289; revolution, 173
Documentary, 77; medical, 74; semi, 80; sterilization, 130–31

Epidemic: bubonic plague, 94, 100–101, 104; delousing, 97, 99, 110; diseases, 97, 98, 282; typhus, 93; lice, 95
Esch, Sophie, 9
Eugenics, 5, 106; attempts, 100; history, 108; ideology, 97; Mendelian, 92, 93; Malthusian, 104, 105, 107, 108, 111; practices, 131, 132; sterilization, 102; theories, 110
Eugenics Records Office in Cold Harbor, New York, 102
Eugenics Society of Northern California, 102

Fernández, Emilio, 6, 69, 70, 71, 72, 73, 77; adaptation, 82; motif, 78, 79; parable, 83; person, 84n2; works, 84n5
Film: history, 69, 83; Golden Age, 70, 77, 84n2
Ford Foundation, 44–45
*Forgotten Village, The*, 69, 70, 71, 72, 73; companion book, 84n1; connections, 78, 6; Five-Year Plan, 285; meaning, 77, 81, 82, 84; origins, 84n6; scene, 75, 76; trope, 74
Forste, Renata, 10
Fox, Vicente, 45

Gamble, Clarence, 106
Gender: differences, 52, 53, 54, 58–62, 66; depression, 64–65; discrimination, 137, 303, 305; enrollment, 213; inequality, 170; migration, 55; segregation, 97–98
Germ theory of disease, 144
Goethe, C.M., 102
Gonadectomies, 300
Gorgas, William, 145
Guayaquil, 2

Hackensmid, Alexander. *See* Hammid, Alexander
Hammid, Alexander, 62, 84n1
Health, 5; department, 96; disparities, 125; enrollment, 212–13; literacy, 122; mental, 51, 53; migration, 55, 62; outcomes, 56; public, 5; programs, 45, 147; sterilization, 104; women, 203
Healthcare, 3, 5; class-based, 98; level, 45; migrants, 54; practice, 80; public, 66n1; universal, 6, 279; workers, 79, 123–24; working class, 95
Hippocrates, 23, 26
Hirschfeld, Katherine, 8
Hispanic, 118, 126n1; community, 121; disparities, 122, 124; education, 123. *See also* Latino/a/x
Homeopathy: group, 28, 34; school, 31, 33. *See also* medical
Huerta, Luis Miguel Barbos, 2
Hurricane, 157–58, 161, 165; damage, 166

*I, Rigoberta Menchú. An Indian Woman in Guatemala*, 169
IMSS General Coordination of the National Plan for Depressed Zones and Marginalized Groups, 34, 44, 45, 46
Indigenous, 2; ancestry, 91; characters, 81; communities, 203, 281, 214, 205, 214; conditions, 45, 66n1; employment, 48; health, 5, 30, 32; inequality, 6; medicine, 36n1; peoples, 10, 23, 34 (*See also* mestizo); programs, 31; women, 206, 208, 209–10
Intersex: sexuality, 296, 303, 304, 306n1; individuals, 297, 298, 301, 305
Intersex Genital Mutilation, 297
Island, the. *See* Cuba

Johns Hopkins School of Public Health, 30
Jordan, Davis Starr, 102

Kirchner, Alberto Fernández de, 289
Kirchner, Cristina Fernández de, 278
Kirchner, Néstor, 278
Kirk, Emily J., 8
Kline, Herbert, 71, 72
Koch, Robert, 26

Language: barrier, 206; services, 121, 125
Latin America: dengue fever, 151; factors, 4, 12; healthcare, 2, 5, 6; neonatal, 170–71; revolutions, 174
Latino/a/x, 1, 4, 6–7; action suit, 110; colonial

care, 99; community, 117, 120, 132; disparities, 122; diversity, 118; healthcare, 91, 119, 124; health outcomes, 123; stereotypes, 104; use, 12n5, 111n1, 126n1, 138n2
León, David L. García, 10
León, Javier E. García, 10
León-Pérez, Gabriela, 6
LGBTQ+: community, 297, 304, 305; gay rights, 149
Liberal: constitution, 27; Mexico, 29; nineteenth century, 28; neo-, 32
Los Angeles County-USC Medical Center in California, 8

Macri, Mauricio, 279, 293n9; plan, 290, 289; campaign, 288
*Madrigal v. Quilligan*, 132
Medical: devices, 82, *83*; profession, 19; pluralism, 20, 35
Medina, Manuel F., 10
Mellinger, Christopher D., 7
Menchú, Rigoberta, 169, 175
Meraulyock, Rafael de J., 28
Mestizo, 23. *See also* Indigenous
Meteoro, 160, 163
Mexica, 21. *See also* Nahua
Mexican Family Life Survey, 51, 55, 56; characteristics, 58; data, 64; origins, 57
Mexican Institute of Social Security, 32, 43, 66n1
Mexican Revolution, 40, 41, 70, 71, 73, 84n3, 93; post-Revolution, 292n4; immigrants, 97
Mexico, 2; artistic movements, 6; condition, 72, 80; constitution, 27, 29, 31, 45; economy, 52; erasure, 102; fertility, 44; gender role, 28, 33; government, 32, 43, 73, 74, 77, 84n3; healing, 19, 20; healthcare, 5, 6, 30, 35, 40, 111; immigrant, 96; immigration, 93; impoverishment, 46; medicine, 32, 34; migration, 51, 53, 56, 57, 64–65; mortality rate, 41–42; occupation, 24, 26–27; pediatric, 43; postrevolutionary, 3, 5, 6, 31; programs, 47, 48; progression, 75; Republic, 78; rural medicine, 82; social stereotypes, 102, 110; sterilization, 131; women, 66n2
Midwifery, 34, 211
Migration, 53, 58, 64

Miklos, Alicia Z., 9
Money, John, 299–300
Morales, Evo, 10, 210
Mortality rates, 170, 203, 204
Movement for Socialism, 10 (Movimiento al Socialismo)

Nahua, 23. *See also* Mexica
National identity, 5
National Polytechnic Institute, 30, 31, 34
National School of Medicine, 27, 30; guidelines, 28
Neoliberal: reforms, 3, 34; era, 281
New Spain, 23, 24, 25
*No más bebés/No More Babies*, 8, 130, 131, 132, 134, 136, 137

Obrador, Andrés Manuel López, 2, 48
*Obra Social*, 290

Pacino, Nicole L., 10
Palma, Tomás Estrada, 145
Pasteur, Luis, 26
*Pearl, The*, 69, 70, 72, 82, *83*
Perón, Juan Domingo, 280, 284–85, 290
Peronism, 280; government, 286; healthcare, 287
Pierce, Claude, 97, 112n12
Pincus, Gregory, 108
Populism, 280, 284, 285
Porfiriato, 26, 29, 51
Positivism, 27, 36n3, 282, 292n2
Puenzo, Lucía, 297, 299, 300, 305, 306n2
Puerto Rico: birth control, 106, 107; health, 104; natural disaster, 8; sanitation, 102; sterilization, 111; stereotypes, 110; trials (science), 104, 108, 109

Quarantine, 101; Cuba, 145; delousing, 97–98; HIV, 149; Station, 99; Typhus, 100
Quilligan, Edward J., 130, 133, 138

Rawson, Guillermo, 282, 292n3
Revolution of 1910, 5. *See also* Indigenous
Ricketts, Ed, 81
*Río Escondido*, 70, 72, 73; meaning, 82; parable, 80; scene, *78*, 79; trope, 74
Rockefeller Foundation, 30, 42, 104

Rural: areas, 56, 214; depression, 65; education, 53, 205; enrollment, 212–13; health, 214; healthcare, 146, 147, 211; pregnancy, 171; population, 57, 66n1; women, 210

Saavedra, Daniel Ortega, 9
Sánchez, Yoani, 152, 154n10
Sanger, Margaret, 104, 108
Sarney, José, 280
SARS-CoV-2, 1; deaths, 12n2; country-by-country response, 12n1
*Sea of Cortez: A Leisurely Journal of Travel and Research*, 70, 82
Secretariat of Public Health and Social Welfare, 32, 43. *See also* Department of Public Health
Southern Cone, 4, 11
Spanish: colonial rule, 144, 165; colonizers, 5, 22; Conquest, 2, 9; conquistadors, 21
Steinbeck, John, 6, 69, 70, 72, 73, 77; adaptation, 83; motifs, 79
System for Social Protection in Health, 46, 47, 48

Tajima-Peña, Renee, 8, 130, 131, 132; editing, 138; claims, 133, 134
Tenochtitlan, 21, 23
The Spanish Crown, 23, 24, 25

Torres, Carmelita, 98
Tribunal of the Protomedicato, 24; licensing, 27; regulations, 25, 26
Tubal ligation, 130, 133

United States: natural disaster, 8; Mexico, 20; public health, 96
Urban, 52; areas, 204, 214; depression, 65; education, 53; healthcare, 146; population, 57; pregnancy, 171; urbanization, 55, 282; women, 210

Vaccination: infant, 204–5; smallpox, 99, 103
Vargas, Getúlio, 286, 287
Vargasism, 286, 287
Vásquez, Teodora del Carmen, 169
Venezuela: healthcare, 211; Maduro, Nicolás, 10; mortality rates, 206, 207
Virgin of Guadalupe, 78, 81

Western hemisphere shortcomings, 1
Western medicine, 82, 91, 172
Wilde, Eduardo, 282
World Health Organization, 48, 117, 157, 205; obstetric violence, 171

*XXY*, 11: "corrective surgery," 300; film, 297, 298, 305, 306n2; narrative structure, 299

www.ingramcontent.com/pod-product-compliance
Lightning Source LLC
Chambersburg PA
CBHW030740230426
43667CB00007B/784